CONVULSIVE THERAPY:
THEORY AND PRACTICE

Convulsive Therapy:
Theory and Practice

Max Fink, M.D.

Professor of Psychiatry
Department of Psychiatry and
Behavioral Sciences
Health Sciences Center—School of Medicine
State University of New York at Stony Brook
Stony Brook, New York

Raven Press ▪ New York

Raven Press, 1140 Avenue of the Americas, New York, New York 10036

© 1979 by Raven Press Books, Ltd. All rights reserved. This book is protected by copyright. No part of it may be reproduced, stored in a retrieval system, or transmitted, in any form or by any means, electronic, mechanical, photocopying, recording, or otherwise, without the prior written permission of the publisher.

Made in the United States of America

International Standard Book Number 0–89004–221–7
Library of Congress Catalog Card Number 77–074618

For

Martha, Jonathan, Rachel, and Linda

Some of the studies reported here were acknowledged in the Annual Award of the Electroshock Research Association in 1956, the A. E. Bennett Award of the Society for Biological Psychiatry in 1958, and the Samuel W. Hamilton Award of the American Psychopathological Association in 1974.

Preface

Convulsive therapy was introduced to clinical psychiatry in 1935. After more than 40 years of experience and documented reports of efficacy, its usefulness is still unclear and the methods are only incidentally taught in psychiatric training programs. Electroconvulsive therapy (ECT) is usually discussed apologetically, and the mode of action is lamented as obscure. When legislative and legal criticism is focused on psychiatric practice, the convulsive therapies, psychosurgery, and behavior modification are uncritically restrained together.

I first used ECT during a psychiatric residency in 1952, when a psychiatric supervisor selected some patients to receive ECT and others to receive psychotherapy or insulin coma. When I asked him to explain his choices, he answered, as he tapped his nose with his right index finger and nodded his head sagely, that I should trust his judgment and experience. My first systematic study of ECT was of predictors of outcome, and as a reward for my interest, I was asked to direct the somatic treatment unit at the hospital. For nine years, I was responsible for the treatment of patients with biologic therapies—convulsive, insulin coma, and drug therapies—as well as the teaching of these subjects to psychiatric residents.

During this period, my associates and I studied both ECT and insulin coma therapies. We examined the physiologic changes, particularly the electrical changes in brain function, the predictors of outcome, and the social and psychological factors affecting treatment. We varied the induction of seizures, assessing subconvulsive currents, suprathreshold stimuli, megimide, and flurothyl. When the antipsychotic and antidepressant drugs became available, we examined the relative efficacy of these drugs, insulin coma, and ECT. The studies were supported and encouraged by grants from the National Institute of Mental Health and from private, nonprofit agencies. From 1954 to 1958, I maintained a clinical practice, treating private patients with ECT in an office setting. In 1966, following the pioneering studies of multiple monitored ECT by Blachly and Gowing (1966) and of unilateral electrode placement by Cannicott (1962), a second series of studies of ECT was undertaken, supported by the National Institute of Mental Health and the International Association for Psychiatric Research. These studies were done at Gracie Square Hospital in New York.

In 1971, Dr. Milton Greenblatt invited me to edit a volume on convulsive therapy for the series *Seminars in Psychiatry*. That volume (IV, No. 1, February 1972) focused on both theoretical and clinical aspects of the convulsive therapy process.

In April 1972, Dr. Seymour Kety, Dr. James McGaugh, Dr. Thomas Williams, and I chaired a conference on the *Psychobiology of Convulsive Therapy*. A volume of the conference papers was published in 1974 by V. H. Winston & Sons, Washington, D.C. The meeting and volume examined three aspects of convulsive therapy: neurophysiologic effects, biochemical changes, and decrement in memory performance.

In the fall of 1975, the American Psychiatric Association responded to the many legal and judicial challenges to psychiatric practice, particularly in California, by convening a Task Force on Convulsive Therapy with Dr. Fred Frankel of Boston as Chairman. As a member of the Task Force, I was charged with reviewing the neurophysiologic consequences and the theories of the mode of action of convulsive therapy.

ECT provides an interesting window into the problems of brain and behavior and the psychopathology of the endogenous psychoses. Considering the recent interest in the convulsive therapies, it is timely to review the studies in my laboratories, to relate these to the experimental and clinical literature, to describe the present practice of the seizure therapies, and to examine the theories of their mode of action in the hope that the findings will stimulate a more effective use of ECT and a more active search for its mode of action. ECT remains our most effective treatment for depressive psychosis; an understanding of its central effects should lead to a clearer view of the pathogenesis and prophylaxis of mood disorders, depressive psychosis, and suicide.

Max Fink, M.D.
Great Neck, New York

Acknowledgments

This volume is derived from the studies of convulsive therapy from 1954 to 1962 at the Hillside Hospital in New York. The initial interest was in neurophysiologic and behavioral interrelationships, for the then-current theory ascribed the therapeutic efficacy of seizures in psychoses to altered brain function. Studies included the neurophysiologic effects of electrical and inhalant seizures (flurothyl Indoklon), the differences between convulsive and subconvulsive currents, the relationship between ECT and insulin coma, the effects of seizures on memory, perception, and speech, and the predictors of outcome, particularly psychological and physiologic predictors.

From 1962 to 1966, some studies of the biochemical effects of seizures were continued at the Missouri Institute of Psychiatry. In 1967, systematic studies at Gracie Square Hospital in New York were designed to define the differences in efficacy of the locus of electrodes (unilateral versus bilateral ECT) and multiple seizures.

In the studies at Hillside Hospital, my co-workers were Martin A. Green, M.D., Joseph Jaffe, M.D., Robert L. Kahn, Ph.D., Max Pollack, Ph.D., Hyman Korin, Ph.D., Ira Belmont, Ph.D., Eric Karp, Ph.D., and Nathaniel Siegel, Ph.D. The studies were encouraged by the Medical Director, Dr. Joseph S. A. Miller, and by the hospital founder, Dr. Israel Strauss. The theoretic structure of those studies was derived from the lectures of Dr. Morris B. Bender and Dr. Edwin A. Weinstein of Mount Sinai Hospital.

In the studies at the New York Medical College, my collaborators were Rhea Dornbush, Ph.D., Jan Volavka, M.D., Stanley Feldstein, Ph.D., and Richard Abrams, M.D. The encouragement of the chairman, Dr. Alfred Freedman, and Mr. Irvin Schwartz was essential to the success of the studies. The clinical studies were made possible only by the cooperation of the physicians and nurses at Gracie Square Hospital, and, of these, I am particularly indebted to Dr. William Karliner and Dr. Lothar Kalinowsky.

In organizing the 1972 conference on the psychobiology of convulsive therapy, I am indebted to the support of the cochairmen, Dr. Seymour Kety of Harvard and Dr. James McGaugh of the University of California at Irvine, and of Dr. Thomas A. Williams of the Clinical Research Branch of the National Institute of Mental Health.

Throughout the years, Dr. Jonathan O. Cole has been a principal supporter of the electrophysiologic studies of drugs, which have paralleled these studies of convulsive therapies. He has encouraged and supported the search for a common basis between the central effects of psychoactive drugs and seizures, facilitating many of the studies reported here.

These studies would not have been possible without extensive support from the National Institute of Mental Health in numerous grants in support of my research since 1954 (MH-927,* 2092,* 2715, 4798, 7249, 7432, 11380, 11381, 13358,* 15561,* 18172, 20762,* and 24020). The studies at Hillside Hospital were also supported by the Dazian Foundation, the Foundations Fund for Psychiatry, and the National Foundation for Infantile Paralysis. The encouragement and material support, both financial and in drug supplies, of many in the pharmaceutical industry was instrumental in providing the mortar for the governmental bricks. I am indebted to the officers and physicians of Smith, Kline and French Laboratories, Geigy Pharmaceuticals, A. H. Robins, and Burroughs-Wellcome Laboratories who, among others, supported the studies at Hillside Hospital and New York Medical College. Lately, the encouragement of the physicians of Organon, BV (Holland) and Fisons Pharmaceuticals (England) has been most helpful.

I am beholden to the directors of the International Association for Psychiatric Research—Arnold B. Canter, Henry Feiwel, Martin A. Green, Theodore J. Israel, Jr., Melvin Muroff, Donald M. Shapiro, and Joshua S. Vogel—who have actively supported the studies of convulsive therapy since 1967. And I am particularly indebted to my family, for their patience during these and many other academic labors that often took me away from home, and for their encouragement that this work was worthwhile.

The text has been typed and checked by Robin Canter Allendorfer, Barbara Cardella, and Linda Fink.

M. F.

---

* Principal ECT studies.

Contents

Chapter 1 Introduction 1
Chapter 2 History of Convulsive Therapies 5

CLINICAL STUDIES

Chapter 3 Clinical Efficacy 21
Chapter 4 Risks of Convulsive Therapy 41
Chapter 5 Risk-Benefit Analysis 51
Chapter 6 Predictors of Outcome 59
Chapter 7 ECT Usage 73

EFFECTS OF SEIZURES

Chapter 8 Electrophysiology of ECT 85
Chapter 9 Neuropsychology of ECT 107
Chapter 10 Behavior, Language, and Attitudes 131
Chapter 11 Biochemical Effects of Induced Seizures 143
Chapter 12 Vascular Effects: Cardiac and Cerebral 155

THEORIES OF CONVULSIVE THERAPY

Chapter 13 Review of Theories 161
Chapter 14 A Theory of Convulsive Therapy 171

TECHNICAL ISSUES

Chapter 15 Methods of Seizure Induction 189
Chapter 16 A Manual for Convulsive Therapy 215
Chapter 17 L'Envoi 235

References 239
Index 284

"*First Thesis:* Our knowledge is vast and impressive. We know not only innumerable details and facts of practical significance, but also many theories and explanations which give us an astonishing intellectual insight into dead and living objects, including ourselves, and human societies.

"*Second Thesis:* Our ignorance is boundless and overwhelming. Every new bit of knowledge we acquire serves to open our eyes further to the vastness of our ignorance.

"Both of these theses are true, ..."

Karl R. Popper, 1963

Chapter 1

Introduction

Convulsive therapy is effective in alleviating the symptoms of endogenous depression. When the available methods of administration are used, it carries as little risk as other treatments. It has been modified since its introduction more than 40 years ago and now bears little resemblance to the early procedures. It was first heralded as a panacea and applied widely; its use was soon criticized. With the introduction of the antidepressant drugs in the late 1950s, its death knell was sounded; but unlike its sibling therapies—insulin coma and leucotomy—convulsive therapy continues to be used.

ECT is undergoing an extensive reassessment, in part because the alternate therapies for the depressive illnesses—the tricyclic antidepressants and the monoamine oxidase inhibitors—are limited in therapeutic efficacy and in safety, and the catecholamine theories of depression, used as explanations for their mode of action, have not been supported by experimental data.

Another factor in the reassessment is political. The libertarian movements, fueled by the excesses of war and conscription, turned to the mental hospitals and asked whether these agencies may not be abusing the rights of patients—the right to treatment and the right to decide (consent) to what treatment will be given. The movement reached a pinnacle in legislation in one state limiting the practice of medicine by restricting the application of three treatments: behavior modification, lobotomy, and electroshock therapy. The limitation in the use of electroshock sparked reexaminations of its efficacy and safety to provide a basis for appeals to raise the legal restrictions.

This volume has been in preparation for a decade. Convulsive therapy provides a model of the interaction of brain functions and behavior and allows a variety of experimental studies, including the relationship of changes in brain chemistry and brain electrical activity to mood, vegetative functions, performance, language, and memory, as well as to the pathology of mood disorders. Since 1954, my associates and I have studied the convulsive therapy process. Recent demands of medical school teaching and service on commissions established to examine convulsive therapy provided the stimulus to bring together our experience. The volume distills the data from two complementary arenas: the theoretic and basic science studies of laboratory scientists seeking an explanation of the mode of action of convulsive therapy, and the practical clinical studies, which seek to improve treatment by the better selection of patients and a safer and more rapid treatment course. This volume seeks to answer four main questions:

1. *What is the evidence for the efficacy and usage of ECT?* Reviews of the indications, risks, and risk-benefit analysis are followed by descriptions of recent usage and the data of studies of predictors of outcome. (Chapters 2 to 7).

2. *What are the experimental findings, particularly the relationships between changes in brain functions and behavior?* Reviews of the extensive studies in electrophysiology and neuropsychology are followed by some descriptions of the biochemical, vascular, and language and attitude effects (Chapters 8 to 12).

3. *What is a viable theory of ECT?* The many theories are reviewed, and a new theory is presented, based on data from electrophysiology, the clinic, and neuroendocrine studies. It was not possible to encompass the diverse actions of ECT in a single theory, so the formulation discusses the specific effects of ECT in patients with endogenous depression. Secondary suggestions are made for its effects in catatonia, mania, and schizophrenia (Chapters 13 and 14).

4. *What is essential in the ECT process, and how can treatment be applied safely and effectively?* Chapters 15 and 16 present a review of the treatment parameters and a detailed manual of the therapy.

No review is complete without the writer donning the seer's hat, and Chapter 17 is a view into the future, an assessment of tests of the present theory that may extend it; and suggestions for the improvement of teaching and practice of convulsive therapy that may enhance the opportunity for patients to receive the best treatments available, particularly the proper use of convulsive therapy in the severe mentally ill, the suicidal, and the depressed.

DEFINITION OF TERMS

There is some confusion about terminology. Convulsive therapy is the use of controlled grand mal seizures, usually at intervals of days, to achieve a change in a psychotic patient's abnormal mental state. Many names have been given to this process: convulsive therapy, ECT, shock therapy, electroshock, electrostimulation, seizure therapy, electroseizure therapy, EST, electroplexy, electrotherapy, and clonotherapy. The term shock therapy was often used by the psychiatric pioneers. It is derived from the German *Insulinschockbehandlung,* the treatment that preceded the convulsive therapies and with which it was initially confused. Shock, either in its electric (shocking currents), medical (as in surgical or hemorrhagic shock), or psychologic (as in frightening) connotations, bears no relation to the therapeutic process of the convulsive therapies. Since "to shock" or "shock therapy" are not descriptive of this therapy and may be frightening to patients and their families, these terms should not be used (Fink, 1973).

The significant part of the process is the *seizure* in the central nervous system, and not the *motor convulsion.* For this reason, I have recently used the terms "seizure therapy," "electroseizure therapy," and "EST" in discussing these treatments. However, the Task Force of the American Psychiatric Association, recognizing the conventional (if less accurate) use of "convulsive therapy," "electroconvulsive therapy," and "ECT," recommended the preferential use of these names. These terms are used interchangeably in this volume.

Electric currents are also used to induce convulsions in animals. Location of electrodes, strength of currents, frequency of seizures, and use of adjuvants (such as anesthesia or muscle relaxants) are unstandardized, and few studies are comparable. It is customary to refer to these inductions as "electroconvulsive shock." In this volume, references to animal studies will continue to use the terms "electroconvulsive shock" and "ECS" interchangeably. The terms "convulsive therapy," "EST," and "ECT" refer to seizures induced in patients.

The treatments described as "ECT" or "EST" are distinguished from the "shock treatments" allegedly used in military and repressive political societies to instill fear and compliance in populations. Such "shock treatments" usually involve the application of sustained, painful, nonseizure-producing currents to genital or other sensitive body areas in awake individuals. The confusion between "shock treatments" as used in military and political circles and the medical uses of seizures is regrettable. The distinction among these different uses of electric currents will become clear in this monograph.

"Electroshock" is a term also used to describe experiments undertaken by psychologists to assess compliance and coercion. A recent headline in *Science*, "Electroshock Experiment at Albany Violates Ethics Guidelines," referred to social psychological experiments in volunteers in which painful electric charges were given to subjects to assess their tolerance for pain under different instructional sets (Smith, 1977). A similar confusion is engendered by scientists who equate studies of implanted electrodes in animal brains and stimulations with increasingly larger currents to induce convulsions as analogs of convulsive therapy. One repugnant example is seen in the reports by Pinel and Van Oot (1977), who summarize such brain stimulation experiments with:

> Repeated electroconvulsive shocks (ECSs) administered once every 3 days to rats . . . [find] . . . a treatment–drug interaction which could have hazardous consequences for patients undergoing electroconvulsive therapy.

Such a lack of discrimination illustrates a profound ignorance of the parameters of ECT, which in turn leads to misjudgments of the risks of ECT since the hazards that they cite are clearly prevented by anesthesia, forced ventilation, and surface electrodes used in clinical practice (Fink, 1977*a*).

Convulsive therapy is also to be distinguished from other biological treatments for the mentally ill: insulin coma therapy, lobotomy (psychosurgery, leucotomy), sleep therapy, and behavior modification techniques using aversive electric currents. In insulin coma, up to 50 daily hypoglycemic comas are induced by larges doses of insulin. Seizures may occur during the treatment but are generally considered as complications and not part of the therapeutic process. It is a treatment with a proclaimed efficacy in schizophrenia. Because modern antipsychotic drugs were found to be therapeutically as successful with greater safety and greater ease of administration, insulin coma has been universally replaced by pharmacotherapy.

Psychosurgery involves the cutting of selected brain tissues for a behavioral effect. It, too, was largely advocated for patients with schizophrenia and has been replaced by pharmacotherapy, except in selected cases of obsessional states. Sleep therapy requires a drug-sustained sleep for days and is no longer recommended. Behavior modification, usually of neurotic behavior, is a procedure in which painful (aversive) stimuli, often using electric shocks to extremities, are associated with the behaviors to be extinguished. There is no loss of consciousness, no seizure, and no amnesia in these treatments. In their indications, procedures, modes of action, efficacy, and safety, these therapies are clearly distinguished from the convulsive therapies. Their continued juxtaposition, particularly in legal and judicial discussions, is not helpful, and their separation as unique processes is to be encouraged.

Chapter 2

History of Convulsive Therapies

> The history of science is one long series of tournaments, of champions and challengers, of pledges and surrenders and rewards beyond compare in chivalry. The conquests and captures of the knights errant of natural history, the feats of backroom squires and laboratory heroes, are also legendary. But they are less ephemeral than those of romance, because the scene of the scientist adventurers is an expanding one and their purpose endless and unchanging. The Round Table of Science, moreover, has room for all who can find their way to it—the rim of it is a snowflake curve.
>
> Grey Walter, 1956
> The Curve of the Snowflake

The origin of convulsive therapy[1] is ascribed to the use of electric eels by the Romans, to experiments with electricity by Italian natural philosophers, and to the experiments of Mesmer. Such views are based on the belief that electricity is the essential component of modern convulsive therapy (Alexander and Selesnick, 1966). Others emphasize the convulsion, with either its physiologic or symbolic consequences, as the basis for treatment. I hold that these views are not correct. A different source is seen in an early treatise on mental illness (Battie, 1758):

> The eighth remoter cause of Consequential Madness, viz Muscular Constriction, gradual, gentler and uniform, but more obstinate may sometimes be relieved or as it were diverted by convulsion, that is by an alternate motion of muscular fibres artificially excited in some other part of the body. On which account vesicatories, vomits, rough cathartics, errhines, and the most poinant amongst the medicines called nervous, may in this particular case of spasm become even antispasmodic. For, ignorant as we are and perhaps shall always be of the reason, experience has shown that, although many parts of the body may be convulsed together, one species of spasm however occasioned seldom fails to put an end to that other which before subsisted.

Even today, medical folklore includes tales that gross bodily stresses can alleviate mental illness. Such beliefs were an integral part of nineteenth century beliefs and were the basis for clinical trials with fever, convulsions, and surgery in the treatment of the mentally ill.

A second root for the biological psychiatric therapies is the belief that mental illnesses arise from disorders of the brain. Griesinger and Maudsley described connections between abnormal mental states and brain pathology. The neurolo-

---

[1] Modifications of ECT and studies of efficacy are intimately bound to concepts of its mode of action. Attempts to separate reports of efficacy, changes in treatment, selection of patients, and predictors or other clinical aspects of the treatment from concepts of the mode of action of ECT must be artificial. In a historic review, however, it is useful to distinguish the evolution of the treatment from changes in the concepts of its actions, since guesses about the former have been combined with some errors regarding the latter. A detailed review of the theories of ECT is presented in Chapter 13.

gists Fritsch, Hitzig, Jackson, Westphal, Wernicke, Meynert, and Alzheimer described a diversity in the functions of specific brain areas, and developed concepts that dysfunctions in these areas could be the basis for abnormal behavior. In dementia paralytica (neurosyphilis) the lesions were thought to involve many brain areas, and this concept and a belief in the therapeutic efficacy of fever led Wagner-Jauregg to attempt a fever cure of this mental illness. The apparent success of that effort encouraged other pathologic theories of the mental illnesses and their alleviation by similar drastic therapies. The convulsive therapies are a development of this period (Marti-Ibanez et al., 1956). An outline of the developments in the past decades is presented in Fig. 2.1.

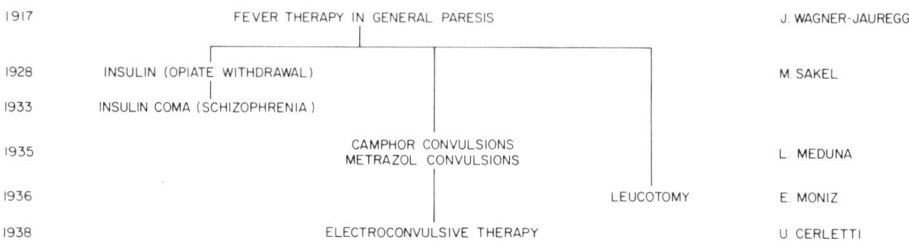

FIG. 2.1. Historic tree: Somatic therapies in psychiatry.

THE PIONEERS

Fever Therapy and General Paresis: Julius Wagner-Jauregg (1917)

Nineteenth century medical experience included many observations that improvement in chronic ailments, including the psychoses, followed a severe infection.[2] One such report was that syphilis in Russian troops improved after an epidemic of typhus. Among the early observers to seriously consider fever as a therapy, Wagner-Jauregg (1857–1940) began to induce fevers in the mentally ill in 1886. He tried many agents, including tuberculin in 1907 and typhus vaccine a few years later, with encouraging results. To stimulate a greater bodily response, he selected tertian malaria, an active febrile illness that could be checked with quinine. In 1917, nine patients with general paresis were treated. Blood from patients with active malaria was injected intramuscularly, and each patient was allowed to have fever for a few days. Such episodes were repeated for 10 to 12 bouts of fever. Three patients recovered and returned to work; three showed temporary symptomatic relief; and three failed to improve (Dattner, 1944; Kalinowsky, 1970).

The favorable results of the first experiments in a disease with a notoriously poor prognosis were soon confirmed, and fever therapy became a principal treatment for neurosyphilis until it was replaced by penicillin in the 1940s. Despite

---

[2] This idea has been active in psychiatric writings up to the present. See Terry, 1939.

its radical nature—the alleviation of one illness by inducing another—fever therapy was heralded by the scientific community; and in 1927, Wagner-Jauregg received the Nobel Prize for Medicine, "for his discovery of the therapeutic value of malaria inoculation in the treatment of dementia paralytica" (Liljestrand, 1962).

Prior to Wagner-Jauregg's success, the prevailing attitude among alienists responsible for the care of the mentally ill was one of psychological optimism and biological nihilism. Sakel (1956) summarized the status of the teaching in Vienna in the early 1900s:

> In my time as a medical student, those of us who chose to specialize in psychiatry were taught to deal with all nervous-emotional diseases by employing the scholastic remedies of a psychological handling of the symptoms. For lack of knowledge of a more scientific medical technique, the sicknesses themselves remained untreated. Consequently, by emulation of teachers and by force of habit, one generation of doctors after another went on thinking in terms of symptoms, mistaking them for illnesses, instead of attacking fundamental causes.

Fever therapy showed that a mental syndrome could be alleviated through biological procedures, and that not all therapies need be directed against mental or psychological operations. The modern biological therapies, insulin coma, pentylenetetrazol (Metrazol), electroconvulsive therapies, and even leucotomy, are derived from these observations and the optimistic philosophy that they spawned.

An early development was the introduction of continuous sleep treatment for the functional psychoses by the Swiss psychiatrist Klaesi in 1922. Patients were maintained in continuous somnolence for 10 days or more by the repeated administration of sedative drugs. Cardiovascular and renal complications, drug withdrawal seizures, and delirium, however, limited the usefulness of this treatment (Kalinowsky and Hoch, 1961).

Insulin Coma: Manfred Sakel (1933)

Insulin coma therapy was developed by Manfred Sakel (1900–1957), who graduated from the University of Vienna Medical School in 1925. At the time, psychoses were thought by some to be the symptoms of a cerebral disorder, and Sakel (1956) sought:

> . . . a physiological approach to influence the center of the autonomous nervous system, the hypothalamus, which appeared to be the bridge between physiologic functions and mental manifestations.

The identification of insulin by Banting, Best, and McLeod in 1922 provided a means to alter hypothalamic functions. Insulin-induced hypoglycemia was found to have autonomic effects, to impair consciousness, to reduce motility, excitement, and insomnia, and to induce weight gain. Insulin was soon used as a sedative for psychiatric patients (Wortis, 1959).

As a staff physician in a private psychiatric hospital in Berlin from 1927 to 1933, Sakel used insulin to treat the hypermotility, irritability, insomnia, and weight loss of morphine-dependence withdrawal (Sakel, 1956). Although the long-term effects of insulin in morphine dependence were not impressive, the short-term behavioral gains were significant. Some patients convulsed after insulin, and at first Sakel sought to prevent seizures by adding barbiturates to the intravenous doses of insulin. As the population sample broadened, he reported favorable results after insulin in other mental illnesses, including schizophrenia. In 1933, he returned to Vienna as a physician in the University Psychiatric Hospital, where he was encouraged by Wagner-Jauregg's successor, Professor Otto Poetzl, to use insulin in the psychiatric clinic. On Novemeber 3, 1933, he reported to the Vienna Medical Society that the repeated induction of hypoglycemia, often with coma and occasionally with convulsions, had prolonged favorable behavioral consequences in patients with schizophrenia (Sakel, 1938, 1956). In 1936, he came to New York to demonstrate the "Sakel Shock Treatment," and he remained, first as a physician in the Department of Mental Hygiene, and later in private psychiatric practice until his death in 1957 (Bowman, 1966).

Insulin coma and insulin subcoma therapy were important treatments of patients with schizophrenia during the 1940s. Many specialized insulin coma treatment units were built throughout the world. The hazards of the therapy, its unpredictable efficacy, and the need for a large professional staff led many physicians to try to simplify the Sakel regimens. Because of the greater ease of application, ECT became a preferred treatment of the severely mentally ill. With the introduction of chlorpromazine, the early comparative trials in the mid-1950s found the drug therapies safer and equally effective; insulin coma therapy was rapidly abandoned.

Convulsive Therapy: Laszlo Meduna (1934)

A Hungarian psychiatrist, Laszlo Meduna (1896–1964), is credited with developing modern convulsive therapy. Following medical school graduation in 1921, he was an active member of the neurological (1924–1927) and psychiatric (1927–1939) research institutes in Budapest. He surely was acquainted with the philosophy and the achievements of the Viennese school of psychiatry. Much of his research was in the neuropathology of schizophrenia, in a school where schizophrenia was thought to be an incurable, endogenous, hereditary disease in which cerebral neurons were preferentially attacked (Meduna, 1956). Other mental syndromes, particularly the epilepsies, were considered exogenous in origin and hence curable. Meduna noted that glial hyperplasia was common in the brains of epileptics:

> . . . Working upon biopsy material of the primary convulsant foci in several cases of so-called genuine epilepsy, I observed the extreme hyperplasia of the glia system in epileptic brains, in contrast with the apparent torpor of the glia system in schizo-

phrenic brains. To explain the difference . . . I developed the hypothesis that the noxa causing epilepsy has a stimulating effect upon the growth of the glia cells, while the noxa producing schizophrenia has an opposite, a paralyzing, effect of the glia system. Thus, fairly early, I developed an idea of some sort of antagonism between the behavior of the glia system in epilepsy and the behavior of this system in schizophrenia.

Meduna became acquainted with studies (Nyirö and Jablonsky, 1929) that reported that:

> . . . in those cases of schizophrenia which later became combined with epilepsy, the epileptic attacks either had disappeared completely or had occurred only infrequently. In cases . . . of epilepsy which later developed a schizophrenic disease, the epileptic attacks had . . . become less frequent and had later disappeared completely.

Belief that the schizophrenic process had a curative effect in epilepsy led to unsuccessful attempts to transfuse the blood of schizophrenic patients to treat those with epilepsy.

Meduna sought to achieve the reverse, to use the epileptic process to treat schizophrenia. His determination was supported in part by reports that among more than 6,000 patients with schizophrenia, only about 20 had a history of epileptic attacks. Some authors had suggested that typical epileptic attacks, if they occur at all in true schizophrenia, were so rare that the correctness of a diagnosis of schizophrenia could be doubted. Another had reported two patients with catatonia in whom spontaneous epileptic attacks developed, after which they recovered from both the epileptic and the schizophrenic forms of the disease. Meduna compared the beneficial effect of the epileptic attack on the schizophrenic process to the beneficial effect of high temperature on the course of general paresis. From these observations, Meduna concluded that:

> From that time on, I was convinced that there is a biological antagonism between the process which produces epileptiform attacks and the process which produces schizophrenia. I had only to find a convulsant drug which could be used safely in human beings, which would produce epileptic attacks by acting upon the nerve cells of the brain, and which would leave the cerebral blood vessels intact.

Camphor and Pentylenetetrazol

Of the many convulsants known, Meduna first injected camphor into guinea pigs to establish its safety. He treated his first patient on January 23, 1934, and published his observations in the first 26 cases in January, 1935. He reported a successful influence on the course of the illness in 10 of 26 patients. In the improved group, each patient had an average of 6.2 seizures; in the unimproved group, the average was 2.0 seizures. The difficulty in inducing seizures with camphor led to trials with pentylenetetrazol (Metrazol, Cardiozol); by 1936 he wrote:

> . . . the effect of the epileptic convulsions is that they change the chemical constituents in the organism in a way suitable for the cure of schizophrenia.

A monograph was published in 1937, followed by additional reports in 1938 and 1939.

Antagonism developed between the proponents of insulin coma and pentylenetetrazol therapies, an antagonism which he deplored, describing the sequential use of the two treatments in patients who had not responded well to either treatment alone (Meduna, 1937). As a therapeutic optimist, he anticipated modern pharmacotherapy when he wrote:

> . . . that schizophrenia is not a biological catastrophe; that it is caused neither by a sudden strike of the endocrine system nor by a sudden block of the mesenchyme; that it originates as a consequence of a logical chain of chemical processes; . . . that when these pathologic reactions have reached a definite . . . intensity, the patient becomes schizophrenic; that both insulin and metrazol treatments break . . . up this process; [and] . . . in the future . . . we should be able to . . . apply only those slow chemical processes that are produced by the explosive actions of both treatments and that are responsible for recovery.

Meduna (1956) reports some earlier uses of camphor in the treatment of mental illness. Von Auenbrugger, who is credited with the auscultatory percussion method of examining the chest, used camphor to induce seizures in patients with "mania virorum;" and Weickhardt had recommended epileptogenic doses of camphor for delusional states. The first reports of the use of Metrazol in depressive psychoses appeared in 1937 (Verstraeten, 1937).

After emigrating to the United States in 1939, Meduna continued his interest in convulsive therapy. He also developed carbon dioxide therapy (Meduna, 1950). In his explanation of the mode of action of ECT (Meduna, 1956), he anticipated our present views:

> In the therapeutical convulsions there may be some components . . . that are germane to the means whereby the convulsions are produced . . . [which] may be nothing other than the severity of the convulsion, which may be the factor responsible for the different qualities of improvement achieved by the different convulsive therapies.

Electroshock: Ugo Cerletti (1938)

The next development in the convulsive therapies was the introduction of electric currents to induce seizures. By 1935, Ugo Cerletti (1877–1963), Professor of Neuropathology and Psychiatry in Rome, had used electrical methods to induce experimental seizures in animals. Reports of the clinical efficacy of insulin coma and pentylenetetrazol convulsive therapies led Cerletti to send assistants to Vienna and Budapest to learn the new techniques and to introduce them into Rome. Because many patients who received intravenous Metrazol experienced painful and frightening experiences, he thought to replace Metrazol with the electrical inductions of experimental epilepsy. After extensive studies in animals failed to demonstrate any additional pathology after electrical seizures, he undertook to treat a psychiatric patient (Cerletti, 1956).

In April, 1938, a 39-year-old man who had been found wandering the streets of Rome was sent to the psychiatric clinic. He spoke in neologisms of being telepathically influenced, and his mood was indifferent to his environment. He had responded to pentylenetetrazol therapy 1 year earlier. He received 11 electrical applications, responded well, and 1 year later was working regularly in his old job. The first demonstration and report of this new method of induction was made to the Medical Academy of Rome in May, 1938 (Cerletti and Bini, 1938). The new method soon spread to other countries and by 1939 was accepted in the United States, despite warnings against possible electrocution by the editors of the *Journal of the American Medical Association* (Kalinowsky, 1970).

Cerletti continued his research attempts to improve the treatment and to understand the mode of action of electroshock. He determined that the cerebral seizure was essential to the clinical results, while neither the currents used to elicit a seizure nor the motor aspects of the convulsion were significant.

> I have always maintained that in the therapeutic mechanism of electroshock the electricity itself is of little importance: it is only an epileptogenic stimulus, while the important and fundamental factor is the epileptic-like seizure, no matter how it is obtained. Therefore, maintaining that only the convulsive attack induced with the minimum stimulus is the essential therapeutic factor, I have never paid much attention to the different variations of the electric machine proposed.

Anticipating some of the recent interest in hormonal effects of seizures, he suggested (Cerletti, 1956) that:

> . . . the anatomicofunctional substratum of the vegetative syndrome induced by electroshock is to be localized in the diencephalic section of the cerebrospinal axis.

Psychosurgery: Egas Moniz (1935)

The eventful years of the 1930s saw yet another new treatment for the severely mentally ill. Neurosurgery had made many strides in the decades since Horsley, Dandy, and Cushing demonstrated the safety of neurosurgical approaches on the brain. Fulton, Bucy, and Jacobsen had shown that cutting the "silent" frontal brain areas resulted in changed behavior in animals—less aggressivity and decreased psychomotility and tension. In 1935, Egas Moniz (1874–1955) performed the first surgical intervention on the frontal lobes of a schizophrenic patient. The success of his intervention was heralded by many, but it was Freeman and Watts (1942) in the United States who simplified the procedure and made its use commonplace. Psychosurgery was used often in patients with schizophrenia, aggressivity, or mania. In 1949, Moniz was awarded the Nobel Prize for Medicine for "his discovery of the therapeutic value of leucotomy in certain psychoses."

Many of the clinicians saw similarities between the types of cases responsive to leucotomy and to convulsive therapy, suggesting that either their sites or modes of action were similar (Hemphill and Walter, 1941).

THE HOMESTEAD YEARS: 1939-1958

By 1939, two decades after the successful treatment of general paresis by fever therapy, the convulsive therapies were accepted as successful treatments for dementia praecox. Therapeutic optimism succeeded psychiatric pessimism, and, as psychiatrists became acquainted with the safety and efficacy of convulsive therapy, almost all types of mental illness were treated. Successful results in patients with schizophrenia led to trials in other conditions. The value of the convulsive therapies for patients with depressive psychoses (Bennett, 1938, 1939; Weigert, 1940), involutional depression (Bennett, 1940; Weigert, 1940; Hamilton and Ward, 1948; Huston and Locher, 1948a, b; Fishbein, 1949), and mania (Bennett, 1939; Zeifert, 1939; Ziskind et al., 1943, 1945) was soon recognized. The success of short courses of ECT for patients with involutional and endogenous depressions was described, and the specificity of induced seizures among clinical syndromes was emphasized (Myerson, 1941; Kalinowsky, 1943; Savitsky and Tarachow, 1945; Savitsky and Karliner, 1947). The special usefulness of the therapies in patients with suicidal thoughts and intentions was realized (Huston and Locher, 1948a). Trials were soon reported in patients of all ages, from childhood to the senium, and in all mental conditions, including the neuroses, psychopathies, drug dependence, and organic psychoses. Some observers noted the progressive rise in seizure threshold with repeated seizures and suggested that ECT be used in the treatment of uncontrolled epilepsy (Androp, 1941).

The interest in the convulsive therapies increased with the demands of war. Many physicians were trained in clinical psychiatry by the military, and the convulsive therapies were a significant part of their education and their military clinical experience. As patients failed to respond to one therapy, insulin coma and seizure therapy were combined. Some increased the number and frequency of seizure inductions and found efficacy, particularly in schizophrenia, to be related to dose (number and frequency of seizures).

Much attention was paid to the complications. Death, fractures, panic, fear, memory loss, postseizure delirium, spontaneous seizures, and cardiovascular complications were described for both pentylenetetrazol and electrical inductions. By 1940, Bennett had introduced curare (Intocostrin) to reduce the incidence of fractures (Bennett, 1941, 1946, 1968). Its usefulness was immediately recognized, but difficulties in its administration led to trials with other relaxants. Gallamine triethiodide (Flaxedil) and then succinylcholine (Anectine) replaced curare, and the ease of use and safety of succinylcholine led to its widespread acceptance in standard treatment regimens.

Incomplete or partial seizures, described as petit mal convulsions, occurred frequently. The experiences were frightening and painful and often resulted in the refusal of further therapy. Barbiturate premedication and anesthesia were introduced, with thiopental (Pentothal) and later methohexital (Brevital) usually used. The ease and safety of their administration led to their acceptance, and their use not only relieved anxiety but also reduced the incidence of death, postseizure delirium, and spontaneous seizures.

Texts appeared with the publication of *Physical Methods of Treatment in Psychiatry* by Sargant and Slater in 1944 in Great Britain. *Shock Treatments, Psychosurgery and Other Somatic Treatments* by Kalinowsky and Hoch, *L'Électro-choc* by Delay and *Šokové Léčeni Duševnich Chorob* by Roubicek appeared simultaneously in 1946 in the United States, France, and Czechoslovakia. In 1951, these were followed by *Die Moderne Psychiatrische Schockbehandlung* by von Baeyer in Germany.

Throughout this period, much interest was shown in the mode of action of ECT. Pathological, psychological, biochemical, and physiological theories were proposed, each depending on the author's view of the origin of mental illnesses and the emphasis placed on specific aspects of the convulsive therapy process. In 1948, Gordon listed 50 theories, most of which were incomplete and inadequate. A detailed review of the theories is presented in Chapter 13.

Modified Convulsions

By 1950 and after 10 years of treatment exploration, seizures modified by muscle paralysis and anesthesia were in common use. The course of treatments was accepted as four to 12 seizure inductions in depressed patients and 12 to 20 in schizophrenic. Insulin coma and convulsive therapy facilities were available in many private and public mental hospitals. Matters of concern were no longer the efficacy of the convulsive therapies but ways to improve the delivery of the treatment to reduce complications. Some clinicians sought to improve the currents used to elicit seizures (Liberson, 1948), while others increased the frequency of treatments, developing regressive therapy (Kennedy and Anchel, 1948; Rothschild et al., 1951). Some continued low electric currents after the seizure, as in electronarcosis (Frostig et al., 1944), and others used subconvulsive currents alone to avoid the risks of the convulsion (Alexander, 1953).

ECT was widely used after World War II, and allegations that its use was promiscuous led American psychiatrists to examine these concerns. A single page report, issued by the Group for the Advancement of Psychiatry from Topeka, Kansas, in 1946 and again in 1947 stated:

> ... Both the extravagant claims as to its efficacy made by its proponents and the uninformed condemnation of its use at all by its opponents indicate the emotional aura which surrounds the whole topic.

After surveying the practice in different communities, the committee concluded:

> Abuses in the use of electro-shock therapy are sufficiently widespread and dangerous to justify consideration of a campaign of professional education in the limitations of this technique, and perhaps even to justify instituting certain measures of control.

FIG. 2.2. GROUP FOR THE ADVANCEMENT OF PSYCHIATRY

Report No. 1 3617 W. Sixth Ave., Topeka, Kansas September 15, 1947

SHOCK THERAPY

In view of the reported promiscuous and indiscriminate use of electro-shock therapy, your Committee on Therapy decided to devote its first meeting to an evaluation of the role of this type of therapy in psychiatry. Both the extravagant claims as to its efficacy made by its proponents and the uninformed condemnation of its use at all by its opponents indicate the emotional aura which surrounds this whole topic.

Your Committee bases its conclusions and recommendations on data gathered by the members of the Committee from their personal experience, reports from the literature, reports from the Army, Navy, Veterans Administration, University Hospitals, Canadian Army and Veterans Affairs, private hospitals and other sources. The Committee is grateful to Dr. A. E. Bennett who sat with us as an invited expert and gave freely of his extensive experience in this field. The conclusions and recommendations which follow have the unanimous concurrence of the Committee members and of the invited expert.

1. There is as yet no adequate theory of the mode of action of electro-shock therapy. All indications are that it operates on a symptomatic rather than an etiological level.

2. The preponderant weight of the evidence points to the conclusion that electro-shock therapy materially shortens the majority of depressive episodes, especially those which occur in the involutional period. It may or may not aid in shortening or controlling individual manic episodes. No evidence has been found to indicate that it has any effect in altering the cycles of manic-depressive psychosis.

3. The evidence is conflicting as to its efficacy in the schizophrenias. Good results have been reported in some cases of severe catatonic and acute paranoid reactions, but these conditions may respond also to appropriate psychotherapy and good hospital care. Any improvement which occurs appears to be due to modification of the affective components. The schizophrenic personality is not altered by electro-shock therapy.

4. The preponderance of evidence indicates that the use of electro-shock therapy is contra-indicated in the psychoneuroses, with the possible exception of severe, resistant, neurotic depressions, in which symptomatic relief may at times be obtained.

5. The complications and hazards in its use should be re-emphasized, since they appear to have been minimized by some workers. Some workers have reported that such pre-shock measures as curarization or sedation with barbiturates offer a safeguard against traumatic complications.

6. In view of the foregoing considerations, electro-shock therapy should be administered only by psychiatrists who are trained in treatment techniques, and then only as an adjuvant in a total psychiatric treatment program.

7. Electro-shock therapy should be restricted to hospitalized patients. The only possible exception would be its use as part of a treatment program under competent supervision in selected outpatient departments. The Committee unitedly opposed the use of shock therapy in the private office because of its indiscriminate use; there were a very few members of the Group who were in disagreement with this point.

8. Your Committee deplores certain widespread abuses of electro-shock therapy, amongst which are:
   a. Its use in office practice.
   b. Its indiscriminate administration to patients in any and all diagnostic categories.
   c. Its immediate use to the exclusion of adequate psychotherapeutic attempts.
   d. Its use as the sole therapeutic agent, to the neglect of a complete psychiatric program.

9. Your Committee feels that the overemphasis and unjustified use of electro-shock therapy short-circuits the training and experience which is essential in modern dynamic psychiatry.

10. In spite of a voluminous literature on the subject, your Committee feels that active research is still indicated in many areas. Some of these are:
    a. Establishment of uniform criteria for evaluation of results.
    b. Combined physiological and psychodynamic studies which would lead to a greater understanding of the basic problems.
    c. Adequate, long-time, follow-up studies, with careful psychological and electroencephalographic investigations, leading to a better evaluation of the patient's clinical status during a remission or after an apparent recovery.
    d. Better application of statistically valid methods in surveying results.
    e. Definitive studies as to the possibility of irreversible brain damage, and correlation between such sequellae and the intensity and number of shock treatments administered.

11. Abuses in the use of electro-shock therapy are sufficiently widespread and dangerous to justify consideration of a campaign of professional education in the limitations of this technique, and perhaps even to justify instituting certain measures of control. However, the research studies suggested in number 10 should be available to provide a sound basis for inaugurating such a campaign.

Report formulated by Committee on Therapy. Approved by the entire Membership of G. A. P. Circulated originally as Circular Letters No. 9, November 8, 1946, and No. 18, January 22, 1947.

The committee was concerned not only with its widespread use but also with the impact that such use had on the acceptance of psychotherapy, then in the first flush of postwar enthusiasm (Fig. 2.2).

Impact of Pharmacotherapy

The introduction of reserpine and chlorpromazine in the early 1950s dramatically changed the course of modern psychiatric therapy. The drug therapies were heralded as the solution to the problems of mental illness, and as their efficacy and safety were confirmed, interest in other therapies waned.

When insulin therapy was a mainstay in the treatment of schizophrenia, no single course of coma therapy was defined. The numbers of treatments and dosages of insulin varied widely, and the risks of death, spontaneous seizures, and prolonged coma interfered with acceptance of the treatment. The introduction of convulsive therapy generated controversies about the relative significance of the coma and of convulsions in insulin therapy and the comparative efficacy of the treatments (Meduna, 1956; Sakel, 1956). Questions were raised as to whether coma therapy was specific for schizophrenia or a nonspecific amelioration of hypermotility, excitement, insomnia, and irritability. Comparative studies of insulin with barbiturate coma (Ackner et al., 1957) and with chlorpromazine (Boardman et al., 1956; Fink et al., 1958) found the chemotherapies as effective as insulin coma and safer, less expensive, and easier to use. By 1960, most of the specialized insulin coma units had closed (Brill, 1966).

While direct comparisons between leucotomy and the drug therapies were not done, it was so clear that the psychotropic drugs were easier to use and safer to administer that by 1960, leucotomy had been virtually abandoned. At present, it is occasionally used in special cases of unresponsive seizure disorders and obsessive-compulsive neuroses (Bridges and Bartlett, 1977; National Commission, 1977).

Psychotropic drugs replaced ECT in the treatment of most cases of schizophrenia. The efficacy of tricyclic antidepressant drugs, the monamine oxidase inhibitors, stimulants, and lithium in depressive and manic disorders further reduced the interest in and use of ECT. Many ECT facilities were closed, and it was only in the mid-1960s, as the limitations of the antidepressant drug therapies were recognized, that interest in ECT was rekindled.

In 1956, the discovery of the epileptic properties of a halogenated ether, hexafluorodiethylether (flurothyl, Indoklon) led to its trial as a substitute for electroconvulsive therapy (Krantz et al., 1957; Kurland et al., 1959). In subsequent years, its use was explored as a pharmacologic replacement for ECT, but difficulties in its administration and the lack of any material advantage over ECT led to its disuse.

YEARS OF CONSOLIDATION: 1959–1978

Despite the decline in the clinical use of the convulsive therapies, some scientists continued their studies, although in reduced numbers of subjects. They examined the relative safety and efficacy of the antidepressants and ECT, the usefulness of the sequential use of ECT followed by pharmacotherapy, and the combined use of drugs and ECT not only in the treatment of depression but also in schizophrenia. Some studies found that psychotic depressed and some chronic schizophrenic patients who did not respond to pharmacotherapy improved after ECT.

Much research was devoted to understanding the seizure process and improving its safety. The location of the stimulating electrodes was changed to one side of the head; it was found that unilateral placement elicited a seizure that was therapeutically effective with less effect on memory functions. Multiple seizures in one sitting were introduced with both an EEG control and hyperoxygenation. This modification was termed multiple monitored ECT (MMECT), the patients showing a rapid clinical response without the severe memory deficits noted in regressive ECT treatments. The usefulness of intensive treatments in severely ill schizophrenic patients was reexamined, with those receiving intensive ECT showing better follow-up results in residual symptoms, work records, and rehospitalization rates than those treated with pharmacotherapy alone (Murillo and Exner, 1973a; Exner and Murillo, 1977). The significance of the seizure in convulsive therapy was demonstrated by studies of subconvulsive and convulsive therapies, with the finding of limited efficacy for subconvulsive treatments (Ulett et al., 1956; Fink et al., 1958a, b).

Public concerns with the safety of ECT, problems of consent, and complaints about its misuse have led to a renewed public and professional interest. Insulin coma, leucotomy, and the convulsive therapies are viewed as clinically and legally equivalent by many. Whereas insulin coma and leucotomy have been virtually abandoned, convulsive therapies continue to be used, with an incidence of from 1 to 5% of admissions to general psychiatric hospitals in the United States. In some private hospitals the incidence of its use is considerably higher, ranging to 40% (Chapter 7).

There is much concern that ECT may cause irreparable damage to the brain and that its use may contravene or deny patients' rights to knowingly decide what is done to them. These concerns led to judicial and legislative challenges to its use, as exemplified by its virtual proscription in California in 1974. The profession responded to these concerns with conferences to assess its psychobiology (Fink et al., 1974) and efficacy (Fink, 1972b, c, 1977c, 1978b; Squire, 1977; Salzman, 1977; Greenblatt, 1977; Friedberg, 1977; Frankel, 1977). In 1975, the American Psychiatric Association appointed a Task Force on Convulsive Therapy; its report appeared in November, 1978. Similar anxieties concerning the role of ECT were voiced in Great Britain, Scandinavia, and Holland, resulting in additional evaluations (Editor, 1975, 1977a, b,; Royal College of Psychiatrists, 1977; Kendell, 1978; Parliamentary correspondent, 1978). Responses to some of the editorials have been clarifying (Fink, 1976; Eastwood and Peacocke, 1976c).

A coincident concern regarding the continued use of psychosurgical procedures for patients with epilepsy and mental illness led to the appointment of a National Commission for the Protection of Human Subjects of Biomedical and Behavioral Research in 1973 and the publication of its report in 1977.

The continuing assessment of the convulsive therapies in the 1970s has elicited reviews of its safety and efficacy (Catalano-Nobili and Cerquetelli, 1972; Ilaria and Prange, 1975; Eastwood and Peacocke, 1976a; Turek and Hanlon, 1977; Fink, 1978b), conferences with published proceedings (Fink et al., 1974; Editor, 1977c), continuing education programs dedicated to the administration of ECT, and suggestions as to the research needs (Frankel, 1978). And scientists again considered the biochemical aspects of ECT more seriously. New theories of its mode of action were proposed (Modigh, 1975, 1976; Bolwig et al., 1977; Grahame-Smith, Green and Costain, 1978), and the biochemical aspects were included as a topic for a main symposium at the Vienna meeting of July, 1978 of the CINP—an international organization of scientists dedicated to the study of the effects of drugs on brain function.

As the experience with the biologic therapies matured, a number of editors invited the principal contributors to describe the accomplishments and conditions that led to their contributions (Marti-Ibanez et al., 1956; Ayd and Blackwell, 1970). Goldman (1962) and Bennett (1972) described their experiences with convulsive therapy, as did Kalinowsky in his periodic texts (Kalinowsky and Hoch, 1952, 1961; Kalinowsky and Hippius, 1972) and in reviews (Kalinowsky, 1964).

The continuing interest in ECT holds some promise for the future. With improved techniques of treatment and equipment, clarification of the indications, and better education, the incidence of adverse reactions should decline even further. With studies of the hormones derived from the hypothalamus and hypophysis, it is probable that we will come to understand the pathogenesis of the endogenous depressions. It is also likely that the complex and difficult procedures of the convulsive therapies will soon be replaced by a simpler pharmacologic substitute and by both social and genetic programs of prophylaxis of the mood disorders. An important legacy of this unique period of experimental psychiatry will be a better understanding between brain function and behavior achieved in the studies of convulsive therapy.

CLINICAL STUDIES

The principal justification for the use of convulsive therapy lies in its efficacy in relieving some psychotic disorders with equal or better results than alternate therapies (Chapter 3) and with lesser or equal risk (Chapter 4). The practice of ECT has undergone many modifications, and its application is complicated by an ignorance of its efficacy, fears about its risks, and legal, economic, and ethical concerns which modify its usage (Chapter 5). Much has been learned about the clinical predictors in selecting patients for treatment (Chapter 6). Clinical experience, particularly the evidence of efficacy and risks, guides to the selection of suitable patients, and patterns of usage provide the basis for a comparison of the convulsive therapies and alternate therapies (Chapter 7).

Chapter 3

Clinical Efficacy

ECT was introduced for the treatment of dementia praecox. Its initial clinical success and apparent safety led to trials in other conditions; thus, by 1939 it was also recommended for the manic and depressed phases of manic-depressive psychoses (Bennett, 1939). The early reports were largely uncontrolled clinical case records of diverse samples with a variety of treatments. As clinicians experimented to develop optimal results, they varied the number and frequency of seizures and modes of induction. Clinical evaluations of convulsive therapy in the first decades of its use (1938–1958) were done as the treatment rapidly changed. A troublesome question in assessing these early records is the extent to which we can rely on evaluations done in frightened patients, without anesthesia or muscle relaxants, with apnea and cyanosis as accepted parts of the therapy for an understanding of the efficacy of modern ECT, which depends on the routine use of anesthesia, muscle paralysis, and hyperoxygenation.

Not only have the treatment methods changed, but the diagnostic criteria, methods of selection and evaluation, and concurrent treatments also differ (Blum, 1978). Modern diagnosis depends on behavioral, familial, genetic, and historic factors, and less on the psychodynamic formulations that were current at the time ECT was introduced. Populations labeled "schizophrenic" in early studies may have included patients now labeled "manic" or "acute confusional psychosis," leading to clinical results different from those we may find today. The wide variation in efficacy of ECT in schizophrenia reflects differences in the sample treated, those with larger numbers of catatonic and manic patients having better outcome statistics than those with fewer numbers of these responsive patients. In addition, today's widespread use of alternate treatments, such as antidepressants, antipsychotic drugs, and lithium, selectively parcels out therapy-responsive populations, leaving groups of nonresponsive patients for ECT. Furthermore, few clinical studies of ECT meet the present standards for the evaluation of therapeutic efficacy. There is little description of previous or concurrent therapy, follow-up studies are infrequent, and defined contemporaneous controls or comparison groups are lacking (Riddell, 1963).

Yet the clinical literature and practice define mentally ill populations for whom induced convulsions elicit salutary changes in behavior. The benefits of convulsive therapy are directly related to clinical diagnosis. It is most effective in psychotic depressive syndromes and in mania where success rates are reported for 60 to 90% of cases selected. Although ECT is often used in acute and chronic schizophrenia, the data in these populations are less compelling. Improvement rates vary from 20 to 50% of selected populations with few differences among ECT, drug therapies, and milieu treatments in comparative studies.

The methods of assessment are another important caveat in assessing the efficacy of the convulsive therapies. In the initial years, only the more seriously incapacitated patients were given ECT, and any favorable response was considered "improvement," often despite such treatment-induced complications as memory loss and panic (Fink and Kahn, 1961). In the treatment of the depressive and manic syndromes, indices of improvement rapidly evolved, and patients were considered improved who stopped being suicidal, or who could be returned to home care, or who returned to work. The accompanying deficits in memory and difficulties in self-perception often made the assessment of improvement difficult (May, 1968; May and Tuma, 1976). In the past decade, the issues of evaluation of improvement have been considered, but the application of modern rating scale evaluations, observer- and self-ratings, and the other paraphernalia of modern controlled assessments, as exemplified by the NIMH volume on principles in establishing the efficacy of psychotropic agents (Levine et al., 1971), have yet to be applied to the assessments of the convulsive therapies.

Some confusion is generated by the occasional use of subconvulsive currents, and unless populations are clearly specified, efficacy rates may be erroneous. Various authors have found subconvulsive currents and partial seizures ineffective in depressive psychoses and acute schizophrenia (Androp, 1941; Kalinowsky et al., 1942; Ulett et al., 1956; Fink et al., 1958*b*). Others report some success in uncontrolled studies, particularly in patients with neurotic depression and anxiety, syndromes with a high incidence of nonspecific response (Alexander, 1953).

DEPRESSIVE PSYCHOSIS

Depressive psychosis, almost regardless of subtype, is the principal indication for convulsive therapy. Patients with diagnoses of bipolar, unipolar, and involutional depression, and depression in the elderly, respond rapidly, usually requiring two to eight seizures spaced at 48-hr intervals to elicit an elevation of mood, the relief of suicidal preoccupation and agitation, and a reversal of the symptoms of hypothalamic dysfunction (Sargant and Slater, 1944, 1972; Kalinowsky and Hoch, 1952; Alexander, 1953; Riddell, 1963; Kalinowsky and Hippius, 1972; Ilaria and Prange, 1975; Turek and Hanlon, 1977; Greenblatt, 1977; Kiloh, 1977; Barton, 1977; Fink, 1978*b*). In most instances, a total of six to eight seizures are given. This number seems constant regardless of whether seizures are induced electrically using bilateral or unilateral electrode placements or by flurothyl (Kalinowsky, 1943; d'Elia, 1970*a*, 1974; Laurell, 1970; Barton et al., 1973). Increasing the frequency of seizures may reduce the time needed for a therapeutic response (Blachly and Gowing, 1966; White et al., 1968). This result is only occasionally seen, however, and at some additional risk to the subject (Bidder and Strain, 1970; Abrams and Fink, 1972; Abrams, 1974).

Many open clinical studies report that depressed psychotic patients treated with convulsive therapy show greater improvement, fewer relapses, and shorter hospitalization periods than historical controls (including patients' own prior episodes) or patients receiving no therapy (Bennett, 1938, 1939, 1944; Tillotson and Sulzbach, 1945; Feuillet, 1948; Hamilton and Ward, 1948; Huston and Locher, 1948a; Fishbein, 1949; Karagulla, 1950; Oltman and Friedman, 1950). Special interest was shown in the response of patients with involutional depression where favorable clinical results were reported (Ewald and Haddenbrock, 1942; Bennett and Wilbur, 1944; Huston and Locher, 1948b; Hamilton and Ward, 1948; Fishbein, 1949). Prior to convulsive therapy, many of the patients were treated with estrogens, with limited success. Bennett and Wilbur (1944) describe the use of convulsive therapy in 41 cases of involutional therapy with a 90% social or full recovery in 4 to 6 weeks with an average of eight seizures (range, 3 to 22). In a detailed report, Huston and Locher (1948b) compared the effects of ECT in 61 involutional patients treated in 1941–1943 with 93 patients treated by psychotherapy and other means in 1930–1939. Of the control group, 46% had recovered after an average of 49 months' hospitalization, 18% were ill after 10 years; 13% had died by suicide; and 23% had died from other causes. In the ECT-treated group, 77% recovered with follow-up periods to 4 years and a mean hospitalization period of 6 months. Patients with melancholia did considerably better than patients with the paranoid form. Although 31% of ECT-treated patients relapsed within 6 months, they responded rapidly to a second course, with an 80% recovery rate with a median hospitalization of 6 weeks.

In comparative studies, depressed patients receiving ECT show greater reduction in symptom scores, better discharge evaluations, and shorter periods of hospitalization than those treated with placebo (Tillotson and Sulzbach, 1945; Kiloh et al., 1960; Wilson et al., 1963; Greenblatt et al., 1964; Shepherd, 1965; McDonald et al., 1966), psychotherapy (Huston and Locher, 1948a, b; Appel et al., 1953), or simulated ECT or subconvulsive treatments (Fink et al., 1958b; Sainz, 1959; Ulett et al., 1956; Wilson et al., 1963).

ECT and Drugs

In comparison with antidepressant drugs, ECT is either more effective or equal to thymoleptics in efficacy (Bruce et al., 1960; Kristiansen, 1961; Norris and Clancy, 1961; Robin and Harris, 1962; Fahy et al., 1963; Hutchinson and Smedberg, 1963; Wilson et al., 1963; Greenblatt et al., 1964; Shepherd, 1965; Greenblatt et al., 1966; McDonald et al., 1966). It is more effective than the monoamine oxidase inhibitors phenelzine (King, 1959a; Stanley and Fleming, 1962; Hutchinson and Smedberg, 1963; Shepherd, 1965), iproniazid (Kiloh et al., 1960), isocarboxazid (Corsellis and Meyer, 1954; Cotter, 1967), or phenelzine and amitriptyline combined (Davidson et al., 1978). Bratfos and Haug (1965) compared the discharge evaluations of 207 manic-depressive patients treated with ECT with 215 patients who received a variety of antidepressant drugs; they found the ECT group to respond better and in a shorter time than the drug-treated group. In an evaluation of studies of the clinical efficacy of various antidepressants, Cole and Davis (1967) cited six studies comparing ECT and imipramine; in three, ECT is more effective than imipramine, and in three the treatments are equal. In no study was ECT less effective than imipramine.

When ECT is combined with imipramine (Seager and Bird, 1962; Wilson, et al., 1963; Imlah et al., 1965) or amitriptyline (Kay et al., 1970), there is no difference in the number of seizures needed to obtain improvement; but follow-up results are better or equivalent for the combination compared to ECT alone (Seager and Bird, 1962; Wilson et al., 1963). Similarly, ECT combined with phenelzine is equivalent to ECT combined with imipramine (Imlah et al., 1965); but ECT and amitriptyline together are superior to ECT and diazepam (Kay et al., 1970). The combination of ECT and chlorpromazine was not superior to convulsive therapy alone (Arfwiddson et al., 1973), nor was ECT combined with *l*-tryptophan (d'Elia et al., 1977*a*). In a comparison of *l*-tryptophan and ECT, the patients who received ECT were significantly better on a number of behavioral scales and global assessments (Herrington et al., 1974).

Subsequent treatment with antidepressant drugs sustains improvement better than sedative drugs (Kay et al., 1970) or no maintenance drugs (Seager and Bird, 1962; Imlah et al., 1965). The efficacy of lithium in reducing relapse rates in depressive illness is still a matter of debate, but the evidence is favorable (Schou, 1973; Gerbino et al., 1978). In one controlled trial of prophylactic lithium, 16 of 37 depressed patients receiving maintenance placebo therapy were referred for ECT, whereas none of 28 patients receiving lithium required this treatment (Coppen et al., 1971). A recent open, uncontrolled study is reported by Bennie (1978), who notes that whereas 22 depressed patients had received ECT before lithium therapy, only one required ECT during an average of 2.8 years of maintenance therapy with lithium.

Controlled Comparisons

A frequent question is the efficacy of ECT compared to a control treatment in which raters and patients were unable to distinguish whether they received ECT or a sham procedure. ECT is too complex a treatment to allow a simple scheme for a satisfactory sham control (Riddell, 1963; Barton, 1977). Patients receiving modified ECT have been compared to patients receiving (a) anesthesia alone (Miller et al., 1953; Brill et al., 1959*a, b;* Sainz, 1959; Harris and Robin, 1960; Robin and Harris, 1962; Heath et al., 1964; McDonald et al., 1966; Freeman et al., 1978), (b) subconvulsive treatments (Ulett et al., 1956; Fink et al., 1958*a, b*), (c) treatments modified by agents that reduce the duration of the seizure (Cronholm and Ottosson, 1960), and (d) no treatment (Naidoo, 1956; Goller, 1960). In studies comparing drug therapies with ECT, the presence of a placebo-treated group allows comparisons of ECT and a no-treatment group

(Bruce et al., 1960; Kiloh et al., 1960; Harris and Robin, 1960; Wittenborn et al., 1961, 1962; Greenblatt et al. 1962, 1964; Robin and Harris, 1962; Wilson et al., 1963; Shepherd, 1965; McDonald et al., 1966; Robin, 1978). Many of the studies examined the results in schizophrenic patients or mixed populations, and it is not easy to relate their observations to the issues in the treatment of depressive psychoses (Miller et al., 1953; Naidoo, 1956; Brill et al., 1959a, b; Goller, 1960; Heath et al., 1964).

ECT was more effective than anesthesia alone in the treatment of depressed patients (Sainz, 1959; Robin and Harris, 1962; McDonald et al., 1966; Freeman et al., 1978). Sainz (1959) selected 20 patients with psychotic depression and treated half with modified ECT and half with anesthesia alone. Of the 10 patients who received ECT, nine were rated as much improved in 3 weeks; of the 10 who received anesthesia alone, three were worse, six unchanged, and one improved. Nine received ECT as a continuation of their therapy, and seven of these were rated as improved. Robin and Harris (1962) divided a group of 31 depressive patients into two samples; 15 received modified ECT and placebo imipramine tablets, and 16 received anesthesia without seizures and active imipramine medication to 300 mg/day. Of the ECT-treated group, 14 completed the trial; 10 were rated as markedly improved and two as moderately improved at the 3-week evaluation. Of the comparison group, 12 of 16 completed the trial; one was rated as markedly improved and two as much improved; four failed to complete the trial of anesthesia and imipramine; and only one was withdrawn from the ECT trial (Robin, 1978). These authors (Harris and Robin, 1960) reported similar results in an earlier comparison of phenelzine, ECT, and hexobarbital anesthesia.

In a recent assessment of simulated ECT, 40 patients were randomly assigned to either modified bilateral ECT or a course in which the first two treatments were sham—the pretreatment steps were carried out in the same manner with electrodes applied to the head but without any current. The third and subsequent treatments were bilateral ECT (Freeman et al., 1978). The reduction in Hamilton scores (total, depression, and anxiety scores) did not differ for the two groups after the fourth, sixth, and final ratings, although the change was less for the sham treatment group than the treated group after the second treatment. The total number of treatments was greater for the sham ECT group (mean, 7.2) than the treated group (mean, 6.0).

Convulsive-Subconvulsive Comparisons

In convulsive-subconvulsive comparisons, depressive patients receiving grand mal seizures fared better than those receiving subconvulsive treatments (Ulett, 1953; Ulett et al., 1954, 1956; Fink et al., 1958b). In the study of convulsive photoshock, ECT, subconvulsive photoshock, and a control, all patients received secobarbital sedation; the control was thus comparable to the anesthesia-alone group in the other studies (Ulett et al., 1954, 1956). Both convulsive photoshock and ECT were superior to subconvulsive photoshock and to the control treatments in immediate and long-term assessments.

Our study of the efficacy of subconvulsive treatments was part of a continuing evaluation of ECT as successive samples were assigned to unmodified, modified, or subconvulsive treatments. We found the results in 24 patients who received modified bilateral convulsive ECT better than those in 27 patients who received the same treatments except that the currents were subthreshold and did not elicit a seizure (Table 3.1) (Fink et al., 1958b). (In two patients, seizures were elicited; these patients were not included in the assessments as they continued to receive convulsive ECT.) All patients received a minimum of 10 treatments, with most receiving 12. Assessments were done in the 2 weeks following the last treatment, except that 19 patients, who were assessed as unimproved at the end of the treatment trial, continued after 3 to 7 days to receive a course of convulsive ECT. Of these, 14 were rated as much improved (Table 3.1). A case illustration from this series was reported by Jaffe et al. (1961).

TABLE 3.1. Efficacy of convulsive and subconvulsive ECT[a]

Treatment	N	Ratings of improvement		
		Much improved	Improved	Unchanged
Convulsive ECT	24	11	6	7
Subconvulsive ECT	27	1	3	23
Convulsive after subconvulsive ECT	19	14	2	3

[a] Data from Fink et al., 1958b.

A singular study was reported by Cronholm and Ottosson (1960). Following the observation that intravenous lidocaine reduced the duration of the seizure, modified its EEG pattern, and abolished the clonic phase of the convulsion in ECT (Ottosson, 1960), depressed patients were divided into three groups to receive suprathreshold or threshold currents to induce ECT, or threshold ECT after lidocaine. The lidocaine-modified treatments were significantly less effective than the unmodified treatments, indicating that duration of seizure was a feature of the therapeutic process.

Most comparisons of the antidepressant effects of ECT and placebo in a drug-placebo-ECT comparison found ECT more effective than placebo (Harris and Robin, 1960; Kiloh et al., 1960; Greenblatt et al., 1962, 1964; Fahy et al., 1963; Wilson et al., 1963; Shepherd, 1965; McDonald et al., 1966). ECT was also more effective than the drug treatments, although in many the differences were not significant. In comparisons of ECT, placebo, and antidepressant drugs, Davis (in press) carried out statistical analyses of the probability of the differences in ratings occurring by chance by combining the observations in various studies. ECT was calculated as more effective than simulated ECT or placebo in 10 studies ($p = 5 \times 10^{-17}$), and more effective than tricyclic antidepressant drugs in six ($p = 4 \times 10^{-19}$).

ECT and Suicide

Depressed patients have a higher death rate than the general population, from both suicide and nonsuicide causes (Avery and Winokur, 1976); this rate is reduced by ECT. Both Huston and Locher (1948a, b) and Ziskind et al. (1945) found suicides to be lower in ECT-treated patients compared with those treated by psychotherapy alone. There were nine deaths in 109 patients treated by psychotherapy, compared to one death in 88 patients treated with ECT (Ziskind et al., 1945). Mortality from nonsuicide causes was also reduced. In a historical review of depressed patients treated by conservative means (1900–1948) or by convulsive therapies (1940–1948), Karagulla (1950) found that the suicide rate was reduced by ECT during treatment but was not reduced after discharge from the hospital, suggesting a limited persistence for this therapeutic effect of ECT.

In a careful, 3-year follow-up study of 519 depressed patients treated from 1959 to 1969 either by ECT alone, by antidepressants in "adequate" or "inadequate" dosage, or by neither ECT nor antidepressants, Avery and Winokur (1976) found a lower fatality rate for the ECT-treated group, compared to both the drug-treated patients and those treated neither by drug nor ECT. Their findings support the clinical observation that ECT is effective in reducing mortality and morbidity in depressive patients exhibiting agitation, exhaustion, inanition, fever, infections, or cardiotoxicity.

In a second follow-up study, Avery and Winokur (1977) reviewed the hospital course of 609 hospitalizations for depression from 1959 to 1969. Improvement rates for patients treated by ECT were greater than for those treated by either adequate or inadequate dosage antidepressant therapy. Furthermore, at the end of 7 weeks of hospitalization, 74% of the ECT group had been discharged, significantly more than the adequate antidepressant treatment group (54%). Delusional patients responded more frequently to ECT than to drugs, confirming reports by Hordern et al. (1963), Glassman et al. (1975), and Davidson et al. (1977).

Significance of Diagnosis

These recent evaluations of the efficacy of tricyclic antidepressants in patients with endogenous depressions find the drugs of limited clinical value in patients with delusions. The patients, however, are responsive to ECT. Hordern et al. (1963) found an 82% overall response rate to amitriptyline and a 54% rate to imipramine in depressed patients. The response rate in deluded patients, however, was less than 20%, with none of 17 imipramine-treated and four of 10 amitriptyline-treated deluded patients improving. Glassman et al. (1975) found that depressed patients with delusions were markedly unresponsive to tricyclic drugs; 10 of 13 so treated failed. When these were retreated with ECT, nine of the 10 failures had a sustained response to convulsive therapy. In a study comparing the efficacy of imipramine and phenelzine, Davidson et al.

(1977) treated 10 unipolar depressed women with monitored dosages of the drugs. Adequate plasma levels were achieved; five patients responded rapidly, and five failed to respond. The nonresponders were those with nihilistic delusions, lacking in insight, and believed that they would never recover and that treatment was futile. Four of the five delusional patients responded rapidly to ECT. Kantor and Glassman (1977) support a special distinction between delusional and nondelusional patients with depression. They cite the analyses of Aubrey Lewis that before the introduction of pharmacotherapy, most depressed patients eventually recovered; almost all of those who did not respond came from the delusional group. After the introduction of ECT, the distinction was lost as both groups were equally responsive to this treatment. With the recent studies showing unipolar depressed delusional patients as less responsive to tricyclic antidepressants than nondelusional patients, they conclude that the presence of delusions in depressions should influence the choice of therapy.[1]

The distinctions between psychotic and neurotic depression (depressive neurosis), among the endogenous, vital, and somatic (S-type) depressions on the one hand and the exogenous, personal, and justified (J-type) depressions on the other, are blurred and confusing. The very multiplicity of terms reflects the confusion among psychopathologists and clinicians who use the terms to denote the severity of the syndrome, its etiology, or a mechanism of development. The efficacy of ECT is greatest in more severely ill cases with the greatest number of symptoms, particularly those described as vital, somatic, or endogenous. While some authors suggest that the milder forms of depression may also respond, the response may be reduced if the patient also exhibits anxiety. The more that tremulousness, sweating, tachycardia, and defined fears of imminent death dominate the syndrome, the less likely is ECT to be a specific therapy and the more likely that the outcome will be unfavorable. The diagnostic issue is further distorted by the use of diagnostic labels for social purposes, e.g., the use of the term depressive neurosis, to minimize the stigma of the illness and enhance the likelihood of coverage by insurance funds. Few reports make these distinctions clear, but the efficacy of ECT in depression is related to the severity of the depression, with the greater the number of endogenous or vital features, the better the clinical result (Chapter 6).

Clinical studies of different methods of inducing the seizure also reflect the efficacy of convulsive therapies in depressive illnesses. Comparisons of ECT using unilateral or bilateral electrode placements find the two methods effective

---

[1] In a re-analysis of data from an earlier random assignment imipramine-chlorpromazine-placebo study, Quitkin et al. (1978) extracted the data for the imipramine-treated depressed patients and found that the delusional patients had responded as well as the nondelusional. They cite their dosage of 300 mg/day as a probable factor in the success. This observation is consistent with that of Simpson et al. (1976) who found better improvement in depressed patients, including those with delusions, with imipramine at 300 mg/day than at 150 mg/day. Sweeney et al. (1978) provide another explanation, finding that delusional patients have lower urinary MHPG and higher CSF HVA levels than nondelusional patients. Another recent report finds that 12 of 13 delusional depressed patients responded well to the combination of antipsychotic and tricyclic antidepressant drug therapies (Nelson and Bowers, 1978).

in reducing symptoms and shortening hospitalization (Abrams et al., 1972; d'Elia, 1974; d'Elia and Raotma, 1975). d'Elia and Raotma (1975) examined 29 studies in which the results of unilateral electrode placements were compared to those of bilateral placements. The results were equal in 14 studies, bilateral was more effective in 13, and unilateral placements were more effective in two. Comparisons of seizures induced electrically with those induced by the inhalant flurothyl also find the results equivalent (Laurell, 1970; I. Small, 1974). The efficacy of ECT is related more to clinical diagnosis than to the mode of seizure induction (Kalinowsky, 1943; Scholz, 1951; Rose, 1963; Fink, 1978b).

Therapeutic Window

The efficacy of ECT is related to the number of seizures and to their duration. Since missed or incomplete seizures are less effective than complete seizures, some therapists have ascribed the lesser efficacy of unilateral ECT to the greater frequency of incomplete seizures and have suggested that seizures be monitored for better therapeutic results (Small and Small, 1968; Laurell, 1970). Better clinical results are seen with longer durations of seizures (Green, 1960; Ottosson, 1962a, c; Maletzky, 1978). Maletzky (1978) found that seizure durations of less than 210 sec are much less effective than courses of ECT with 210 to 750 sec of cerebral electrical seizure activity, as recorded on an EEG monitor. Finner (1954) noted that the duration of seizures was longer in schizophrenic patients than in those with other diagnoses and in the first and second seizure than in subsequent seizures. The observation, combined with the evidence of an elevation in threshold in successive seizures, makes it likely that unmonitored seizures may yield less than optimal therapeutic results (Huddleson and Lowinger, 1945; Finner, 1954; Brockman et al., 1956; Green, 1960). These observations support the concept of a therapeutic window for ECT and suggest that other comparisons with pharmacotherapy may be fruitful.

MANIA

Defining mania is a significant problem in assessing the efficacy of ECT. Delineation of the syndrome of manic-depressive illness, manic type, is ascribed to Emil Kraepelin, who separated it from dementia praecox by differences in the course (periodicity versus progressive mental deterioration) and the presence of familial and hereditary factors. But the diagnosis in the individual instance is made difficult if one must rely on family history and clinical course. The symptom picture is the only verifiable basis for classification that is usually available. Thus, in individual instances, it is difficult to separate the excitement of a schizophrenic patient with catatonic features from an acute schizophrenic episode or from that of a manic patient with manic-depressive illness. To these different diagnoses might be added the similarity in syndromes of patients with delirium and drug-induced excitement states, who may superficially appear to be manic. As a result of the changing nomenclatures and diagnostic criteria for mania, the reported incidence has varied greatly, as have the criteria to separate mania from other syndromes that may mimic it. Mania is also characterized by spontaneous and rapid remissions, which make the evaluation of treatment even more difficult (Fink, 1978, *d*).

Pentylenetetrazol and Mania

The efficacy of seizure therapy in mania was reported soon after pentylenetetrazol seizures were introduced. Bennett (1939) found mania to improve in eight of nine patients treated with an average of four pentylenetetrazol seizures given in 16 days. He reported full remission in four patients, with remissions lasting 3 to 18 months, and social remissions in four others. Of these, two relapsed, with one recovering subsequently. One patient died of an intercurrent infection while under treatment. Numerous reports from 1938 to 1939 described successful treatment of mania with pentylenetetrazol seizures (Ebaugh and Shanahan, 1939). These authors also described the successful treatment of five cases of mania and found subconvulsive treatments to be ineffective. Zeifert (1939) described two manic patients who required 20 and 30 grand mal reactions to Metrazol for recovery. Küppers (1939) reported that most manic-depressive patients required between two and eight seizures for clinical improvement, the majority requiring six to seven. When patients required more seizures, Küppers suggested that another diagnosis be entertained. Other investigators were less sanguine, noting that some manic patients relapsed rapidly and showed a refractory period early in the illness in which pentylenetetrazol was ineffective (Cronick et al. 1940).

Ziskind et al. (1943, 1945) observed 20 cases of mania, with 14 receiving pentylenetetrazol treatment and six who either refused this treatment or their symptoms were too mild to warrant treatment with a new therapy. In their follow-up, 86% of the treated and 67% of the untreated group were found to have recovered. They believed their sample to be biased in favor of the untreated group and concluded that manic patients responded as well as depressives, particularly that "the treatment prevents death from suicide and exhaustion." Of their total sample of manic and depressive psychoses, 20 patients died, 16 in the control group (nine suicides, four from exhaustion, and three in follow-up), and four in the treated group (one suicide, two during treatment, and one in follow-up). The authors suggested that ECT was a defense against morbidity in manic-depressive psychoses.

ECT and Mania

Reports for electric inductions are similar. Epstein (1943) successfully treated nine of 13 manic-depressive manic patients; Rennie (1943) reported a 75% improvement rate; and Bianchi and Chiarello (1944) found that 68.6% of treated manic patients had successfully left the hospital. Similar findings were reported by Bowman-Barany (1942), Kalinowsky (1943), Geoghegan (1946), and Kino and Thorpe (1946). By the late 1940s, more intensive treatment, as much as two to three times daily, was recommended in patients with acute excitement. Thorpe (1946), for example, emphasized the need for intensive treatment in severe excitement. He noted the need for frequent fits during the first few days of treatment, with a decreasing frequency when the excitement was contained. In his series of 12 cases, eight to 50 seizures (mean, 19) were necessary.

Schiele and Schneider (1949) summarized a number of reports describing the treatment of 466 patients. They suggested that clinical efficacy varied with the type of mania, the best results occurring in manic patients with acute onset and good premorbid adjustment (absence of schizoid or psychopathic overlay or paranoid features). Acute excitement, assaultiveness, and exhaustion responded well to ECT. They also noted the importance of multiple treatments, up to three per day, in contrast to depressive cases. They cautioned, however, that relapse was frequent when treatment ended.

Few comparisons of ECT and the phenothiazines provide data regarding their relative efficacy in mania. Langsley et al. (1959) reported the results of a comparison of ECT and chlorpromazine in schizophrenic and manic patients and found their efficacy to be similar in the degree of improvement attained. Hospital stay was shorter for the chlorpromazine-treated patients than for those treated by ECT. This study is confounded, however, by diagnostic considerations and the possible bias in the assignment of therapies.

The role of ECT in the treatment of mania has recently been examined. In a retrospective chart review, McCabe (1976) compared the course of 28 manic patients treated with ECT in Iowa between 1945 and 1949 with that of control patients admitted during the same period, matched for age, sex, the presence of mania, and not treated with ECT. The follow-up methods were those of the Iowa 500 studies (Morrison et al., 1972). The outcome variables of condition at discharge, duration of hospitalization, and social recovery were significantly improved in the ECT-treated group compared with the untreated control group. For example, 96% of the ECT-treated patients were discharged home compared with 44% of the untreated.

In an extension of this study, McCabe and Norris (1977) compared ECT, chlorpromazine, and no active treatment in matched groups of manic patients. They found that both chlorpromazine and ECT were superior to no active treatment in shorter duration of hospital stay, better discharge evaluations, and a lower mortality rate.

Aden (1976) described identical twins with recurrent manic episodes treated with ECT, lithium, and phenothiazines. He found that ECT or lithium together with phenothiazines were more effective than phenothiazines alone. To determine whether there was an interaction between ECT and maintenance lithium therapy, Small et al. *(personal communication)* reviewed the records in their hospital and identified 25 patients who received the combined treatment. They matched their records with patients who received ECT alone by number of ECT, age, and duration of illness. The patients who received ECT and lithium had less clinical benefit, more memory loss and confusion, more atypical neurological features, and longer hospitalizations than the comparison group.

SCHIZOPHRENIA

The assessment of the therapy of schizophrenia is particularly difficult since the diagnosis of schizophrenia is highly subjective, varying with the education of the physician who identifies the case, selects the treatment, and assesses the outcome (Taylor and Abrams, 1978). The schizophrenias may be divided into heuristically useful acute and chronic types, which reflect the duration and severity (intensity) of the disturbances in motility and thought processes. Chronic schizophrenia is often described by such terms as hebephrenic, paranoid, catatonic, and simple, but these have less utility as outcome predictors.

The number, frequency, and type of seizures induced are important variables in assessing the efficacy of ECT in schizophrenia where more seizures, more frequently induced, are usually needed than are needed in treating depressed patients. Adequate therapy in schizophrenic patients is often precluded by some popular dicta (Redlich and Freedman, 1966):

> Electric convulsive therapy is still employed in the treatment of schizophrenia. It has not been very effective. Even critical proponents of the method do not recommend it in general, but specifically for the treatment of stuporous and hyperactive catatonic patients. Remissions in pure catatonics may occur after a few shocks, but experienced therapists generally suggest a full course of treatment, consisting of twelve to twenty shocks. Very massive treatment with one or more shocks daily in our opinion, is not justified. It regresses the patient, makes him apathetic, and produces temporary deficit states.

This opinion contrasts with that of Kalinowsky (1943), who summarized an experience with 1,500 patients:

> Stress is placed on the efficacy of electric convulsive therapy in cases of acute schizophrenia where a sufficient number of convulsions is administered; discontinuation of treatment after the usual early improvement leads almost invariably to relapse and is the most important reason for failure of this method in treatment of schizophrenia.

ECT is recommended for the treatment of acute and chronic schizophrenia (Paterson, 1963; Sargant and Slater, 1954, 1963; Detre and Jarecki, 1971; Kalinowsky and Hippius, 1972). The efficacy varies with the patient's length of illness (Zeifert, 1941; Kalinowsky and Worthing, 1943; Danziger and Kindwall, 1946) and the number and frequency of seizures (Kalinowsky, 1943; Baker et al., 1960a). ECT is effective in illnesses of less than 2 years' duration and acute in onset; but in illnesses of longer duration with a slow and insidious onset, the results are inverse to the length and severity of the illness (Ross and Malzberg, 1939; Kalinowsky, 1943; Miller et al., 1953; Naidoo, 1956; Brill et al., 1959a, b) and the intensity of the treatment (Kennedy and Anchel, 1948; Glueck et al., 1957; Jacoby and van Houten, 1960; Baker et al., 1960a; Murillo and Exner, 1973a; Exner and Murillo, 1977).

In the treatment of schizophrenic patients, symptomatic changes after ECT vary with the presenting symptoms. Hyperactivity, catatonic withdrawal and posturing, and hallucinations often resolve rapidly, but changes in ideation occur more slowly, often requiring 10 to 20 seizures. Withdrawn, apathetic behavior (the so-called "burned out" stages of schizophrenia) is generally unresponsive and may require even more seizure inductions.

Acute Schizophrenia

In open clinical studies done before the advent of psychotropic drugs, improvement rates averaged 75% of cases treated, based on a reduction in symptoms and shorter hospitalization (Guttman et al., 1939; Zeifert, 1941; Danziger and Kindwall, 1946; Kino and Thorpe, 1946; Baker et al., 1960b; Goller, 1960). The findings are similar in some recent uncontrolled studies in patients, some of whom had not responded to drug therapy (Folstein et al., 1973; Wells, 1973; Sullivan, 1974).

Zeifert (1941) found improvement rates of 84% with pentylenetetrazol and 80% with ECT. In comparisons of ECT with psychotherapy, milieu therapy, and sedatives, ECT-treated samples showed better discharge rates, improved symptom evaluations, and fewer relapses (Goldfarb and Kieve, 1945; McKinnon, 1948; Palmer et al., 1951; Wolff, 1955). In studies using a historical control, ECT exhibited better improvement rates compared to those for an earlier period (Ellison and Hamilton, 1949; Gottlieb and Huston, 1951; Currier et al., 1952; Bond, 1954). In a follow-up of 317 hospitalized patients treated by psychotherapy, ECT, or insulin coma therapy, Rachlin et al. (1956) found shorter hospitalization periods and better discharge rates for ECT.

With the advent of psychotropic drugs, the interest in assessments were mainly in comparisons of ECT and drug therapy, either alone (Langsley et al., 1959; Ayres, 1960; Baker et al., 1960b; Childers, 1964; May and Tuma, 1976; May et al., 1976a, b) or combined (King, 1960; Childers, 1964; Smith et al., 1967; Weinstein and Fischer, 1971). In controlled comparisons of ECT and phenothiazines in first admission of acute schizophrenic patients, the treatments were found to be equivalent in short-term results (Langsley et al., 1959; Baker et al., 1960b; King, 1960; Childers, 1964; May, 1968). Patients receiving 12 to 20 ECT treatments or chlorpromazine from 300 to 1,200 mg/day showed an equivalent reduction in symptom ratings as evaluated by blind raters on nurses' ward observations and improved discharge evaluations (Langsley et al., 1959; May et al., 1976a).

Many authors combined drug therapy with ECT, initially finding favorable effects (Ford and Jameson, 1955; Kinross-Wright, 1955; Foster and Gayle, 1956; Borowitz, 1959; Ayres, 1960; Ollendorff, 1960). Others, however, did not find the combination more effective (Berg et al., 1959) or cautioned that the combination carried additional risks (Weiss, 1955; Foster and Gayle, 1956; Gaitz et al., 1956; Bross, 1957; Grinspoon and Greenblatt, 1963). Hypotension and cardiovascular complications were a factor in patients treated with reserpine. The combination of ECT and chlorpromazine, however, was not associated with these difficulties (Berg et al., 1959; Rhode and Sargant, 1961; Gonzalez and Imahara, 1964). In some instances of poor response to neuroleptic drugs, schizophrenic patients given ECT showed a striking improvement in disordered thought processes (Witton, 1962).

Two studies compared the efficacy of the combination of ECT and phenothiazines with ECT alone (Childers, 1964; Smith et al., 1967). Childers (1964) found no difference between ECT alone and chlorpromazine with ECT in changes in symptom ratings. However, in comparing ECT (with or without chlorpromazine) with fluphenazine (20 mg/day) or chlorpromazine (1 g/day) alone, the ECT-treated group showed more improvement than either drug treatment alone. Smith et al. (1967) found greater short-term (1 and 3 weeks) improvement scores for patients treated with ECT and chlorpromazine (400 mg/day) than those treated with ECT alone. In later assessments (6 weeks, 6 months, 1 year), the therapies were equivalent.

The efficacy of unilateral ECT in the treatment of schizophrenia has only occasionally been assessed. El-Islam et al. (1970) found the efficacy of unilateral ECT to equal bilateral ECT in their effects on schizophrenic delusions and hallucinations; they further noted that the clinical results bore no relationship to the memory retest results. Similar findings were reported by Abrams (1967) in an open study and by Doongaji et al. (1973). No difference between the treatments was found by Wessels (1972), who compared unilateral and bilateral ECT combined with thioridazine in acutely ill schizophrenic patients.

Catatonia

The response of patients with catatonia is of special interest. It is a syndrome of diverse etiology that is often responsive to convulsive therapy (von Angyal and Gyarfas, 1936; Roubicek, 1948; Sargant and Slater, 1954). In periodic catatonia, there are indications that the syndrome reflects metabolic disorders in nitrogen metabolism; the patients may also exhibit EEG abnormalities (Hamilton, 1976). Although catatonia is usually classified as a type of schizophrenia, some patients with acute illnesses of known etiology may exhibit catatonic symptoms (Roth and Rosie, 1953; Bernstein et al., 1977; Breakey and Kala, 1977; Weinberger and Kelly, 1977). It is a syndrome with high risk, often with a fatal outcome, and unresponsive to the usual medical therapies (Penn et al., 1972; Regestein et al., 1977). Pernicious catatonia is a special variety of excitement and self-mutilation in which ECT is recommended as lifesaving (Hamilton, 1976). Mutism, a symptom of catatonia that may dominate a clinical picture, is particularly responsive to ECT, usually with as few treatments as are needed in patients with psychotic depression (Roubicek, 1948).

Roth and Rosie (1953) described the rapid response of eight patients with clouding of consciousness to short courses of ECT. The sample was heterogeneous, with infection or metabolic toxicity as the basis for five of the cases. They could not find clear evidence of such an etiology in three cases, but the severity and rapid resolution led them to infer a similar etiology in these cases as well. In an interesting recent report, Breakey and Kala (1977) described 12 patients in whom catatonia developed following a severe infection with typhoid fever. The catatonia was distinct from the delirium of typhoid fever and lacked the characteristics of schizophrenia. ECT produced a rapid and lasting resolution of the syndrome. A patient with catatonia and a persistent high fever, who had failed to improve with different drug regimens, improved rapidly with ECT (O'Toole and Dyck, 1977). Another unusual application of ECT was reported by Bernstein et al. (1977), who noted that a mute, delusional, and resistant 24-year-old patient in catatonic withdrawal following a kidney transplant responded dramatically to four ECT after failing to respond to pharmacologic and psychotherapeutic treatments. Not all such trials, however, are successful (Penn et al., 1972).

Taylor and Abrams (1977) report symptoms of catatonia to be prevalent among patients with affective disorders, suggesting that the syndrome is nonspecific for schizophrenia and may occur in a variety of psychiatric states. Catatonia may accompany neurologic syndromes and may appear with signs of parkinsonism in response to phenothiazines and haloperidol (Gelenberg and Mandel, 1977; Weinberger and Kelly, 1977; Weinberger and Wyatt, 1978). Catatonia may also be a feature of viral encephalitis, lesions of the globus pallidus and thalamus, and some metabolic and toxic conditions (Gelenberg and Mandel, 1977).

Chronic Schizophrenia

Open clinical studies find ECT effective in discharging 10 to 20% of the long-term mentally ill (Kalinowsky, 1943; Shoor and Adams, 1950; Brussel and Schneider, 1951). Symptom reduction, particularly decreases in excitement and the need for restraints, is often described. In open comparative studies of ECT with milieu, drug, and insulin coma therapies, little differences among the treatments are reported (Cheney and Drewry, 1938; Chafetz, 1943; Gottlieb and Huston, 1951; Funk et al., 1955; Roudeau et al., 1955; Hoenig et al., 1956; Stinson et al., 1972). A comparison of ECT, insulin coma, and psychotherapy found no difference in short-term evaluations of improvement (Gottlieb and Huston, 1951), whereas a follow-up study showed better clinical results for ECT than for insulin coma or psychotherapy alone (Rachlin et al., 1956). Some found insulin coma or electronarcosis superior to ECT in chronic schizophrenia (Paterson and Milligan, 1947; Tietz, 1947; Rees, 1949); Salzman (1947) reported that:

> . . . shock therapy increases the frequency of readmission and thus raises the question of whether the time saved in the hospital in the first admission is not lost by the

early readmission following shock therapy. This is particularly significant since it seems likely that shock therapy does produce deterioration and personality changes which may explain this increased readmission frequency.

Others (Apo and Achte, 1966; Achte and Apo, 1967) reported that the duration of hospitalization for first admission schizophrenic patients remained less than 2 years, regardless of which somatic treatment—ECT, insulin coma, or neuroleptics—was used. The relapse rates however, were also equivalent, being about 40% readmissions in 3 to 5 years. In a similar historic survey, Pritchard (1967a, b) found that ECT-treated patients remained out of hospital longer than those treated by psychotropic drugs. Better long-term results were associated with the shorter duration of illness; he concluded that the two treatments were essentially equivalent in readmission rates or duration of stay. Others found ECT superior to psychotropic drugs in reducing relapse rates (Ayres, 1960) or the reverse, a reduction in relapse rates after drugs were introduced (Rovere, 1967; Skoda et al., 1968; Lassenius et al., 1973). In an early clinical study, Androp (1941) treated 50 moderately chronic psychotic patients with either convulsive or subconvulsive currents. Patients receiving convulsive currents had a 60% improvement rate, 10% relapse in 1 year, and required fewer treatments than patients receiving subconvulsive currents, who had a 46% improvement rate and 18% relapse rate. Results were better in patients with affective components.

ECT: Drug Therapy Comparison

Controlled clinical trials of ECT and alternate treatments find little difference among the treatments (Riddell, 1963; Heath et al., 1964). Miller et al. (1953) compared the effects of ECT, anesthesia alone, ECT and anesthesia, and subconvulsive currents in chronic mentally ill and found each equally ineffective. Brill et al. (1957, 1959a, b) compared the effects of ECT alone, ECT and succinylcholine, ECT and thiopental, thiopental alone, and nitrous oxide in chronic, hospitalized veterans and found no difference among the treatments. They concluded that ECT was ineffective in chronic schizophrenia. May and his co-workers (1968, 1976a, b) assigned middle prognosis schizophrenic patients, many of whom were readmissions, to ECT, milieu therapy, psychotherapy, psychotropic drugs, or psychotherapy and psychotropic drugs. The short-term results for both drug therapies were superior to ECT and other therapies; in more recent reviews, however, they found that patients treated with ECT or drug therapies had shorter stays in the hospital before discharge and shorter rehospitalization periods after their initial release (May, 1968; May and Tuma, 1976; May et al., 1976a, b).

Combinations of neuroleptic drugs and ECT are frequently used in treating chronic schizophrenia. Aside from the issues of safety discussed earlier, the evidence for efficacy for the combination is not compelling, since few studies are controlled. Improved clinical results with shorter hospital stays are reported by some (Rohde and Sargant, 1961; Kelly and Sargant, 1965; Roth et al., 1966; Smith et al., 1967), whereas others found the single treatment, either drug alone or ECT alone, as effective as the combination (Gambill and Wilson, 1966). The studies comparing combinations of drugs and ECT are criticized as being uncontrolled (Turek, 1973; Abrams, 1975*a, b*).

Regressive Therapy

The number and rate of treatments and the duration of illness affect the efficacy of ECT in chronic schizophrenia. The longer the duration of illness, the poorer the therapeutic results and the greater the number of treatments needed for symptom relief. Relief is estimated as 50 to 70% in patients who have been ill for less than 1 year to less than 20% in patients who have been ill more than 3 years (Ross and Malzberg, 1939; Kalinowsky, 1943; Kalinowsky and Worthing, 1943; Danziger and Kindwall, 1946; Palmer et al., 1951; Miller et al., 1953; Naidoo, 1956; Brill et al., 1959*a, b*). Courses of treatment with less than 20 seizures are usually less effective than longer courses (Kennedy and Anchel, 1948; Glueck et al. 1957; Baker et al., 1960*a*; Jacoby and van Houten, 1960; Murillo and Exner, 1973*a*). Baker et al. (1960*a*) compared the efficacy of 12 with 20 ECT treatments and found greater benefits with the latter.

Some authors increased the frequency to daily treatments or a few treatments a day leading to regressive therapy (Tyler and Lowenbach, 1947; Kennedy and Anchel, 1948; Shoor and Adams, 1950; Koenig and Feldman, 1951; Glueck et al., 1957; Jacoby and van Houten, 1960). In this therapy, many treatments are given within a short period until a persistent, acute, organic mental syndrome has developed. In the early reports, efficacy was deemed superior to treatments given three times weekly (Danziger and Kindwall, 1946; Kennedy and Anchel, 1948; Shoor and Adams, 1950; Koenig and Feldman, 1951; Rothschild et al., 1951; Garrett and Mockbee, 1952; Glueck et al., 1957). Others failed to find improved therapeutic results (Tyler and Lowenbach, 1947; Valentine, 1949; Weil, 1950; De Wet, 1957; King, 1958, 1959*b*, 1960). In the ensuing decades, the availability of antipsychotic drugs contributed to the disuse of regressive therapy, although sporadic favorable (Cameron et al., 1962; Drooby, 1972) and unfavorable (Jacoby and van Houten, 1960; Graber and McHugh, 1960) reports appeared. Murillo and Exner (1973*a*) reexamined the role of multiple ECT in chronic relapsing schizophrenic patients. In their initial report, they found greater improvement in ratings of psychopathology, self reports, and social adjustment for patients treated with ECT compared with those treated with psychotropic drugs. In a follow-up study, Exner and Murillo (1977) found the difference in psychopathology to be maintained after 3 years. They failed to find evidence of defects in memory function and EEG measures suggestive of brain damage. The initial study was criticized, however, for not controlling the drugs given the drug-treated patients (Spensley, 1973; Murillo and Exner, 1973*b*).

OTHER DISORDERS

The initial success of the convulsive therapies in schizophrenia and depressive disorders led to trials in other psychiatric conditions. In the main, the reports lack adequate controls, and it is unclear whether or not convulsive therapy is useful. The range of conditions includes patients with organic mental syndromes and medical conditions of diverse origin, personality disorders, epilepsy, and intractable pain (Moore, 1947; Sargant and Slater, 1963; Geller, 1965; Detre and Jarecki, 1971; Kalinowsky and Hippius, 1972).

ECT has been found useful in reducing both depression and the motor symptoms of Parkinson disease (Savitsky and Karliner, 1953; Brown, 1975; Lebensohn and Jenkins, 1975; Dysken et al., 1976; Asnis, 1977) and tardive dyskinesia (Price and Levin, 1978); the excitement and confusion of senile dementia (Roth and Rosie, 1953); the syndrome of general paresis (Heilbrunn and Feldman, 1943; Tomlinson, 1943; Solomon et al., 1948; Savitsky and Karliner, 1953; Dewhurst, 1969); and the depression in progressive muscular dystrophy (Zeidenberg et al., 1976). ECT has been recommended in intractable epilepsy, particularly as a maintenance treatment for patients who have seizures under controlled conditions to reduce the incidence of spontaneous seizures (Kalinowsky, 1945; Caplan, 1946; Taylor, 1946; Wolff, 1956). Intoxications, particularly when delirium occurs, have been reduced (Roth and Rosie, 1953; Roberts, 1963; Arneson and Ourso, 1965; Muller, 1971; Dudley and Williams, 1972), as has a case of organic stupor after head injury (Silverman, 1964). Catatonia after typhoid fever has responded rapidly to ECT (Breakey and Kala, 1977).

ECT and Medical Illnesses

Some patients with medical diseases of unknown etiology have been treated by ECT. Thus, some improvement in physical symptoms as well as mood has been reported in lupus erythematosus (Malamud and Sands, 1954; Guze, 1967; Allen and Pitts, 1978), multiple sclerosis (Savitsky and Karliner, 1951, 1953; Hollender and Steckler, 1972), mental symptoms in pernicious anemia (Ende et al., 1950), intractable pain (Hohman and Wilkinson, 1953; Boyd, 1956; von Hagen, 1957; Weinstein et al., 1959; Mandel, 1975), mania accompanying cerebral spastic paralysis (Lowinger and Huston, 1953), porphyria (Lemere, 1954), myxedema (Pitts and Guze, 1961), and anorexia nervosa (Gallinek, 1952a; Laboucarie and Barres, 1954; Balduzzi, 1955; Bernstein, 1964). Although the presence of a brain tumor is considered an absolute contraindication to the use of ECT by some authors, Dressler and Folk (1975) reported the successful treatment of depression in such a patient.

Some clinicians cite the successful use of ECT in the treatment of patients with acute confusional states, pseudodementia, toxic delirium (as in bromide intoxication), and senile agitation (Mitchell, 1952; Roth and Rosie, 1953; Roberts, 1963; Silverman, 1964; Salzman, 1977), although a recent note found a case of bromide psychosis not to respond to ECT (Davis et al., 1978). Such usage presents a problem, since the precipitation of an organic type psychosis and spontaneous seizures are among the complications of convulsive therapy (see Chapter 4). Systematic assessment of the use of ECT in patients with an organic psychosis is needed.

Although ECT has been sporadically reported as helpful in the neuroses, such patients usually do badly and represent the principal contraindication to ECT. This was recognized in the first GAP report on convulsive therapy (Fig. 2.2, p. 14) and is probably true for cases of hypochondriasis, hysteria, obsessive-compulsive neurosis, and phobias. There are sporadic reports that patients with depressive neuroses may respond (Sargant and Slater, 1963; Kalinowsky and Hippius, 1972; Carney and Sheffield, 1974), as may patients with acute grief reactions (Lindemann, 1944; Meyerson, 1944; Barnacle, 1949; Lynn and Racy, 1969), but such successful applications are uncommon. Patients with personality disorders have been treated without success (Darling, 1945; Thompson, 1949).

ECT and the Military

The convulsive therapies were used frequently during World War II, where cases of acute psychoses in the military were treated (Grinker and Spiegel, 1943; Solomon and Yakovlev, 1944; Ross, 1946). In one report, Funkhouser (1948) reported an improvement rate of 68%, with the best results in patients with acute onset of symptoms and the greatest degree of psychomotor excitement, refusal of food, mutism, soiling, depression, and waxy flexibility of the extremities.

In more recent military campaigns, the convulsive therapies have found less use, being replaced by the psychoactive drugs (Bourne, 1970). Some military psychiatrists found ECT useful in psychoses following illicit drug use (Black et al., 1974). An unusual and unconventional use of convulsive therapy was described by Cotter (1967). In a Vietnam community hospital during the Vietnam war, Cotter used operant conditioning methods to induce the return of patients to their home community. Convulsive therapy and witholding of food were both used as reinforcers, with some apparent success in discharging patients from the hospital. This experience is often cited as a particular abuse of convulsive therapy; it is clear that at the time Cotter was using this method of aversive conditioning, the proper experimental demonstrations of the efficacy of the method had not been done, and he failed to provide the necessary control data to substantiate this use of ECT.

ECT in Children

ECT has been used in children and adolescents. Studies of indications, efficacy, and safety of ECT in children are few, and none are controlled. Bender (1973) reviewed her experience in a follow-up of 80 psychotic children treated with

ECT and found little benefit for ECT above the 32% "adequate adjustment" for the whole group. Her experience is often quoted (Fish, 1967; Campbell, 1973), while others report single cases (Arajarvi et al., 1964; Gillis, 1955). Heuyer et al. (1947) describe their experience with 29 psychotic children in uncontrolled studies and report that the use of ECT was symptomatically helpful in depressed, manic, or confusional syndromes in children but without sustained benefits. Hift et al. (1960) found no successes in the ECT treatment of 23 psychotic children after 2 years. Despite this record, a recent survey found ECT to be used frequently in childhood disorders in Massachusetts (Frankel, 1973), although the use fell off rapidly when reporting requirements were imposed (Grosser et al., 1975).

Maintenance ECT

Another application of ECT is its use as a prophylactic or in maintenance therapy (Moore, 1943; Kerman, 1945, 1957). Geoghegan and Stevenson (1949) observed 13 manic-depressive patients who received monthly treatments for 5 years after a course of ECT. In 3 years, there were no rehospitalizations in this group compared to 11 readmissions among 11 patients who did not agree to receive prophylactic treatments. In the next 2 years, two of the 13 were readmitted, despite continued treatment (Stevenson and Geoghegan, 1951). Karliner and Wehrheim (1965) offered maintenance treatment to 210 patients. Of these, 57 accepted and received an average of 1 treatment a month, and 12% relapsed. Of 153 patients who received no maintenance treatments, 79% relapsed within a 6-year observation period. These observations are supported by additional open clinical reports (Hastings, 1961; Holt, 1965).

Barton et al. (1973) compared the effects of two extra treatments to those who ended a course as soon as improvement was established and found no additional benefit at 2-, 6-, and 12-week evaluations.

Chapter 4

Risks of Convulsive Therapy

Complications of ECT are infrequent and are usually limited to memory impairment and spontaneous seizures. Brain damage is alleged, and death is rare. These complications are similar to those seen after head trauma, to which ECT has been compared (Fink, 1966). Fracture (particularly of the spine) was an important hazard of the early inductions, but this hazard has been relieved by the use of muscle paralytic agents, such as succinylcholine (Anectine). Fear and panic were frequent in early treatments; with pretreatment sedation and short-acting barbiturate anesthesia, however, this hazard is uncommon. Postseizure headache, delirium, and skin burns at the electrode sites are also reported with sufficient frequency to be considered risks of ECT.

The early treatments with intravenous camphor and pentylenetetrazol were the most hazardous of the seizure therapies. Patients were treated without anesthesia or muscle relaxation; anoxia was a standard part of the treatment; and fracture, panic, posttreatment amnesia, delirium, and spontaneous seizures were frequent. The introduction of electrical induction (ECT) in 1938, barbiturate anesthesia soon thereafter, and curare for muscle relaxation in 1939 served to reduce fractures, postseizure delirium, panic, anxiety, and missed seizures to negligible levels. For a while, anesthesia and muscle relaxation were not well accepted because of the risks inherent in their use (Kalinowsky and Hoch, 1946, 1952). With improved techniques, better education, and better instrumentation, the safety of the modified induction was accepted and the incidence of missed seizures was reduced. Since 1960, the principal complication of ECT has been a persistent memory deficit. The introduction of unilateral electrode placements reduced its incidence and severity. In 1966, Blachly and Gowing described multiple seizures under hyperoxygenation, and as the value of forced ventilation and oxygen saturation was accepted, the incidence and severity of post-ECT memory deficits were further reduced.

The principal studies of the complications of ECT and pentylenetetrazol were done when the treatments were first introduced and before the general use of anesthesia, muscle relaxation, forced ventilation, and modified electrode placements. Among recent studies, Havens (1958) found equivalent therapeutic benefit and patient acceptance of ECT when it was modified or unmodified by pretreatment anesthesia. Those patients receiving unmodified treatment had a higher incidence of fractures (28% versus none), organic psychotic reactions (3 versus none), and spontaneous seizures in follow-up (1 versus none). Furthermore,

Havens notes that the treatment in 39% of the patients assigned to unmodified treatment was changed to the modified procedure because of complications.

The following discussion describes the complications, mostly for unmodified seizures. The complication rates under the conditions of modified seizure induction in common use today may be significantly different (Table 4.1) (Fink, 1972a, 1977a).

TABLE 4.1. Principal risks of modified ECT

Risk	Incidence (patients)	Prophylaxis[a]
Amnesia, prolonged	< 1/100	4,5,6
Organic psychosis	< 1/200	4,5,6
Spontaneous (tardive) seizures	< 1/500	1,4,(5)
Death	< 3/10,000	1,2,3,4
Fracture	?	1,2
Panic, fear	?	1
Post-ECT delirium	?	1
Prolonged apnea	?	7
Missed seizures	?	8

[a] Prophylaxis measures: 1, anesthesia; 2, succinylcholine; 3, atropine; 4, oxygenation; 5, unilateral electrode placement; 6, threshold currents; 7, succinylcholine sensitivity test; 8, monitoring seizure duration.

BRAIN DAMAGE

The evidence for sustained pathologic changes of the brain after convulsions comes from examinations of brain tissues from three sources: (a) patients who died after convulsive therapy, (b) epileptic patients who died in status epilepticus, and (c) animals subjected to experimentally induced seizures. Evidence for brain damage may also be inferred from changes in psychologic and physiologic tests, which are usually interpreted as measures of brain function in man (Fink, 1977a).

Human Brain Tissue

An assessment of the pathology of convulsive therapy is made difficult by the time elapsing between treatment(s), death, and autopsy. In some studies, tissues were examined under conditions in which the seizures were clearly proximal to the event of death, whereas other tissues were examined and changes ascribed to ECT where the ECT was an event distant to the death. The pathologic data may or may not have been related to the treatments. With this caveat, brain tissues after ECT have been reported to show increased gliosis (Ebaugh et al., 1943), diffuse degeneration (Gralnick, 1944), petechial hemorrhages in the midbrain and evidence of fat embolism (Meyer and Teare, 1945), capillary hemorrhage (Martin, 1949), and edema and subarachnoid hemorrhage (Alpers and Hughes, 1942; Alpers, 1946; Larsen and Vraa-Jensen, 1953; Liban et al.,

1951). Will et al. (1948) found the brain of a patient who died 15 min after the twelfth convulsion to be swollen and edematous with neuronal damage and increased lipofuscin pigmentation. Madow (1956) examined the autopsy data in four subjects and found one with intraventricular hemorrhage and three who died of cardiovascular disease.

Various experimental studies in animals sought to define the parameters of electric current which resulted in clear evidence of tissue damage during and after induced seizures. Weeks and Alexander (1939) and Alexander and Löwenbach (1944) studied the effects of currents on peripheral nerve and brain. They noted that reversible changes were found when nerve (to 10 mAmp/mm^2 of tissue) and brain (15 to 18 mAmp/mm^2) were stimulated, but that irreversible changes were observed when currents exceeded 14 mAmp/mm^2 for nerve and 20 mAmp/mm^2 for brain. In ECT, they calculated that the conventional treatments utilized 300 to 900 mAmp for 0.1 to 0.3 sec through electrodes that ranged from 2,000 to 3,000 mm^2, a current density of 0.02 to 0.15 mAmp/mm^2. Although this evidence is inferential, it is consistent with the data from autopsy studies.

The risks to the integrity of the brain from induced seizures were recently reexamined (Beresford, 1978; Garcia and Cervos-Navarro, 1978). The principal risk was to the brain vasculature rather than directly to the brain parenchyma. Hypertension may be severe during the convulsion, but the effects may be minimized by adequate ventilation and anesthesia. The compensatory mechanisms to increase cerebral blood flow are ordinarily sufficient to meet the metabolic demands of the brain, although if ventilation is not maintained, injury may follow. Cerebral spasm may occur. Protein permeability increases, with an accompanying alteration in the metabolism and distribution of nucleic acids. The latter may be demonstrated in rigidly controlled studies using ultrastructural (electron microscopy) methods, but these changes are transient, lasting less than 1 hr. The authors (Garcia and Cervos-Navarro, 1978) conclude that ECT ". . . induces mostly reversible changes in the vasculature-circulation of the brain parenchyma."

Deaths in Status Epilepticus

The cerebral pathology of repeated seizures may be inferred from studies of patients with idiopathic epilepsy. It is difficult to separate the lesions that may be the basis for the epileptic state from the changes that result directly from repeated convulsions. Epileptics may show sclerosis of the pyramidal cell layer of Ammon's horn after a long history of seizures (Marjerrison and Corsellis, 1966). Others find diffuse necrosis, neurophagia, and gliosis (Scholz, 1951; Norman, 1964).

One source of the pathologic changes may be an impaired blood and oxygen supply with the pathologic changes secondary to hypoxia (Norman et al., 1974). This theory has been the subject of experimental study (Meldrum and Brierly,

1973; Meldrum et al., 1975). Baboons were subjected to seizures at varying rates, and biochemical and pathologic changes in brain function were measured. It required repeated, sustained seizures over 1.5 hr without muscle paralysis and 3.0 hr with muscle paralysis to produce measurable ischemic cellular changes. The authors compared these findings with the 30 to 60 min required to produce measurable cerebral pathology in febrile convulsions in human infants and 6 hr or more in adults. In these studies, cerebral changes were transient unless hypoglycemia or hypoxia supervened. Similar observations are reported by others (Collins et al., 1970; Wasterlain, 1974; Plum et al., 1974) and were confirmed in patients undergoing ECT (Szirmai et al., 1975).

The pathologic changes described after many seizures probably are the result of cerebral anoxia. A direct measurement of blood oxygenation in patients who received ECT with adequate ventilation and under succinylcholine failed to show evidence of cerebral hypoxemia (Posner et al., 1969). Jugular venous oxygen tension remained constant during treatment, although there was a small decrease in venous pH, which was accounted for by the observed rise in venous CO_2 tension. Lactate levels in the jugular vein rose slightly late in the seizure, with the levels of creatine phosphokinase remaining stable. They interpreted their observations to indicate that the demands of cerebral metabolism are met by the ventilation procedures during induced seizures. The findings were similar in animal studies (Plum et al., 1968; Beresford et al., 1969). Similar studies were done in epileptic patients who had suffered spontaneous seizures less than 3 hr before observation (Brooks and Adams, 1975). In these subjects, CSF levels of lactate rose slightly and a mild transient metabolic acidosis was in evidence in blood samples. The rise in CSF lactate persisted for many hours, but this was not associated with impaired consciousness.

Animal Experimental Data

When animals are subjected to experimental seizures, punctate hemorrhages and subarachnoid bleeding occur (Alpers and Hughes, 1942; Heilbrunn and Weil, 1942). There is also a transient loss of outline of ganglion cells, disappearance of Nissl bodies, and swelling and vacuolization of the cells. Nuclei may be eccentrically located. Such changes were transient, being no longer demonstrable 45 min after the seizure. After multiple seizures, the neuropathologic changes were observable for longer periods (Heilbrunn and Liebert, 1941).

Ferraro et al. (1946) examined brain tissues of monkeys subjected to four to 18 seizures at a rate of three per week and reported the degeneration of cells and gliosis which they termed reversible. Ferraro and Roizin (1949) carried out a more extensive study with a follow-up of 30 min to 18 months for monkeys receiving an extensive course of 32 to 100 seizures. They noted gliosis and cellular degeneration soon after treatment but none after months and concluded that the changes were reversible. Hartelius (1952) examined the effects of seizures in cats and noted disintegration of nerve cells, neuronal loss, and glial reactions that were not extensive and that were related to the age of the animal and the number of seizures.

Other workers (Barrera et al., 1942; Globus et al., 1943; Lidbeck, 1944; Palmer et al., 1951), carrying out as extensive studies, failed to find either vascular or glial reactions to repeated seizures.

Physiologic Indices

Psychologic tests and electrophysiologic measures are measures of the intactness of brain functions. The scalp-recorded EEG, perceptual motor tests, language, memory, and orientation tests are conventional indices whose impairment is interpreted as evidence of brain damage. The persistence of changes in EEG and memory and performance tests are discussed at length in Chapters 8 and 9 with the experimental studies of ECT.

Amnesia is often cited as a measure of persistent brain damage with ECT. Each seizure is associated with an amnesia for the seizure; with successive seizures, the duration of the amnesia is progressively longer. For most patients, performance on memory tests improves progressively after the last seizure; by 4 weeks, performance is equal to or improved over the performance when the patient was ill (Chapter 9).

A similar recovery is seen in EEG measures. EEG changes are central to every seizure, and the interseizure records show a progressive slowing with treatment. EEG slowing resolves rapidly after the last treatment; thus by 4 weeks, the resting EEG no longer exhibits slow waves and is usually filled with well-synchronized, alpha-dominant activity (Chapter 8).

SPONTANEOUS (TARDIVE) SEIZURES

Spontaneous seizures are convulsions that occur outside the treatment setting days or weeks after the last treatment (Pacella and Barrera, 1945). They are also known as "tardive seizures." Until 1955, 51 cases were reported, when Blumenthal (1955) added 12 more. He estimated the incidence of spontaneous seizures after EST to be 0.5%, similar to that recorded for epilepsy in the population. Six additional cases in patients without a history of epilepsy were reported by Karliner (1956). The seizures remitted within 3 years, and Karliner viewed their appearance as evidence of persistent brain dysfunction. More recently, Assael et al. (1967) reported a single case of a 30-year-old woman without a personal or family history of seizures in whom a typical grand mal convulsion developed 2 weeks after the successful treatment of a catatonic stupor with four EST. Seizures recurred once or twice weekly until anticonvulsant drugs were given. Havens (1958) observed one case of spontaneous seizure in a patient receiving ECT without anesthesia. No cases were observed in patients with modified ECT.

It has been suggested that EST may "kindle" an epileptic focus (Pinel and

Van Oot, 1975). Kindling is a phenomenon described in some animal species when small electric currents are passed through implanted electrodes in the brainstem, lowering the threshold to seizures such that incidental stimuli elicit spontaneous seizures (Goddard et al., 1969). Pinel and Van Oot (1975) stimulated male rats with 45 1-sec, 400 µAmp, 60-Hz stimulations, 3 times/day, 5 days/week through electrodes in the amygdala. They then intubated the animals and administered large amounts of alcohol for 45 intubations. When alcohol administration ceased, the withdrawal symptoms were found to be intensified. Similar observations were made using repeated administrations of pentylenetetrazol and subconvulsive amygdaloid stimulations. From these data, they hazard warnings that similar increased sensitivity to seizures may occur in patients receiving EST. They repeated their concerns in a second report, in which a similar design led to similar observations (Pinel and Van Oot, 1977).

ECS was shown to inhibit the development of tardive seizures through repeated stimulation of the rat amygdala (Babington and Wedeking, 1975). These authors stimulated different brain areas daily with 1 min of subconvulsive currents. By 3 to 4 weeks, a stimulus of 5 to 7 sec elicited 45 to 75 sec of seizure. A single ECS (0.25 sec, 60 Hz, 50 mAmp) through the amygdala electrode effectively blocked the subconvulsive-stimulated seizures in a fashion similar to earlier studies with antidepressant drugs (Babington and Wedeking, 1973).

The lowering of the cerebral threshold is inherent in the definition of kindling, which finds seizures to be elicited by subliminal, incidental stimuli. This definition is inconsistent, however, with the observations by Brockman et al. (1956) and Green (1960), each of whom reported that the threshold for the currents necessary to elicit a seizure in EST rises during the course of the treatment. Green found that the current necessary to elicit a seizure rose in 24 of 39 cases and showed no change in 15. In no case did the threshold for a seizure fall in his series. Brockman et al. (1956) found that patients needed greater amounts of intravenous Azozol to induce seizures as the course of treatment progressed. Similar findings were reported earlier by Huddleson and Lowinger (1945) and Finner (1954). Although it is not clear what the mechanism of spontaneous seizures in ECT may be, it is improbable that the pathogenesis is the same as that of kindling. The difference between EST and the animal experiments cited in the studies by Pinel and Van Oot is in the use of depth electrodes, the absence of anesthesia, the large amplitudes of the currents needed to elicit seizures, the frequency the brain was stimulated, the species used to study the phenomenon, and the likelihood that direct brain damage is engendered by the implanted probes and high currents (Fink, 1977a).

ORGANIC PSYCHOSIS

The characteristics of an organic psychosis are impairment in orientation, memory, intellectual functions, and vigilance, with confusion, perceptual defects, lability of affect, and defective judgment as occasional symptoms. Technically, all induced seizures are associated with an organic impairment, since memory loss and change in affect are common. But a severe organic psychosis has been described to occur in some subjects (Polatin et al., 1940; Kalinowsky, 1945; Elmore and Sugerman, 1975). The psychosis usually disappeared within a few days, and the observers suggested that its appearance should not be interpreted as an adverse sign; particularly that the finding should not preclude additional seizures if the depressive symptoms have not been relieved. The attitudes to the organic psychosis after EST may have been conditioned by the earlier experience with insulin coma where a prolonged coma resulted in a prolonged confusional state, often with good clinical results when the confusion resolved.

In one comparison of modified and unmodified ECT, Havens (1958) observed organic psychoses in patients receiving ECT without anesthesia and none in the modified ECT group.

These observations led some authors, notably Kennedy and Anchel (1948), Garrett and Mockbee (1952), Glueck et al. (1957), and, more recently, Murillo and Exner (1973a), to treat severely ill schizophrenic patients three times daily to induce an organic psychosis in a process termed regressive EST. Glueck and his associates noted regression to be complete when a patient manifested memory loss, confusion, disorientation, lack of verbal spontaneity, slurring of speech to dysarthria or muteness, and apathy. In this special form of EST, the psychotic state is reversible with the long-term clinical benefits for schizophrenia equal to or better than those of drug therapy (Exner and Murillo, 1977). A detailed description of the recovery process from a severe dementia due to frequent EST has been reported by Regestein et al. (1975). They noted that with cessation of EST, mental functions and behavior recovered over a period of more than 1 year. Another description of the organic mental syndrome is found in the report by a psychiatrist of his experiences through two courses of EST. He notes in eloquent detail the types of memory effects, particularly the differential impact on recent events, the topographical disorientation, and the changes in mood accompanying these treatments (A Practicing Psychiatrist, 1965).

A modification of regressive EST was suggested by Blachly and Gowing (1966) in which multiple seizures (up to six) are induced daily under conditions of assisted ventilation with high concentrations of oxygen. It is not clear why multiple ECT (MECT) rarely gives the severe organic psychosis noted by the many observers describing regressive ECT, although the maintenance of blood oxygen tensions is believed to be of significance. Abrams and Fink (1972) noted two cases of confusion in a series of 40 cases, and Strain and Bidder (1971) reported a single such case, suggesting that hyperoxygenation or other aspects of present techniques may not fully protect the patient in MECT.

An interesting aspect of the organic psychosis is seen in the syndrome of denial of illness. In neurological patients with brain damage, a syndrome of anosognosia, perceptual distortion, and changed language patterns may be elicited by barbiturates and defined as a measure of brain dysfunction (Weinstein et al., 1952). The same patterns of denial language and perceptual errors are seen after EST, indicating that the post-EST syndrome is qualitatively similar to other forms of diffuse cerebral dysfunction (Kahn et al., 1956).

Some depressed patients, particularly those with manic-depressive illness, may exhibit a manic excitement and continue in a manic phase during convulsive treatment. In schizophrenic patients, ECT may elicit a severe excitement or agitation. These reactions are uncommon and can usually be treated by psychoactive drugs.

DEATH

In the early literature, the incidence of death in ECT varied from 0.04 to 1.1% of patients treated (Kolb and Vogel, 1942; Martin, 1949; Deshaies and Pellier, 1950; Maclay, 1953; Alexander, 1953; Alexander et al., 1956; Lewis, 1956; Impastato, 1957; Barker and Baker, 1959; Arneson and Butler, 1961; Hussar and Pachter, 1968; Beresford, 1971; Kalinowsky and Hippius, 1972; Gomez, 1974; Heshe and Roeder, 1976). Perrin (1961) surveyed the results in more than 40,000 patients and found that one patient in 950 died, and that one treatment in 12,500 was fatal, with more than one-half the deaths of cardiovascular origin. Tewfik and Wells (1957) calculated a mortality rate of one in 2,300 patients treated, while Barker and Baker (1959) estimated the risk as one in 28,000 treatments. Granville-Grossman (1971) reviewed the reported deaths in England and Wales from 1947 to 1966 and found a progressive reduction from 13 to 19 per year from 1949 to 1951 to zero to six in 1963 to 1966. Turek and Hanlon (1977) reported no deaths in 8,500 treatments in 870 patients and cite similar experiences of other therapists.

Three recent surveys of ECT practice include estimates of fatalities. The 1977 American Psychiatric Association survey of psychiatric practice queried a randomly selected sample of 3,000 members of the association. From 1975 to 1976, 22% had either used or recommended convulsive therapy, and 16% had treated at least one patient. The respondents reported 21 deaths in the prior 5 years. Extrapolation from the numbers of patients treated indicated a mortality rate of 0.03% (3.2 deaths in 10,000 persons treated). The majority of the deaths (67%) were ascribed to cardiac complications (Frankel, 1978). In a 1976 survey of the institutional use of ECT in metropolitan New York hospitals, Asnis et al. (1978) cited reports of three deaths in 5 years in their sample. Extrapolating from the numbers of patients treated, the calculated mortality rate is 0.034% (3.4 deaths in 10,000 patients treated). Heshe and Roeder (1976) surveyed the use of ECT with anesthesia in Denmark in 1 year and found one death in 22,210 treatments in 3,438 subjects, a rate of 0.03%.

Death is usually ascribed to cardiovascular complications. The most common time is immediately postseizure during the postconvulsive recovery period (Lewis et al., 1955; Impastato, 1957; Hussar and Pachter, 1968). In 49 of 90 cases described by Tewfik and Wells (1957), 100 of 254 deaths summarized by Impastato (1957), and six of nine cases of Barker and Baker (1959), death was caused by cardiac failure. The death rates are higher in the early reports (Maclay, 1953; Alexander et al., 1956; Barker and Baker, 1959) and decrease in more recent surveys (Granville-Grossman, 1971; Heshe and Roeder, 1976). One cause of cardiac death may be the induction of ventricular arrhythmia, which may be lethal in patients with coronary artery disease (Altschule, 1950; Brown et al., 1953a; Perrin, 1961; McKenna et al., 1970). Cardiac arrest (Arneson and Butler, 1961; Cropper and Hughes, 1964; Barron and Sullivan, 1967; Malik, 1972) and coronary thrombosis have both been reported in ECT (Impastato, 1957; Heggtveit, 1963; Matthew and Constan, 1964; Hussar and Pachter, 1968). Arrhythmias may be prevented by hyperventilation with oxygen (Bankhead et al., 1950; McKenna et al., 1970; French, 1974) or premedication with atropine (Altschule, 1950; Nowill et al., 1954; Barron and Sullivan, 1967). Their incidence may also be reduced by using methohexital rather than thiopental for anesthesia (Pitts et al., 1965). Arrhythmias usually occur after completion of, rather than during, the seizures (Perrin, 1961).

In some of the pathologic reports, the authors note that the patients had been subjected to multiple seizures, since the first application had been unsuccessful and a *missed seizure* had occurred (Will et al., 1948; Larsen and Vraa-Jensen, 1953; Corsellis and Meyer, 1954; Madow, 1956). *Missed* or *incomplete* seizures occur when a current passes between the scalp electrodes without inducing a seizure and its associated amnesia. Patients experience pain, fear, and panic; following such an experience, they can rarely be induced to have another treatment. Missed seizures occurred frequently with pentylenetetrazol, and are still frequent with ECT. They are most damaging in unmodified seizures without anesthesia, where the panic and terror of patients subjected to missed seizures provide the conditions for a cardiac death (Engel, 1976; Dimsdale, 1977). It is probable that an unmodified missed seizure provides a suitable medium for a postseizure death. The modern use of anesthesia is a clear prophylactic for this complication, and the reduction in the incidence of death in ECT may reflect this change in the method of treatment (Lewis et al., 1955).

OTHER COMPLICATIONS

Fractures, particularly of the spine, occurred in up to 40% of examined cases when convulsions were unmodified. Since the introduction of curare and its replacement by succinylcholine for muscle paralysis, the incidence of fractures has become negligible, occurring only in seizures that are unmodified either by neglect or when muscle relaxants are contraindicated by medical considerations in high risk patients (Kalinowsky and Hippius, 1972).

Prolonged apnea is a rare complication (Chessen et al., 1974). Succinylcholine is degraded enzymatically; in some individuals, the levels of pseudocholinesterase are abnormally low, prolonging the action of succinylcholine (Churchill-Davidson and Griffiths, 1961).

Panic and fear reactions occur and are usually seen in patients with syndromes other than endogenous mood disorders. The symptoms were particularly frequent in the first years of the use of ECT but have been reduced by the routine use of pretreatment sedation and general anesthesia (Pitts, 1972). The emergence excitement that is occasionally seen is evidence of the altered mental syndrome and organic delirium and is also responsive to intravenous barbiturate. In some patients, as described in patients with involutional depression, the anxiety can be evidence of the release of repression and may herald a poor prognosis (Freeman and Cameron, 1953; Pollack and Fink, 1961).

Missed or incomplete seizures may still occur in instances in which the seizures are not monitored. In patients who are not anesthetized, the passage of current or the feelings of impending doom associated with intravenous pentylenetetrazol may still occur. Neither missed seizures nor the panic incurred by the sensations of an incomplete treatment need occur in patients who are properly anesthetized and in whom monitoring provides evidence of a sustained seizure following the passage of the current.

ECT has been associated with tardive dyskinesia (Uhrbrand and Faurbye, 1960), but an extensive survey failed to find an association among three kinds of abnormal movements (parkinsonism, akathesia, and facial dyskinesia) with ECT (Demars, 1966). The association of these movement abnormalities with psychotropic drugs has been extensively documented (Demars, 1966; Haase and Janssen, 1965; Schmidt and Jarcho, 1966; Shader and DiMascio, 1970).

The psychological hazards of EST persist. The use of the term "shock therapy" by physicians and the laity conjures up the consequences of uncontrolled electricity and the image of EST as it was described in its first decade of use. The stigma of having received "shock therapy" remains a social and political liability.

Patients receiving EST may also suffer postseizure headache, nausea, skin irritation or burns at the site of electrode placement, and extravasated blood at sites of injection. These risks are now rare in institutions in which trained therapists administer the treatment.

Some concerns about ECT have not been confirmed. Would ECT precipitate labor if given during pregnancy? Neither Smith (1956) nor Forssman (1955) found ECT to precipitate labor; and treatments to the mother were without deleterious effects on the fetus (Gralnick, 1946; Doan and Huston, 1948; Boyd and Brown, 1948; Forssman, 1955; Smith, 1956; Sobel, 1960; Impastato et al., 1964).

Chapter 5

Risk-Benefit Analysis

How can these diverse reports of the efficacy of ECT be related to the risks of intervention? The considerations in a risk-benefit analysis include (a) the efficacy of ECT and the ease of identifying appropriate cases, (b) safety of the treatment and the incidence and ease of prevention of side effects, (c) the alternate therapies, their efficacy and safety, (d) consequence of the nonuse of ECT, and (e) some social factors. There is a stigma in having received "shock therapy," which concerns the families of patients and the therapist, particularly in medical communities where the psychotherapies enjoy enthusiasm and devotion.

Complex economic factors must be considered, such as the direct costs of ECT and of alternate treatments, and the indirect costs of days lost from work, errors in work poorly done, and premature death. Interested readers are referred to the forthcoming analysis by Banta (1978).

EFFICACY

ECT is most effective in the treatment of endogenous (primary, vital, psychotic) depression, regardless of type or duration. It is as effective as and often more so than pharmacotherapy and other therapies used in these conditions. The reduction in mortality from suicide is a particularly compelling observation, making the risk of suicide an important indication for ECT. In addition, among patients with endogenous depression, there are some who do not respond to tricyclic antidepressants but who do respond to ECT. Severely depressed, psychotic patients with somatic delusions are one such subtype.

Patients with catatonia are responsive to ECT. While catatonia is often described as a subtype of schizophrenia, it may also be a feature of a severe infectious syndrome or manic-depressive psychosis. Regardless of these different etiologies, patients with catatonic symptoms unresponsive to pharmacotherapy have often been responsive to ECT.

The efficacy of ECT in mania was defined in the first years of the introduction of the therapy when the number of treatments and the recovery rates were identical to those in patients with depressive illnesses. In succeeding years, the number of treatments used in mania increased until it was equal to the number used in the treatment of schizophrenia. Following the introduction of lithium and antipsychotic drugs, the efficacy of ECT in mania has not been determined in any comparative study, although McCabe (1976) and McCabe and Norris (1977) make compelling observations of the efficacy.

On the other hand, the efficacy of ECT in the treatment of exogenous (secondary, personal, reactive) depression, in addiction and drug dependence, and in patients with organic psychoses is not well demonstrated; nor are the data for its successful use in children and adolescents convincing.

The assessment of the efficacy of ECT in schizophrenia is difficult, since the literature reporting clinical results is largely unacceptable, often lacking adequate criteria for diagnosis and outcome. In acute schizophrenia, ECT produces some symptomatic benefit, usually similar to that produced by psychotropic drugs. This is particularly true for patients with hyperactivity, delusions, confusion, and impulsivity. In chronic schizophrenia, the reports are much less impressive, with most authors finding it no more effective than other treatments that are minimally effective in the long-term mentally ill. In part, its lesser efficacy may be related to the number of treatments given, which is often lower than that recommended by the few therapists who assert that regressive ECT is successful in chronic schizophrenia (Fink, 1978c; *in press*).

SAFETY

The principal risks of ECT are amnesia and an organic mental syndrome. Other risks, such as fracture, fear, panic, and death, are hazards that can be prevented by available treatment procedures.

Amnesia is the principal risk of modern ECT. It accompanies every seizure for the time of the seizure, the anesthesia, and some time before. Memory defects vary in severity and in duration, depending on the age of the subject, location of the electrodes, intensity of the currents, and number and frequency of prior seizures. Usually, amnesia resolves rapidly; thus within 2 weeks of the last treatment patients perform as well or better than when ill. Some patients, however, persist in their concern and complaint. Defects in memory may be significantly reduced by the selection of minimal currents and by unilateral electrode placements, particularly if the electrodes are placed over the nondominant hemisphere, and further reduced by the use of brief stimulation currents (Chapter 9).

Spontaneous seizures are a rare manifestation and may be considered evidence of persistent altered brain function. From a review of various reports, I estimate the post-ECT organic mental syndrome, including amnesia and tardive seizures, to persist in less than one in 200 cases.

Under modern conditions of treatment, death may occur with an incidence of four in 100,000 treatments. More deaths were reported in the early years, when treatment procedures were less well defined, with significantly fewer deaths being reported in recent surveys. The risk associated with anesthesia is a principal factor, although the death rate for ECT is considerably less than that for anesthesia alone. The latter is reported to be from 3.3 to 37 per 100,000 inductions (Campbell et al., 1961; Phillips and Capizzi, 1974; Bodlander, 1975; Collins, 1976). The incidence was less in the decade 1963 to 1972 than in the decade

1953 to 1962; and the incidence is clearly age related (Phillips and Capizzi, 1974). A consequence of the relative safety of modern ECT is the rarity of pathologic material, leaving the issue of persistent brain damage unresolved.

The other complications of ECT are reduced by the proper application of modern treatment procedures. The incidence of fractures and panic is negligible in patients who are treated with ECT modified by anesthesia, muscle relaxation, and oxygenation. Anesthesia is also the prophylaxis for recurrent spontaneous seizures.

ALTERNATE TREATMENTS

The risks and benefits of ECT must be compared to those of alternate treatments, such as tricyclic antidepressants, monamine oxidase (MAO) inhibitors, psychotherapy, and milieu therapy. The risks of tricyclic antidepressants are not well defined, although they may be severe. The onset of the therapeutic response is usually delayed, with the standard reference works suggesting that a minimum of 7 to 14 days is required for antidepressant efficacy. The anticholinergic effects of imipramine and amitriptyline in older patients may be associated with dry mouth and difficulty in urination and vision. Cardiovascular complications may also be severe, particularly the incidence of arrhythmia and hypotension (Klein and Davis, 1969; Hartshorn, 1974; Ayd, 1978; Brewer, 1978; Biggs, 1978; Kantor et al., 1978). Hypotension may be sufficiently severe to cause falls and fractures (Glassman, 1978). Death by suicide using tricyclic compounds is calculable, although surveys are not available. Some of the more recently introduced tetracyclic compounds, such as mianserin, are significantly less cardiotoxic (Peet and Turner, 1978; Crome et al., 1978).

Psychotic disorders in medically ill patients, particularly those with serious cardiovascular, renal, or metabolic disorders, postsurgery or postfracture, or extensive neoplastic disease, present complex conditions for medical management. In such patients, the rapidity of response and the safety of modified ECT compels its consideration (Moore, 1947; Kalinowsky and Hoch, 1961; Shaw, 1977).

The use of MAO inhibitors is restricted by hypertensive crises, cardiovascular and hepatic toxicity, and the interactions of these compounds with common foodstuffs, tricyclic drugs, and some drugs in common medical practice (Hartshorn, 1974). Although few authors consider the risks of psychotherapy and milieu therapy, the inefficacy of these interventions in the condition for which ECT is useful is well documented, suggesting that the risk of their use is that of suicide and persistent illness.

In comparisons of the safety of ECT and antidepressant drugs, Avery and Winokur (1976, 1977) make a strong case for the safety of ECT compared to alternate therapies for the depressive psychoses, finding lower suicide and death rates in ECT-treated patients.

Impairment in memory function may also be a feature of depressive illness, with depressive patients exhibiting improvement in memory performance after treatment with both ECT and tricyclic drugs (Henry et al., 1973; Sternberg and Jarvik, 1976; Sand-Strömgren, 1977). For example, Sternberg and Jarvik (1976) document a decrement in short-term but not in long-term memory in depressed patients. With adequate tricyclic antidepressant drug therapy, short-term memory scores improve. Sand-Strömgren (1977) found an impairment in short-term memory in depression and an improvement with ECT. The resolution was so defined that she suggested that the failure of memory tests to improve in patients with endogenous depression indicated a residual depression and was an indication for further treatment.

Comparisons with alternate treatments for other mental illnesses are more difficult. The efficacy of lithium and the phenothiazines in mania is well defined, as are the risks of mortality, blood dyscrasia, organic psychosis, tardive dyskinesia, and other neurologic sequellae (Klein and Davis, 1969; Gershon and Shopsin, 1975). Lithium therapy has also been associated with adverse effects on memory function (Schou, 1968; Kusomo and Vaughan, 1977). In very manic patients, the practice of giving large parenteral doses of phenothiazines for many days until lithium exerts its clinical effect exaggerates the risk for neurological damage (Cohen and Cohen, 1974; Marhold et al., 1974; Loudon and Waring, 1976; Beck and Reis, 1976). ECT probably is a useful alternative to lithium in patients presenting a problem in management.

The complications of ECT in schizophrenia depend on the number and frequency of treatments. Higher dosages are more effective, but the larger number of treatments increases the probability of persistent mental changes, particularly memory deficits and spontaneous seizures. The hazards of the antipsychotic drugs are well known, particularly the high incidence of tardive dyskinesia, hepatic dysfunction, lenticular opacities, and blood dyscrasias. New concerns in the use of these drugs seem to crop up with increasing frequency, the latest being the concern that elevated levels of prolactin (which accompany the use of major antipsychotic drugs) may stimulate breast tissue growth and carcinogenesis in man, as they may do in rats (Schyve et al., 1978). Despite these hazards, pharmacotherapy has advantages over ECT in the long-term mentally ill, particularly since maintenance therapy is more readily provided by drug therapies.

CONSEQUENCE OF NONUSE OF TREATMENTS

It is useful to consider the natural course of these illnesses in the era before ECT and drug therapies were introduced. During the twentieth century, the number of resident mental hospital patients escalated each decade until 1960; since then, the large mental institutions have been reducing in population. The records of these periods describe many patients with depressive psychosis, mania, and schizophrenia who remained ill for decades. ECT reduced hospitalization periods to less than 6 months and discharge rates to 80% or better (Huston and Locher, 1948a, b). It is difficult to cite suicide rates, but the recent reports of Avery and Winokur (1976, 1977), McCabe (1976), and McCabe and Norris (1977) reviewing the data from earlier periods find greater efficacy, better discharge rates, fewer deaths from natural causes and suicide, and shorter hospitalizations for patients treated with ECT and/or adequate doses of drugs than alternate treatments, usually milieu and psychotherapies, or inadequate drug dosages.

These reports are of special interest in relation to the high incidence of death among depressed patients. In a novel study of the life history of 652 patients who died with a clinical diagnosis of a depressive disorder (cyclothymic depression, periodic depression, involutional depression, reactive depression, and recurrent mania), Taschev (1974) found that 172 (26%) had died by suicide. The percentage of patients who died by suicide is higher among younger persons, indicating the high mortality risk associated with these disorders (Table 5.1). Failure to administer ECT in a seriously depressed patient may have poignant effects on patient and family (D'Agostino, 1975).

TABLE 5.1. Suicides and attempts of suicide[a]

	Men				Women			
Age	Suicides (%)		Attempts (%)		Suicides (%)		Attempts (%)	
Up to 30	7	63.6	0	0	10	71.6	0	0
Up to 40	12	48.0	2	8.0	15	83.3	1	5.6
Up to 50	15	44.1	3	8.8	15	37.5	7	17.5
Up to 60	26	34.2	7	9.2	23	26.7	21	24.4
Up to 70	20	18.2	19	17.3	22	18.5	31	26.1
Up to 80	4	10.3	8	20.5	3	4.7	16	25.0
Over 80	0	0	3	42.9	0	0	1	11.1
Total	84	27.8	42	13.9	88	25.1	77	22.0

[a] Data from Taschev, 1974.
% figures represent % of sample by age and sex succeeding or attempting suicide.

SOCIAL FACTORS IN ECT

ECT still bears the stigma of its first name: "shock therapy." Physicians and psychiatrists refer to the treatment as "shocks" and tell families that the patient will be "shocked." This insensitivity to the nuances of the language, to the imagery elicited by the comparison with the shocks one may have experienced from open electric circuits in the home, or from the violence depicted on television, is enough to frighten the strongest among us.

The social stigma of mental illness is a factor in treatment. The stigma may be particularly severe when the psychiatric community believes that a patient who receives ECT was unsuitable for a less drastic therapy, one that focuses on the core psychological problem, with the implication that psychotherapy would have yielded a better clinical result. The patient who receives ECT is also suspect as to his trustworthiness.

The practitioner who uses this treatment also bears a stigma. It has been at least 2 decades since ECT was widely used in the treatment of the mentally ill. Most physicians who completed their medical and psychiatric training since 1960 have a limited experience with ECT. Few physicians administer ECT, and fewer still utilize the modified ECT treatments introduced in the past decade (Frankel, 1978). ECT is used primarily by older practitioners, reinforcing the image that ECT is outdated and less valuable than the modern psychotherapeutic and pharmacotherapeutic regimens.

This attitude is enhanced by the common practice of assigning the responsibility for administering ECT to new trainees and residents, particularly in public mental hospitals. The students administer ECT rarely and reluctantly, with little skill and minimal supervision. It is no wonder that the recent surveys find ECT used less frequently in public mental hospitals than in university centers. Finally, the medical insurers accept this stigma and, without evidence that ECT bears any additional insurance risk, charge a higher premium to physicians who give ECT.[1]

RISK-BENEFIT RATIO

The benefits of ECT outweigh the risks. ECT is clearly indicated for hospitalized patients with psychotic depression, particularly those with well-defined symptoms of hypothalamic dysfunction; and for those who are suicidal, who refuse food, and who are in stupor, in whom it may be the primary treatment. A recent review of the practical management of patients with affective disorders states the guidelines directly:

> The most severely ill patients and some of those with moderately severe depression should be given [unilateral] ECT as the initial treatment of choice. . . . ECT may be the best initial treatment for patients with cardiac disease or hypertension [Shaw, 1977, p. 440].

ECT may also be a primary treatment for those patients who exhibit somatic delusions or catatonic features; and it should be considered in patients who fail other antidepressant treatments.

A case may also be made for hospitalized patients with mania or catatonia, but the high efficacy of alternate therapies warrants their initial use. In instances where a response to drug treatment is delayed, or where compliance may be compromised, ECT is an effective alternative treatment.

---

[1] In the American Psychiatric Association (APA) survey, 42 of 2,973 respondents reported that they had been involved in litigation in relation to ECT (Frankel, 1978). Assuming the sample reflects a 10-year period, the incidence of suit is 210 suits for the total APA membership, or 21 suits per year. If we accept the number of patients treated annually as 98,000, the annual incidence is 2.1/10,000 patients treated. Among therapists the incidence of suit is 1.4% in a career, or 0.06% (6 per 10,000) therapists a year (calculated as a 25-year career).

There is little justification for the use of ECT in schizophrenia, except in patients in whom pharmacotherapy and other modalities have been unsuccessful. In such instances, ECT dosage should be assessed carefully.

The indications for the use of ECT in other psychiatric conditions is not well documented, and its use in children, adolescents, and patients with neurosis and drug dependence should be undertaken under research protocols.

If the decision to utilize ECT is made, the same care must be given as with any surgical treatment. Treatments should be modified by anesthesia, muscle paralytic agents, oxygenation, and forced ventilation. Nondominant unilateral electrode placements is preferred, and each seizure should be monitored by an objective method to determine whether a bilateral cerebral seizure has occurred. Seizures with durations of less than 35 sec should be repeated. Treatments should be given in settings where both the equipment and trained personnel necessary for the emergency management of the complications of anesthesia are immediately available. In treating depressed patients, subsequent treatment with an antidepressant for at least 4 weeks should be considered.

ECT should be used only by therapists with demonstrated skills and who maintain its active practice. The occasional use of ECT and its unsupervised use by trainees and physicians without special psychiatric skills is too hazardous to patients to be condoned.

Chapter 6

Predictors of Outcome

The empirical nature of ECT led investigators to seek specific predictors of clinical response. Most examined clinical criteria, such as diagnosis, psychopathology, and historical features. Three studies calculated predictive indices based on clinical and historical features (Hobson, 1953; Carney et al., 1965; Mendels, 1965c). Others based their studies on physiological processes believed to be related to improvement with ECT, such as the blood pressure response to methacholine and epinephrine (Funkenstein et al., 1948), the EEG response to a barbiturate (Kiersey et al., 1951; Roth, 1951; Shagass, 1954), the language changes after amobarbital (Weinstein and Kahn, 1955), and the behavioral response to intravenous methedrine (Roberts, 1959a, b). A third approach examined the personality characteristics as reflected in psychological test performance scores, such as the Rorschach test (Kahn and Fink, 1960), figure-ground tests and the California F-scale (Kahn et al., 1960a, b), and personality typology (Kahn and Fink, 1959; Fink et al., 1959b).

PSYCHOPATHOLOGIC INDICES

An early attempt to delineate behavioral predictors was made by Gold and Chiarello (1944), who identified a symptom complex of muteness, perplexity, and confusion, fear of an immediate personal threat or danger, depression, and suicidal intent as indicators of good prognosis. They also found that patients after the age of 50, with a stable family history, sudden onset, and a short duration of illness (less than 1 year) had a favorable prognosis. Unfavorable signs were a gradual onset of illness, negativism, restlessness, ideas of reference, grandiose delusions, and neurotic personality traits.

To develop a predictive index, Hobson (1953) examined the records of 150 patients treated with ECT and recorded 121 clinical items for each case. Improvement scores were assessed 2 weeks after the course of therapy was ended. Of the sample, 23 cases were excluded because of their refusal of treatment, occurrence of complications, or change in diagnosis. In the final assessment, 78 of 127 cases (62%) were rated as good clinical improvement and 49 (38%) as poor. Using a correlational method of the phi coefficient (Siegel, 1956), Hobson identified five items that were predictive of favorable outcome and eight that were unfavorable (Table 6.1). Attempts to replicate these findings met varying success. The Hobson score successfully predicted outcome in 80% of cases reviewed by Roberts (1959b) and 78% by Mendels (1965a) but were unsuccessful

TABLE 6.1. Favorable and unfavorable clinical features[a]

Feature	Phi coefficient	p
Favorable		
Sudden onset	+0.31	0.01
Good insight	+0.24	0.01
Obsessional personality	+0.21	0.02
Self-reproach	+0.20	0.05
Duration of illness less than 1 year	+0.19	0.05
Pronounced retardation	+0.14	0.10
Unfavorable		
Hypochondriasis	−0.24	0.01
Depersonalization	−0.24	0.01
Emotional lability	−0.21	0.02
Neurotic traits	−0.19	0.05
Hysterical attitude to symptoms	−0.19	0.05
High intelligence	−0.19	0.05
Fluctuating course	−0.18	0.05

[a] Data from Hobson, 1953.

in the cases reported by Hamilton and White (1960) and in our studies (Abrams et al., 1973a).

Other items were suggested to have predictive value. Endomorphy was considered a favorable predictor in two studies (Roberts, 1959b; Hamilton and White, 1960). Roberts (1959b) also found a favorable response to occur in patients over 40 years of age, whereas Hamilton and White (1960) emphasized the value of a clinical history of less than 6 months and the presence of paranoid symptoms. The difficulty in prediction studies when done in homogeneous population samples is seen in the detailed study by Ottosson (1962a), who examined the following data selected from 44 endogenously depressed patients who received bilateral ECT: age, sex, cycloid personality, precipitating stress, number of previous depressions, previous courses of ECT, and duration and severity of depression. Assessments were made 1 week after four treatments and 1 week after the course. Only the presence of cycloid personality was related to the number of treatments and a satisfactory response. The response tended to appear later in older patients and in those who had recently had a prior course of treatments, and the final outcome tended to be less favorable after a greater number of preceding courses of ECT; these findings, however, were not statistically significant. The reason for the paucity of the correlations may lie in the fact that the treatment results were favorable in 41 patients within four treatments, thus restricting the range of discriminations possible in the data.

Carney et al. (1965) carried out a sophisticated and detailed analysis of the records of 135 depressive inpatients who had received ECT and who could be evaluated in follow-up at 3 months ($N = 129$) and 6 months ($N = 108$). They identified 35 items that correlated best with outcome and diagnosis, and constructed two weighted scales—one useful for the separation of endogenous and neurotic depression and one as a predictor of outcome with ECT (Table 6.2). Using the ECT item weights, a final score of one or more was said to be predictive of a good clinical outcome and zero or less of a poor clinical result with ECT. (Similarly, the diagnostic score of six or more is likely to be a case of endogenous depression, and five or less, of neurotic depression.)

Mendels (1965a–c, 1967) reviewed the records of 50 depressed inpatients who had received ECT and were seen in follow-up after 1 and 3 months. He found that the Hobson score successfully predicted outcome in 72 to 78% of cases (Mendels, 1965a), as did the diagnostic separation based on endogenous and reactive features (Mendels, 1965b). To improve these criteria, Mendels (1965c) examined the relationship of 21 factors to outcome and presented a weighted scoring system that increased the prediction to 90% (Mendels, 1965c, 1967). Four items were significantly related to outcome (emotional lability, precipitating factors, neurotic traits in adult life, and inadequate personality—all negative factors); yet he combined 13 items in a linear regression analysis to provide weights for a predictive score in which a final weighted score of less than 5.9 was considered favorable (Table 6.3).

A concurrent effort at prognosis was published by Nyström (1964), who also calculated partial regression coefficients for 25 items obtained from the records in two samples of 188 and 254 patients. Predictions were successful in 76% of 129 patients in whom sufficient data were available, but it was not possible to use the scale in 31% of the sample, indicating its severe limitation.

In our assessment of clinical predictors, we calculated the Hobson, Carney, and Mendels scores for 76 depressed patients receiving either unilateral or bilat-

TABLE 6.2. Diagnostic and ECT prediction indices[a]

Trait	Index weights	
	Diagnostic	ECT
Adequate personality	+1	
No adequate psychogenesis	+2	
Distinct quality	+1	
Weight loss (> 7 lbs.)	+2	+3
Pyknic habitus		+3
Previous episode	+1	
Early awakening		+2
Depressive psychomotor activity	+2	
Anxiety	−1	−2
Nihilistic delusions	+2	
Somatic delusions		+2
Paranoid delusions		+1
Worse in p.m.		−3
Blame others	−1	
Hypochondriacal		−3
Hysterical		−3
Guilt	+1	

[a] Data from Carney et al., 1965.

TABLE 6.3. Prognostic factors for ECT[a]

Factor	Weight
Presence of	
Neurotic traits in childhood	2.7
Neurotic traits in adulthood	1.1
"Inadequate" personality	1.1
Precipitating factors	0.6
Hypochondriasis	0.5
Emotional lability	0.4
Hysterical attitude to illness	0.1
Absence of	
Early morning awakening	1.4
Previous ECT	1.3
Good insight	0.7
Family history of depression	0.3
Psychomotor retardation	0.3
Delusions	0.3

[a] Data from Mendels, 1967.

eral ECT and found no relationship between any of these scores and our assessment of outcome 1 day after the fourth to sixth treatment (Abrams et al., 1973a). The post-ECT depression score was adjusted for the severity of the depression at the onset of treatment. We also examined the predictive value of 22 individual clinical items; again we failed to find any correlation with short-term outcome. Our failure to confirm the reports of others was probably due to methodologic differences: our short-term assessment of outcome, number of ECT given, and older mean age of our population.

Two recent studies are of interest. Using a 57-item behavioral assessment scale, Pilowsky and co-workers (Pilowsky et al., 1969; Pilowsky and Boulton, 1970) divided depressed patients into two taxonomic groups, based on the rules of information theory. They examined the items according to the response of subjects to convulsive therapy and reported that of the 20 items related to the diagnosis of neurotic depression, 11 changed significantly with ECT; of the 28 items identified with psychotic depression, all changed with ECT, indicating that it is more likely for the endogenous features of depression to respond (Pilowsky and McGrath, 1970).

An analysis of the predictive value of behavioral, physiological, and psychomotor tests was undertaken in 170 depressed patients referred for ECT, psychotherapy, and drug treatment in a general hospital (Weckowicz et al., 1971). Tests were done before treatment, and outcome was determined after 3 weeks using only "succeeded" and "failed" as treatment assessments. The authors note that the assignment of patients to treatment groups was not random. They carried out extensive factor, discriminant function, and canonical correlation analyses and concluded that the best therapy predictors for ECT were the presence of self-depreciation and guilt feelings, retardation, loss of libido, low salivation and galvanic skin response, and previous hospitalizations (Table 6.4). They failed to replicate the predictive value of the sedation threshold. In their discussion of their findings, they conclude:

> . . . that ECT is a specific treatment for retarded psychotic depression due to somatic causes. This depression is characterized by low activity and reactivity of the sympathetic nervous system due to disturbance of catecholamine . . . metabolism that affects the autonomic nervous system . . . [p. 26].

In a study of the prognostic significance of the symptoms of depersonalization among depressed patients, Ackner and Grant (1960) were unable to find any relationship to outcome with ECT. In a chart review of 118 consecutive patients with various diagnoses who received ECT, Folstein et al. (1973) found that patients with symptoms of hopelessness, worthlessness, and guilt, or a family history of mood disorder or suicide, improved after ECT, regardless of the diagnostic label. Another recent study (Kukopulos et al., 1977) found that 20% of depressed patients did not respond to ECT. Failure to respond occurred in depression lasting longer than 6 months. The authors reach the cynical conclu-

TABLE 6.4. Therapy predictors in depressive patients[a]

Predictors		ECT	Energizing drugs	Tranquilizing drugs	Psychotherapy
Sex	M	+			
	F		+		
Age	Old	+	+		
	Young				+
Previous hospitalization	Yes	++	+		
	No				+
Self-deprecation and guilt feelings	Yes	++			
	No			+	++
Retardation	Yes	++	+		
	No			+	+
Anxiety	Yes		+	+	++
	No	+			
Agitation	Yes		+	+	
	No	+			
Crying spells	Yes		+	+	+
	No	+			
Loss of libido	Yes	++	+		
	No				+
Fatigue	Yes	+	+		
	No				+
Salivation	High		+	+	+
	Low	++			
Galvanic skin response (GSR)	High			+	++
	Low	++	+		

[a] Data from Weckowicz et al., 1971.
+ Weak indicator; ++ strong indicator.

sion "... that ECT is effective only when given within 6 months of the spontaneous end of the depression."

Summarizing these efforts, it is now clear that the more that endogenous features are present, the better the prognosis; the more that neurotic features predominate, the poorer the prognosis. The items identified by the many reviewers include retardation, early morning awakening, somatic delusions, severity of depressed mood, and guilt as favorable predictors; hypochondriasis, hysteria, anxiety, emotional lability, crying, and depersonalization as unfavorable predictors.

PHYSIOLOGIC PREDICTORS

Tests of autonomic reactivity were a feature of many studies of the pathogenesis of psychosis (Altman et al., 1943; Gold, 1943; Funkenstein et al., 1948; Hill et al., 1951; Gellhorn, 1953, 1956). A common index in these studies was the fall in blood pressure after subcutaneous or intramuscular methacholine (Mecholyl) (cholinergic stimulation) or its rise after intravenous epinephrine (adrenergic stimulation). The rate of change, the peak change, and the rate at which blood pressure returned to baseline were measured. Funkenstein et al. (1948, 1950, 1952) examined consecutive series of state hospital admissions and divided the population into six groups, based on the blood pressure response to epinephrine and methacholine and whether the tests precipitated symptoms of anxiety. The responses of two groups of patients were correlated with improvement after ECT: those in whom a chill developed after methacholine (97% improved with ECT), and those who exhibited a blood pressure rise greater than 50 mm Hg after epinephrine and a fall after methacholine that did not return to baseline within 25 min (89% improved with ECT). These observations were confirmed in part (Blumberg et al., 1956; Roberts, 1959b; Hamilton and White, 1960; Rose, 1962; Fukuda and Matsuda, 1969), but many of these observers concluded that the correlation could be explained by age and the level of the basal blood pressure, the findings being most clear in older patients with hypertension. The reliability of the test was also criticized (Feinberg, 1958; Rose, 1962; Thorpe, 1962).

The inflection point in the increase in EEG beta activity (and onset of nystagmus and slurring of speech) to a calculated intravenous administration of amobarbital (0.5 mg/kg/40 sec) was defined as the sedation threshold and related to both clinical diagnosis and outcome with ECT (Shagass, 1954, 1957; Shagass and Naiman, 1956; Fink, 1958b). Patients with low thresholds were usually diagnosed as suffering from psychotic depression with a good prognosis to ECT; those with high thresholds were found to have schizophrenia, neurosis, or high degrees of anxiety, and a poor prognosis with ECT. These findings were confirmed by some observers (Nymgaard, 1959; Perris and Brattemo, 1963) but not by others (Ackner and Pampiglione, 1959; Roberts, 1959b). Modifications of the test included EEG burst suppression by a barbiturate (Kiersey et al.,

1951) and the sleep threshold (Shagass et al., 1959), but neither were considered better prognostic tests for ECT.

Roth (1951) found a better prognosis with ECT for patients in whom an enhancement of delta activity developed to intravenous thiopental given a few hours after the first, second, or third seizure. In a replication and follow-up study, Roth et al. (1957) reported that the enhanced slowing after pentothal was not related to short-term evaluations of outcome but to the likelihood of relapse at 3 and 6 months, with higher relapse rates found in patients with low EEG slow wave values. In this context, we (Fink and Kahn, 1957) found that the early and sustained enhancement of EEG slow wave activity during ECT was a good prognostic sign (Chapter 8).

Although these physiological tests are of considerable theoretic interest, their low correlation with outcome, covariance with age, and difficulty in assessment preclude their routine clinical use (Thorpe, 1962; Kiloh, 1977).

PSYCHOLOGICAL TESTS

Few authors have examined the role of psychological tests to outcome in ECT. This is surprising since ECT was developed at a time when such psychological tests as the Wechster-Bellevue, Rorschach, TAT, Bender-Gestalt, word-association, and figure-drawing tests were widely applied for classification purposes. Much of the interest of psychologists was in defining the changes in brain function, particularly the degree and persistence of amnesia and tests of "organicity" (Chapter 9).

Patients with organic brain disease were found to evince a variety of syndromes, grossly defined as denial or anosognosia for illness. The administration of amobarbital exaggerated this syndrome and elicited additional aspects, such as explicit denial of illness, displacement and minimization of symptoms, and ludic behavior (Weinstein et al., 1953, 1954a, b; Weinstein and Malitz, 1954; Weinstein and Kahn, 1955). Similar changes in language and behavior occur in patients during a course of convulsive therapy, and the observations led to suggestions that denial of illness was a psychological adaptation which was the basis for improvement in ECT (Weinstein et al., 1952). Since improvement (or denial of illness) was not seen in all patients in whom organic mental changes developed with ECT, differences in psychological structure—the presences of a denial personality—was proposed as an explanation (Weinstein and Kahn, 1953, 1955). As a test of this hypothesis, we undertook studies of the amobarbital test and various personality and psychological tests in patients receiving ECT (Kahn et al., 1956, 1960a, b; Fink, 1957, 1962; Fink et al., 1959b; Kahn and Fink, 1959, 1960; Kahn and Pollack, 1959).

Amobarbital Test

The amobarbital test is one of adaptation, language, and neurophysiological integrity. Patients are first asked questions of orientation and awareness of illness, then given amobarbital at a rate of 0.05 g/min until nystagmus and slurred speech occur; the questions are then repeated. Errors, changes in reference, minimization, and displacement are identified; their occurrence defines a positive test. (Fig. 10.1, p. 136). Patients without brain disease give the same answers after amobarbital as before. Psychiatric patients show more transient disorientation and denial, withdrawal, ludic behavior, and more changes in syntactic speech than do medical and surgical patients in a general hospital (Kahn et al., 1955, 1956).

In patients treated with modified bilateral ECT, positive amobarbital test responses occur in some patients after the first three treatments; with more treatments, more patients exhibit positive responses. Some patients, however, receive up to 12 treatments, and a positive amobarbital test fails to develop (Kahn et al., 1956). In one study, we determined the effects of amobarbital in 24 patients treated with ECT. Based on their clinical status 2 months after their last treatment, they were classified as much improved ($N=11$), moderately improved ($N=6$), or unimproved ($N=7$). Of the markedly improved patients, almost one-half had positive amobarbital tests after three treatments, and all had positive tests after seven to nine treatments. Among the unimproved cases, positive amobarbital tests were infrequent and did not increase during the course of treatment. In addition to the specific positive responses, the improved patients exhibited more changes in verbal responses (evasion, second and third person syntax) and nonverbal behavior (euphoria, withdrawal, selective inattention) than did the unimproved patients. These changes in orientation and in verbal and nonverbal language were identified as the language of denial and associated with the behaviors defined as improved (Chapter 10) (Kahn and Fink, 1958).

Denial Personality

Weinstein and Kahn (1955) described a personality prone to use denial language, both explicit and implicit (verbal and nonverbal). To determine the relationship between such a typology and the response to ECT, the relatives of ECT patients were interviewed in a semistructured interview to answer questions related to 15 aspects defined as characteristic of the "explicit verbal denial" personality (Kahn and Fink, 1959). Items were rated on a scale of 0, 1, and 2. The denial personality scores ranged from 0 to 25 (mean, 11) in 47 patients who received ECT. Patients with scores between 11 and 25 were considered the "high denial" group and patients with scores of 0 to 10 as the "low denial" group. Clinical evaluations were done independently 2 to 6 weeks after the last ECT; more patients who were rated as much and moderately improved on outcome assessments had high denial personality scores than did the patients who were rated as unimproved. These data indicated that patients who respond best to ECT are those characterized as having a denial personality—nonempathic, nonintrospective, highly conventional, and stereotyped.

To further define the characteristics that favored a good clinical outcome, we examined the profiles of ECT-treated patients on the Rorschach and California F-scale tests.

Rorschach Test Criteria

The Rorschach test was given to 87 patients before modified bilateral ECT and in one-half the sample again 2 weeks after ECT (Kahn and Fink, 1960). The Rorschach test was scored according to conventional criteria, and only those items that could be scored quantitatively were studied. Patients were assessed independently 2 to 4 weeks after the last treatment and assigned to one of three groups: much improved ($N = 39$), moderately improved ($N = 35$), or unimproved ($N = 13$).

The relationship of clinical outcome to Rorschach determinants is shown in Table 6.5 and Fig. 6.1. The presence of both human movement and form-color responses was associated with poor outcome and their absence with good outcome with ECT. Again, the absence of human movement and form-color responses is seen in nonempathic, nonintrospective, conventional, stereotyped, and verbally noncommunicative individuals with little imagination or creative capacity. These characteristics are similar to those described from family interviews (Kahn and Fink, 1959).

In 41 patients, the Rorschach test was repeated after the course of treatment; and in 34 patients, the protocols show no change. In four instances, human movement responses disappeared, and in three patients, these were reported only after treatment.

The observations are consistent with other studies that find that psychotic depressed patients show neither human movement nor color responses (Beck, 1943; Pacella et al., 1947). Few studies assess the prognostic value of these criteria for ECT, although some findings have been described for insulin coma therapy where the prognostic criteria differ from those described for ECT (Halpern, 1940; Piotrowski, 1941; Lipton et al., 1951). Lipton and his co-workers

TABLE 6.5. *Rorschach determinants and clinical ratings*[a]

Determinant	Favorable	Unfavorable
Number of responses	Small	Large
% Whole (W%)	High	Low
% Form (F%)	High	Low
% Popular (P%)	High	Low
Human movement (M)	None	Present
Animal movement (FM)	None or few	Present
Color (C)	None; pure C only	None
Form-color (FC)	None	Present
Shading (Sh)	Absent	Present

[a] Data from Kahn and Fink, 1960.

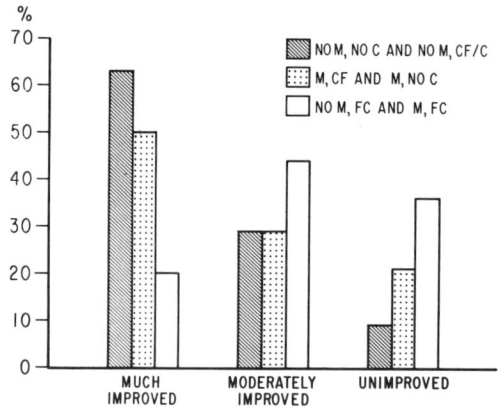

FIG. 6.1. Relationship of Rorschach pattern to clinical response to EST.

(1951) reported that good prognosis with insulin is associated with a large number of responses (> 25), the presence of human movement, three or more whole responses, high color responses, and high form responses.

Social Attitude Scale

The California F-scale was developed as a measure of prejudice and authoritarianism and was thought to reflect the psychological aspects of conventionalism, rigidity, and stereotypy in social attitudes (Adorno et al., 1950). We applied it to study the factors affecting referral for convulsive therapy (Fink et al., 1959; Kahn et al., 1957, 1959, 1960b; Fink, 1961) and as a predictor of outcome (Kahn et al., 1959, 1960b).

We used a 10-item modification of the standard F-scale, as proposed by Gallagher et al. (1957) (Fig. 6.2). In one study, 57 patients receiving ECT responded to the F-scale before treatment (Kahn et al., 1959). The patients evaluated as recovered ($N=8$) had a mean F-score of 53.1, as much improved ($N=26$) an F-score of 41.8, and the group of improved and unimproved ($N=23$) an F-score of 39.7, indicating that patients who recovered with ECT exhibited a greater agreement with the stereotyped statements of the test. We also examined other factors in outcome: age, years of education, and birthplace (Table 6.6). The patients rated as recovered were older, had less education, and a higher percentage were foreign born than the patients rated as improved and unimproved. (All patients referred for convulsive therapy were included in the sample; although the majority were suffering from affective disorders, a significant number were probably classified as suffering from schizophrenia or neurotic depression.)

We explored the significance of the relationship of high F-scale score to outcome in another sample of patients referred for convulsive therapy. In addition

TABLE 6.6. Social factors and discharge ratings in ECT[a]

Rating	N	Mean F-scale	Mean age	Mean years education	Foreign born (%)
Recovered	8	53.1	51.6	9.4	50
Much improved	26	41.8	43.8	10.6	35
Improved and unimproved	23	39.7	32.3	12.3	17

[a] Data from Kahn et al., 1959.

FIG. 6.2. Social Attitude Questionnaire (F-Scale)[a]

Below are a number of statements. For each statement we want to give us your *personal opinion* of whether you agree or disagree, and how much.

Statement	I agree very much	I agree pretty much	I agree a little	I disagree a little	I disagree pretty much	I disagree very much	I can't say
No sane, normal decent person could ever think of hurting a close friend or relation							
Science has its place, but there are many important things that must always be beyond human understanding							
If people would talk less and work more, everybody would be better off							
When a person has a problem or worry, it is best for him not to think about it, but to keep busy with more cheerful things							
What the youth needs most is strict discipline, rugged determination, and the will to work and fight for family and country							
Nowadays when so many different kinds of people mix together so much, a person has to protect himself especially carefully against catching an infection or disease from them							
Sex crimes, such as rape and attack on children, deserve more than mere imprisonment; such criminals ought to be publicly whipped, or worse							
The best teacher or boss is the one who tells us exactly what is to be done and how to go about it							
Young people sometimes get rebellious ideas, but as they grow up they ought to get over them and settle down							
People can be divided into two distinct classes: the weak and the strong							

Scoring:
I agree very much.......... +7
I agree pretty much......... +6
I agree a little............. +5
I can't say................. +4
I disagree very much........ +1
I disagree pretty much...... +2
I disagree a little.......... +3

[a] From Gallagher et al., 1957.

to the F-scale, the patients were given a reverse F-scale—a modification in which the statements are stated as opposite or negative of the original statements, with similar scoring, a high score indicating agreement with the statement. The patients were divided into two groups, as being above or below the median for the conventional F-scale score (Table 6.7). Those patients who made low scores initially (indicating disagreement with the statements) achieved much higher scores on the reverse scale (indicating agreement); those who made high scores on the F-scale also made high scores on the reverse scale, indicating that they agreed with the statements even if their meanings were reversed. Again, the scores suggest that better clinical results are achieved in those patients high in stereotypy and rigidity and low in critical ability and imagination, similar to the findings in the denial personality inventory and the Rorschach test.

TABLE 6.7. Conventional and reverse F-scales[a]

Dichotomized groups	N	Mean score F scale	Mean score reverse scale	Diff.	t
10–37	76	26.3	51.5	+25.2	20.3[b]
38–70	79	47.4	48.1	+ 0.7	0.6

[a] Data from Kahn et al., 1960b.
[b] $p \leqq 0.001$.

COMMENT

None of the predictors of outcome with ECT has been more successful than that of clinical diagnosis. Neither psychopathological symptom complexes, computer-derived weighted indices, nor the physiological or psychological tests examined systematically have been productive. In part, the failure reflects the atheoretic nature of the tasks selected in the psychopathological indices and the physiological tests. In the examination of the significance of denial personality, the theory was clearly stated and the tests were adequate, but the results are confounded by the heterogeneity of the samples studied and by the probability that the personality factors contribute to only a small part of the therapeutic process. The tests that are the best predictors are those that are clearly prominent in patients with severe primary (endogenous, psychotic) depression: weight loss, pyknic habitus, early awakening, somatic delusions, family history of depression, dry mouth, absence of crying and sweating, absence of precipitants, and absence of anxiety. In the physiological tests, the older subjects with hypertension and a sensitivity to the effects of barbiturate are better responders—again, characteristics that can be associated with endogenous depression. The same is true for the psychological tests.

These studies assume direct relationships between diagnosis (or elements of psychopathology that make up a diagnosis) and the clinical response to ECT.

Since the action of ECT is assumed to be physiological or biochemical, there is an implicit assumption of a direct relationship between physical processes that underly behavior and the manifest syndrome or psychopathology. Such an assumption is insecure, however, for many relationships do not follow a tidy association. The protean nature of neurosyphilis, the many precipitants of catatonia, and the overlap of the behaviors that comprise the toxic psychoses, dementia and catatonia, attest to the diversity in the response of the CNS. It is no surprise that behavioral, physiological, and psychological measures, although of some value, are no better predictors than a simpler diagnosis of an endogenous depression. Diagnosis as a predictor is complicated by the subjective elements of the process, as physicians trained in different schools classify quite differently, particularly patients with mood disorders. In a comparison of British, French, and German psychiatrists asked to classify patients from interviews recorded on videotape, Kendall et al. (1974) found minimal disagreement in the classification of patients with schizophrenia, personality disorder, alcoholism, and anorexia nervosa but did find significant diversity in the use of the terms manic-depressive psychosis, affective psychosis, and depressive illness. There is a continuing argument as to whether depressive disorders represent a bimodal distribution or a continuum with a gradual shading of exogenous to endogenous psychoses (Roth et al., 1974; Klerman, 1974; Perris, 1974).

A feature of the difficulties in prediction studies is the difference in the characteristics of the samples selected for initial and verification studies. In the initial study, the sample is apt to be heterogeneous, with many predictors and a range of outcomes. As the therapists become more skilled, the samples used for replication and verification are apt to be homogeneous, and with less divergence in predictors and outcomes. Predictors are relatively easy to identify in the first samples but difficult to validate since both negative predictors and poor results are eliminated (Hamilton, 1974).

In our early studies of ECT and psychotropic drugs, we described a wide range of behavioral reactions to ECT (Fink and Kahn, 1961), imipramine (Klein and Fink, 1962a), and phenothiazines (Klein and Fink, 1962b). We were impressed by the diversity of the response, seemingly occasioned by the heterogeneity of the material recommended for ECT. Thus patients exhibited euphoric-hypomanic, somatization, panic, and paranoid-withdrawal responses to ECT (Chapter 10).

In reviewing the predictors of the ECT response and the results of the clinical efficacy studies of ECT (Chapter 3), we can identify the characteristics of patients responsive to ECT, usually with a few treatments, who exhibit a rapid reversal in disordered mood, alleviation of vegetative symptoms, and, often, denial and minimization of symptoms. These patients exhibit the symptoms variously classified as endogenous depression, manic-depressive illness (either depressed or manic types), bipolar depression, unipolar depression, involutional depression, catatonia, or mania. Their commonality is in their rapid response to ECT with a reversal of mood disorder, withdrawal, psychosis, and vegetative disturbances.

Is it too hazardous to predict that underlying these states is a common psychopathology and pathophysiology that is alleviated by repeated seizures? As a research device and a basis for classification, the response to ECT is as valid as the wide range of phenotypic, symptomatic, and mixed-phenotypic, familial-genetic classification systems based on the Chinese-menu or a decision-tree logic so popular today.

Our failure to better define the predictors of outcome is the result of many factors—samples studied, tests selected, and lack of suitable hypotheses. If the present analysis is meaningful, patients who respond rapidly to ECT will have a common physiopathology, probably in neuroendocrine or neurotransmitter dysfunction, resulting from genetic or familial features in some, and in environmental stresses (probably toxic or inflammatory) in others. Studies of the commonalities of ECT responders will identify genotypic features that will classify patients into more homogeneous clusters than the phenotypic features stressed in present psychopathologies (Fink, 1968, 1974d, 1978a). Tests based on neuroendocrine or neurotransmitter functions or electrophysiologic response to a stressor will yet be more accurate predictors of outcome with ECT. As an example of a probable productive test, the TSH response to intravenous TRH has been found to be decreased in patients with psychotic depression (Chapter 14; Kirkegaard and Smith, 1978; Kirkegaard et al., 1978).

Chapter 7
ECT Usage

Within a few years of the introduction of ECT, its use was believed to be promiscuous and indiscriminate, reflecting its clinical efficacy, ease of administration, and the limitations of the alternate therapies (GAP, 1947). With the introduction of psychoactive drugs, particularly the antidepressants in the late 1950s, usage and interest in ECT waned as drugs were found effective, easy to prescribe, and required little prior training and experience to administer. The use of ECT continued in both private and university hospitals and languished in public mental hospitals.

The recent assessment of consent procedures led some critics to again allege that ECT was needlessly used, particularly among the poor, minorities, and prisoners (Friedberg, 1976, 1977). At the same time, questions about the technical issues of anesthesia, optimum placement of electrodes, and choice of currents encouraged surveys of the use of ECT in clinical practice.

SURVEYS OF USAGE

In response to concerns of the abuse of ECT in Massachusetts in 1972, a Task Force on Electroconvulsive Therapy was established. Among its recommendations was a reporting requirement for institutions licensed in Massachusetts (Frankel, 1973). The first report described the use of ECT in private, public, and VA hospitals for the year 1973–1974 (Grosser et al., 1975). Of 19,040 admissions to 26 reporting hospitals in the state, 2,441 patients (13%) received ECT. The distribution of usage was uneven, however, with 28% of admissions to private hospitals receiving ECT, 3.4% in VA hospitals, and 1.7% in public hospitals (Table 7.1). The variability in use was broad, ranging from 0.6 to 70% of admissions in private hospitals and from 0 to 4.5% among public and VA hospitals. The average number of ECT treatments was 7.4 to 14.3 (mean, 9.4) for private patients and 6.7 to 14.1 (mean, 9.9) for patients in public and VA hospitals. The distribution of diagnoses for which ECT is given varied among the institutions, probably reflecting the differences in the types of patients admitted to each. Thus only 15% of patients who received ECT in the VA hospitals carried diagnoses of primary depression, whereas 44% of patients in private and 40% of patients in public hospitals did so. Nevertheless, after reviewing their data, Grosser et al. (1975) concluded that the discrepancy in usage was not accounted for by differentials in admission rates or by different diagnostic

TABLE 7.1. Usage of ECT, Massachusetts Hospitals, May, 1973–April, 1974[a]

	Private (N = 11)	Public (N = 13)	VA (N = 2)
Admissions (N)	7859	8431	2750
ECT (N)	2207	140	94
ECT (%)	28	1.7	3.4
Range ECT/inpatient admissions (%)	0.6–70	0.0–4.5	1.1–4.4
Median ECT/inpatient admissions (%)	23	1.0	—
Average no. ECT/patient	9.4	9.2	8.7
Diagnosis			
Schizophrenia (%)[b]	24	36	52
Affective (%)	37	24	11
% Total-primary depression	44	40	15
Other (%)	32	24	33

[a] Data from Grosser et al., 1975.
[b] Of patients treated with ECT, not the total hospital sample.

compositions but rather by differences in treatment philosophy, as well as fiscal and administrative concerns.

We undertook a similar survey of the usage of ECT among a sample of metropolitan New York hospitals during 1975–1976 (Asnis, et al., 1978). After determining that 69 hospitals had inpatient psychiatric facilities, we selected a sample of 36 hospitals to reflect the distribution of public and private facilities. We visited these hospitals in the summer of 1976 to ask questions of the senior staff physician and nurse administrator of the ECT section. ECT was used in 30 of the 36 hospitals (83%) with three municipal, two VA, and one private profit hospital not using ECT. Four of the hospitals had discontinued ECT in the prior 10 years, and two institutions were newly opened, the administrators indicating that ECT units would be established when needed.

As in the Massachusetts study, ECT usage varied among the institutions, being used in less than 1% of patients in six hospitals and from 16 to 40% in four hospitals (Table 7.2). Usage was least in public mental hospitals (0.7 to 1.2% of admissions) and most in private profit hospitals (average, 21.3% of admissions). Between 5.2 and 5.4% of patients in university and private nonprofit hospitals received ECT. We did not obtain a picture of the diagnostic spread of the patient populations nor of those who received ECT, and thus we could not exclude the possibility that the usage rate reflected different psychopathologies among the patient samples. Using social class criteria, however, we found a greater utilization of ECT by patients from the middle and upper classes than by those from the lower class.

The psychiatric society in Maryland undertook a survey of the usage of treatments among its members in 1974. A questionnaire was sent to 615 members,

TABLE 7.2. Percentage of patients receiving ECT in Metropolitan New York hospitals, 1975–1976[a]

Percent	Facilities[b]	
	N	%
Less than 1	6	20
1–5	13	43.3
6–15	7	23.3
16–40	4	13.3

Facility type[a]	Patients (%)
Municipal (city and county)	0.75
State	1.0
VA	1.2
Private nonprofit	5.2
Private profit	21.3
University	5.4

[a] Data from Asnis et al., 1978.
[b] $N = 30$.

and 482 (78%) valid responses were tabulated (Dietz et al., 1977). Of the respondents, 29 (6%) used ECT in 513 patients in the prior year. An additional 107 members referred 387 patients to other physicians for treatment. The respondents used intensive individual therapy (85%) and pharmacotherapy (76%) predominantly, while ECT, among similar therapies, was used by a smaller group of therapists who specialized in its use.

The most extensive survey of the use of ECT was undertaken in 1976 by the Task Force on Convulsive Therapy of the American Psychiatric Association (Frankel, 1978). A fixed alternative questionnaire was sent to a random sample of 20% of the membership of the association (4,013 members), and satisfactory replies were received from 2,973 (74%). Sixteen percent of the respondents personally treated 7,300 patients in the prior 6 months, and 22% reported that they had recommended ECT be used in patients treated by resident psychiatrists under their supervision. (The groups were not exclusive.) The annual number of patients treated in the United States in 1975–1976 was estimated at 73,000.[1] The figures of the various surveys allow estimates of the annual usage of ECT in the United States in the years 1973 to 1976, ranging from 1.3 patients/10,000 population in Maryland to 4.6/10,000 in Massachusetts, and a United States rate of 4.4/10,000 (Table 7.3).

In a retrospective examination of the records of three hospitals in Toronto, Canada, Eastwood and Stiasny (1978) recorded the usage of ECT for the 5-

---

[1] At an estimated cost of $200 for each treatment (hospital, anesthesia, and professional fees), a course of nine treatments would cost $1,800, for an annual expenditure for ECT in the United States of $130 million.

TABLE 7.3. Estimates for ECT usage

Country	Year	Treated (N)	Population (millions)	Rate per 10,000
United States[a]	1975–1976	92,965	210	4.4
Massachusetts[b]	1973–1974	2,441	5.3	4.6
Maryland[c]	1973–1974	513	4.0	1.3
Denmark[d]	1972–1973	3,438	4.9	7.0

	APA survey (1975–1976)			
	Sample (6 Months)	Annual APA	Correction (%)[e]	Final
Treated	7,303	73,030	100	73,030
Supervised	2,093	20,930	50	10,465
Referred	2,870	28,700	33	9,470
Total				92,965

[a] Frankel, 1978.
[b] Grosser et al., 1975.
[c] Dietz et al., 1977.
[d] Heshe and Roeder, 1976.
[e] Assumes that supervisees treat one-half patients as recommended, and that two-thirds of referred patients are included in the number "treated."

year period from 1969 to 1973. The institutions were a postgraduate psychiatric research center at a community hospital, a city mental hospital with a high percentage of long-stay patients, and the psychiatric unit of a general hospital (Table 7.4). As was true in the metropolitan New York survey, the usage of ECT varied among the institutions, with the greatest usage at the general hospital and the least in the city mental hospital. In each institution, ECT was used primarily in patients over the age of 35 and with diagnoses of depressive disorders. The differences reflected variations in admission rates of older, depressed patients.

The usage of ECT also varied seasonally, with the greatest usage in the spring and autumn in Ontario, Canada, coinciding with the incidence of successful suicides and hospital admissions for depressive illness (Eastwood and Peacocke, 1976b). These authors note also that while the overall suicide rate is increasing, the increase is greatest for both sexes under the age of 45 years. They suggest that the smaller increase in suicide rate in men over the age of 45 may reflect the "saving" due to ECT.

The principal recent survey of usage of ECT outside the United States is that of Heshe and Roeder (1975, 1976), who sent a questionnaire to 55 psychiatric departments in Denmark, inquiring about practice in 1972–1973. Satisfactory replies were received from 51 departments (93%). They found that 3,438 series of treatments had been given in one year, and they note that some patients may have had more than one course of treatment during the year; thus the actual number treated may be slightly less.

TABLE 7.4. Usage of ECT in three Toronto hospitals, 1969–1973[a]

Hospital	Rate of ECT (%)		By diagnosis (%)	
	Average	5-Year range	Depressive disorder	Other
City Mental (Ontario)	1.2	(0.8–2.2)	4.5	0.4
Community (Clark Institute)	11	(1.6–13.5)	19.8	7.3
General	20	(11 –24.7)	36.5	6.2

[a] Data from Eastwood and Stiasny, 1978.

PRACTICE OF ECT

A principal aim of these surveys is the determination of the methods used for treatment. The questions used in different surveys are not directly comparable, and comparisons can only be made by some adjustment of the data.

The indications for ECT are described in the United States, New York, and Danish surveys. Although there is agreement as to the usefulness of ECT in cases of psychotic depression, differences in usage appear in cases with delirium, schizophrenia, and neurotic depression. Delirium is not considered an indication for ECT by American reporters but is in Denmark, whereas schizophrenia is not a primary indication in Denmark but is in the United States (Table 7.5). These differences may reflect diagnostic practices, particularly as to the differentiation of neurotic and psychotic depression; it is also likely that teaching practices differ in the two countries.

The technical procedures used by therapists are comparable in most respects,

TABLE 7.5. Indications for ECT

Disorder	New York[a]		Denmark[b]	United States[c]
	Any use[d]	Primary use[d]	Departments (%)	Primary use[d]
Endogenous depression	100	47	100	86
Acute depression	—	—	88	2
Mania	60	3	77	42
Hysterical psychosis	—	—	71	—
Reactive depression	37	13	60	6
Catatonia	100	27	50	—
Schizophrenia, acute	87	3	—	25
Schizoaffective depression	83	37	—	—

[a] Asnis et al., 1978.
[b] Heshe and Roeder, 1976.
[c] Frankel, 1978.
[d] Percent of respondents.

TABLE 7.6. Usage of ECT in Scandinavia[a]

Country	Departments using ECT		Use of bilateral and unilateral ECT (%)			
	N	%	Uni	Bi	Both uni and bi	Total uni
Denmark	59/62	95	52	36	12	64
Finland	23/47	49	4	82	14	18
Iceland	2/2	100	0	100	0	0
Norway	46/55	84	2	94	4	6
Sweden	88/95	93	70	19	11	81

[a] Data from Sand-Strömgren, personal communication.

differing only in the use of different electrode placements and the selection of currents for treatments. Unilateral electrode placements are used infrequently in the United States; less than 10% of patients were thus treated in the national survey. Most physicians who used unilateral ECT applied the electrodes over the right hemisphere (9%); less than 1% applied the electrodes to the left hemisphere (Frankel, 1978). In the New York survey, 83% of the therapists used bilateral and 6% used unilateral ECT exclusively, with 10% using either mode in different cases. By contrast, the Danish report cites 25% of centers using unilateral placement and 40% using bilateral placement exclusively; 31% used either method, depending on the severity of the patient's illness (Heshe and Roeder, 1976). In a broader Scandinavian survey, Sand-Strömgren (1977) also found a spread in the use of unilateral ECT among psychiatric departments. Unilateral ECT was used exclusively in 70% of units in Sweden and in none in Iceland; when the use of both unilateral and bilateral placements is considered, the range of usage is from 81% of centers in Sweden to none in Iceland (Table 7.6).

The use of instruments and currents to induce seizures also differed. In the United States, 62% of physicians used a suprathreshold alternating current (Medcraft), 33% used a unidirectional instrument (Reiter), and less than 1% used the brief stimulus alternating current produced by the MECTA (Frankel, 1978). Similar findings were described in the New York survey, where 60% of physicians used the Medcraft and 40% one of the Reiter instruments. In Denmark, the majority of the departments used instruments delivering unidirectional currents (Siemens K622, K3), and only two units used the alternating current (Elema) and one the brief stimulus instrument (Ectron Duopulse) (Heshe and Roeder, 1976).

COMMENT

Two findings stand out in these surveys: (a) differences in the usage of ECT for different populations, and (b) questions concerning electrode placement.

Much of the criticism of ECT is its alleged overuse among patients who may not have the capacity to understand the consequences of the treatment or to consent, particularly patients from the lower social classes. In both the Massachusetts and the New York surveys, the use of ECT was found to be significantly less in patients who were admitted to public mental hospitals, hospitals generally serving patients from the lower social classes. It is possible that these differences reflect different population samples, with patients who are psychotically depressed being selectively sent to institutions that provide ECT. In the absence of comparable diagnostic data from the various institutions, we cannot exclude the possibility that diagnostic differences are the basis for the data, but neither Grosser et al. (1975) nor Asnis et al. (1978) could find merit in this possibility and considered other factors as more compelling.

Considering the usage of ECT in university hospitals as a standard (5% of admissions), we may inquire about the reasons for the underutilization of ECT in the public mental hospitals and the possible exclusion of these patients from an effective therapy. It is more likely that financial, educational, and administrative issues affect the distribution of treatments. In public mental hospitals in the United States, budgetary considerations and therapeutic philosophy limit the availability of trained anesthesiologists and nurses for ECT and other special treatments. Few physicians are experienced in the administration or selection of patients for ECT, since training in ECT is primarily by preceptorship. Where the utilization is already low, training is hampered further. The cost of ECT is frequently paid by insurance carriers, whose contracts limit reimbursement for costs incurred in public mental hospitals compared to the rates allowed private or university hospitals, resulting in adequate reimbursement for costs in one type of hospital and inadequate reimbursement in another. Also, many public mental hospitals are now administered by lay personnel, selected by lay boards who credit criteria other than medical training and experience in their selection. Administrators lacking medical experience are particularly sensitive to the negative image of ECT in the press and the visual media, and their decisions in the allocation of funds for patient care and treatment are easily distorted. An example is seen in the decision by the administration of a large public hospital in New York City to close the ECT treatment facility when general funds for the hospital were curtailed.

ECT and Social Class

The usage of ECT was not always so. In the 1950s, sociologists examined the relationship among social class, diagnosis, type of mental health care, and outcome of treatment. Social class structure was defined for a sample of New Haven residents by weighted criteria of education, occupation, and place of residence (Redlich et al., 1953; Robinson, et al., 1954; Hollingshead and Redlich, 1958). The authors found that patients from upper classes were preferentially treated by intensive psychotherapy, whereas patients in the lower classes received custodial care and the organic therapies predominantly. Social class determined treatment even when psychopathology was held constant. The influence of cost of care could not be excluded as the major determinant, however, since psychotherapy and psychoanalysis were considerably more expensive than organic therapies and therefore available only to the upper classes.

At the time, we at Hillside Hospital examined this problem by surveying the relationship between social class and type of treatment among our patients. Hillside Hospital is a nonprofit private hospital where cost of care was not a factor in the selection of treatment, and all treatment modalities were equally available (Kahn et al., 1957, 1959; Kahn and Pollack, 1960; Pollack et al., 1961; Kahn, 1961; Kaplan and Lefkowits, 1961). We found that older, poorly educated, foreign-born patients were most likely to be referred for ECT. They were also hospitalized for shorter periods and had more favorable outcome ratings than the younger patients, who were referred for psychotherapy. In a test of authoritarianism, the California F-scale, patients referred for ECT had significantly higher scores than patients who received psychotherapy or insulin coma therapy.

In 1958, the study was replicated and two additional samples were studied: patients at the Menninger Foundation Hospital in Topeka, which treated upper class patients primarily, and the Massachusetts Mental Health Center (MMHC), which treated lower class patients preferentially (Siegel et al., 1962; Kahn et al., 1966). The hospitals were selected because all modalities of treatment were said to be equally available to all patients. The study had some special problems in diagnosis, since the hospitals used different classification schemes, with the Menninger Hospital using the more complex and elaborate system and MMHC the simplest. The institutions varied in their treatment patterns, with the longest stay, highest proportion of psychoneurotic diagnoses, more complex diagnostic schemata, lowest use of ECT, and poorest discharge ratings at the Menninger Hospital. The opposite was true at MMHC, where more patients received ECT, and the outcome evaluations were better. These observations suggest that, prior to the widespread use of psychotropic drugs, social class factors affected the use of ECT in the opposite direction to its influence today.

Unilateral ECT

The second question is the wide difference in the use of unilateral ECT. Apparently, in the clinical marketplace in the United States, the efficacy of unilateral ECT is deemed to be less than that of bilateral ECT. Although there is agreement among clinicians that amnesia and confusion are less with unilateral ECT, these favorable findings do not counterbalance, in the clinical risk-benefit analysis, the poorer clinical efficacy seen in many patients. The dissociation between the technical scientist observing the clinical, memory, and physiologic test changes in patients under laboratory conditions and therapists treating patients in a clinical environment is striking.

Perhaps the differences can be understood in the context of the published observations. It is more difficult to induce seizures through unilateral electrodes. Current intensity must be higher; seizure durations are shorter; terminations are less well defined; and patients are alert sooner. Under the usual clinical conditions of modified ECT, with anesthesia, succinylcholine, and forced ventilation, it is difficult to be sure that a patient has had a grand mal convulsion or to determine the length of the seizure. Under laboratory conditions, with research personnel checking each treatment, fewer patients are likely to have missed or abortive seizures; hence the laboratory definition of "equivalence" of the two types of inductions. In clinical settings, however, where therapists usually do not use objective monitoring procedures, missed and aborted seizures are more frequent, and hence the lesser therapeutic assessment of unilateral ECT and the frequent choice of bilateral ECT, particularly in more severely ill patients. d'Elia (1974) comes to a similar conclusion, noting that it is more difficult to establish a maximal seizure with unilateral electrodes. He suggests that too deep a narcosis must be avoided; the distance between electrodes must be sufficiently wide; and the electrode-skin contact must be carefully made to insure that the full current is passed to the brain and is not lost through extracerebral tissues.

In clinical practice, the concerns are so great for patients with severe depressions that the highest priority is given to the most rapid resolution of the dysphoric state, especially if the risk of suicide is material. It is easy to understand the concerns of the physician and the family for a most rapid resolution, even at some cost yet to be measured in a greater risk of amnesia and confusion.

The same factors were also important in the clinical assessment of brief stimulus therapy, for induction with these currents was frequently associated with shorter seizures, early awakening, and a higher incidence of missed seizures. Their lesser efficacy also interfered with their clinical acceptance.

EFFECTS OF SEIZURES

Seizures may be induced in many ways, and the cerebral response is, for the most part, independent of the mode of induction (Chapter 8). Each seizure is a patterned sequence of changes in cerebral, electrical, and biochemical activity which is accompanied by systemic changes in the cardiovascular, respiratory, and musculoskeletal systems. These events elicit biochemical and physiological changes in almost all systems of the body. Although seizures are described as all-or-none phenomena, they vary considerably in type and duration. Effects may be immediate and short lived or develop gradually and be prolonged, as reflected in the psychologic (Chapter 9) and behavioral (Chapter 10) consequences which may persist for years, and the biochemical (Chapter 11) and cerebrovascular (Chapter 12) events, which are measurable only during the seizure and the immediate postseizure period. Some effects, such as those on memory function and EEG, may be measured weeks and even months after the last seizure. To separate the events that are necessary for the therapeutic process and those that are secondary remains an unresolved challenge. We are concerned with some events for an understanding of the convulsive therapy process (Chapter 14) and with others for their relationship to the risks of treatment (Chapter 4).

Chapter 8

Electrophysiology of ECT

The science of electroencephalography developed at the same time as the seizure therapies. The first EEG recordings were published by Berger in 1929. Many studies of the EEG patterns among the mentally ill, the influence of drugs, and the effects of the seizure therapies followed (Brazier, 1950). The early studies sought to find diagnostic patterns, predictors of outcome, criteria for an endpoint to treatment, clues to the mechanism of ECT, and guides to the severity of the side-effects. As new modifications were developed, different techniques were compared to determine their comparability; as a result, there is an extensive experience with EEG in the ECT process. The early descriptive studies were reviewed by Meyer-Mickeleit (1949) and Chusid and Pacella (1952). EEG studies were the basis of the theoretic views of Roth (1951), Fink (1957, 1962, 1966, 1972c, 1974c), and Ottosson (1960, 1968, 1974). Comparisons between ECT and flurothyl were made by Laurell and Perris (1970) and Small and Small (1968), and of unilateral and bilateral ECT by d'Elia (1970a), Volavka et al. (1972), and Sand-Strömgren and Juul-Jensen (1975). Reviews in *Psychobiology of Convulsive Therapy* (Fink et al., 1974) and by Volavka (1972) and Small et al. (1978b) provide the most recent observations.

EFFECTS OF SEIZURES ON EEG

The Seizure EEG

Each seizure in convulsive therapy has characteristics similar to those of the spontaneous seizures recorded from epileptic patients. Immediately after the ECT stimulus, the EEG is isoelectric for 1 to 5 sec (latency period). Beginning in the frontal leads, there is a rapid build-up of diffuse, bilateral, synchronous spike and multiple spike activity which may last from 10 to 25 sec; this activity accompanies the typical tonic muscular contractions of the convulsion. Paroxysmal high voltage slow waves, again bilateral and diffuse, usually follow for 10 to 20 sec; these are associated with the clonic motor movements. Termination of the EEG seizure may be abrupt, with a cessation of all seizure activity and a flat EEG, or it may be gradual, with a decrease in amplitudes and an increase in the EEG mean frequency as slow waves are replaced by faster frequencies (Hughes et al., 1941; Cremerius and Jung, 1947; Meyer-Mickeleit, 1949; Piekenbrock et al., 1956; Piette, 1958; Chatrian and Petersen, 1960; Blachly and Gowing, 1966; J. Small, 1974).

Seizure activity does not follow an all-or-none rule, nor is the seizure pattern independent of the induction. Although the patterns are grossly similar among electric inductions, they may vary in the duration of different phases of the seizure. Latency periods are longer and tonic periods shorter with unidirectional currents than with alternating currents. Total seizure time may also be shorter for unidirectional and brief stimulation (square wave) currents (Proctor and Goodwin, 1943; Liberson, 1953; Alexander, 1953). Such observations are also defined in studies of the seizure patterns and duration in response to the strength of stimulus and repetition rate of seizures in experimental animals, where the type of seizure was determined by the strength of the stimulus. Only at strengths of stimuli from 20% above threshold to 10 times threshold was the typical grand mal convulsive pattern observed (Townsend et al., 1952; Tedeschi et al., 1956; Pollack et al., 1963).

With unilateral electrode placements, seizures may fail to spread to the opposite hemisphere; in such instances, the postictal EEG is similar to the untreated EEG (Blaurock et al., 1950). When seizure activity does spread to the opposite hemisphere and a grand mal convulsion ensues, the EEG is filled with bilateral seizure activity. Toward the end of the seizure and in the interictal period, however, asymmetries have been recorded with relative suppression of the voltages on the side of the application of the currents. Occasionally, voltages are higher. Postseizure isoelectric EEG is infrequent, the seizures usually terminating in an imprecise fashion with a rapid return of alpha activity. (Martin et al., 1965; Valentine et al., 1968; Small and Small, 1971; Abrams et al., 1970, 1972, 1973b; J. Small, 1974; Sand-Strömgren and Juul-Jensen, 1975; Kriss et al., 1977, 1978; Small et al., 1978b).

Seizures following chemical induction also show many differences and vary widely in duration. Flurothyl seizures were longer (120 sec) than after bilateral ECT (45 sec). This observation was accompanied by other differences in EEG: (a) the earlier appearance of continuous delta activity (99 versus 201 sec), (b) the later disappearance of continuous delta (6.6 versus 15.6 min), and (c) the earlier appearance of alpha activity (9.2 versus 24.4 min). During the flurothyl-induced seizure, there was more EEG fast activity and less synchronization than in ECT, and the amount of EEG abnormality from 15 to 30 min after the seizure was also greater after flurothyl than after ECT (Laurell and Perris, 1970). Similar findings were reported by Krantz et al. (1958) and Small et al. (1968b). Some authors find the duration of the seizure activity shorter with unilateral than with bilateral electrodes (Abrams et al., 1973b; J. Small, 1974), whereas others find no difference (d'Elia, 1970a,b).

In recordings from chronically implanted electrodes during seizures induced by flurothyl, pentylenetetrazol, or ECT, the electrical patterns were essentially the same in the prodromal, tonic, clonic, and postictal phases for both chemical inductions (Chatrian and Petersen, 1960). The authors reported that seizures were elicited by recruitment of spike discharges from various parts of the brain and that the three inductions exhibited a similar diffuse stimulatory nature.

Myoclonic jerks are a feature of seizures induced by flurothyl and pentylenetetrazol, occurring usually before the tonic/clonic phase. Incomplete seizures are frequent, with 10 to 20% of the inductions not progressing beyond the myoclonic phase (Knott et al., 1943; Chatrian and Petersen, 1960; Laurell and Perris, 1970).

Similar incomplete, aborted, or petit mal inductions also occur frequently in electric inductions, with the EEG showing some immediate changes in response to the current but failing to develop the progressive recruitment of spikes to a train of spontaneous high voltage spike and slow waves (Pacella et al., 1942; Cremarius and Jung, 1947; Meyer-Mickeleit, 1949; Chusid and Pacella, 1952). Such aborted seizures are usually followed by an immediate return of the pretreatment EEG pattern. Some inductions may be characterized by a prolonged, typical petit mal EEG, with spike and wave configurations of 3 Hz for periods up to 20 sec, without electrical silence or postictal slowing. The postictal EEG in such responses is similar to the untreated EEG (Small et al., 1978b). These, too, may be considered incomplete inductions.

The duration of seizures characteristically varies with the number of inductions, with later seizures becoming progressively shorter. The threshold for the seizure also rises progressively (Finner, 1954; Holmberg, 1954a; Green, 1960; Pollack et al., 1963; Essig, 1969). Termination of later seizures is more likely to be imprecise (Blachly and Gowing, 1966; Abrams et al., 1973b; Small et al., 1978b).

The Interseizure EEG

The principal sequellae to a seizure are a slowing of the mean EEG frequency and an increase in the mean amplitude of the record. After the first seizure, the changes are apparent within a few minutes of the end of the seizure, persisting for minutes to hours. With each successive seizure, duration of slowing is longer, mean frequency is lower, mean amplitude is greater, and burst patterns become prominent. The changes are progressive, symmetric, and appear in all electrode derivations, with amplitudes greater in the bitemporal and frontal electrodes. The duration and extent of EEG slowing are related to the age and psychopathology of the subjects (older, depressed patients exhibit greater degrees of slowing than younger and schizophrenic patients) and to the number, frequency, intensity, and duration of the seizures. With greater numbers of seizures at shorter intervals, EEG slowing is greater and persists longer after the end of treatment. The longer the duration of the seizure, the greater the degree of slowing (Meyer-Mickeleit, 1949; Chusid and Pacella, 1952; Piekenbrock et al., 1956; Roubicek, 1959; Stein et al., 1968). Fast frequencies decrease and disappear (Hoagland et al., 1946). The mean frequency of the prevailing alpha activity decreases, and the mean amplitude increases.

By the fourth treatment in depressed patients, the interseizure EEG remains slow for more than 48 hr. The mean frequency may fall to 4.0 to 5.0 Hz by

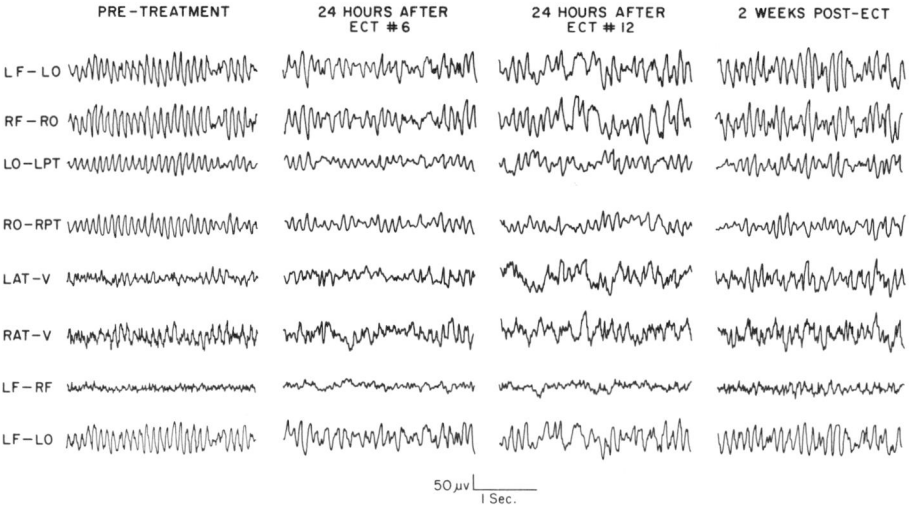

FIG. 8.1. Interseizure EEG in ECT. Male, age 60. All records 24 hr postconvulsion.

the termination of treatment (Roth, 1951; Chusid and Pacella, 1952; Fink and Kahn, 1957; Ottosson, 1960). Examples of the changes in interseizure EEG with ECT (Fig. 8.1) and with flurothyl (Fig. 8.2) show a progressive increase in amplitudes and percent time slowing with treatment and a rapid resolution with a return of higher abundance of alpha activity after the last treatment.

EEG frequency analysis is a technique that clearly defines the changes in EEG slowing with induced seizures. Figure 8.3 shows the changes in frequency patterns in the same patient as represented in Fig. 8.1. Another profile of change is seen in Fig. 8.4.

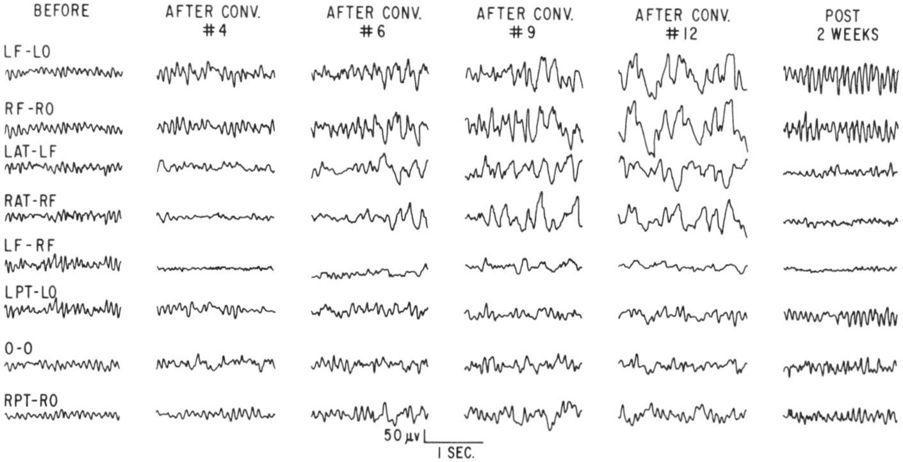

FIG. 8.2. Interseizure EEG with flurothyl. Female, age 44.

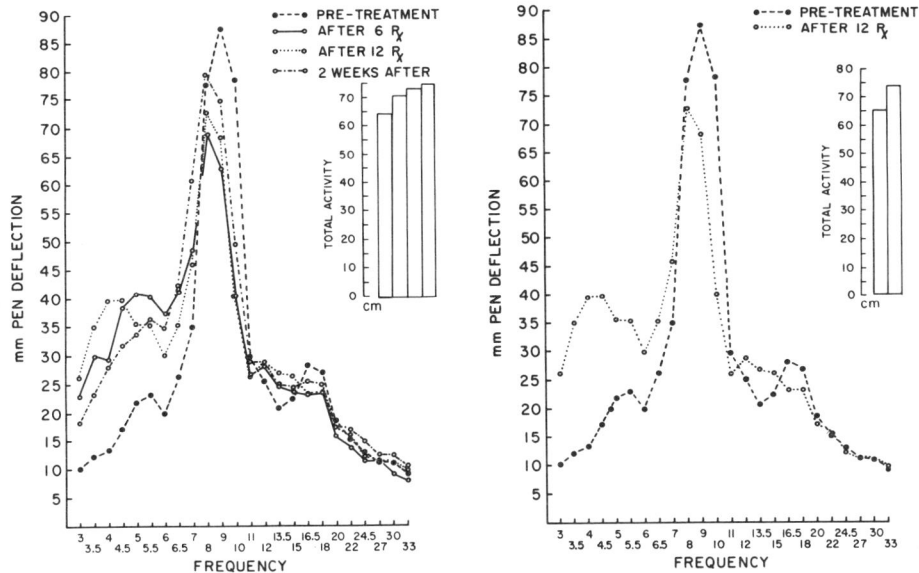

FIG. 8.3. EEG frequency analysis with ECT. Male, age 60. (Same as Fig. 8.1).

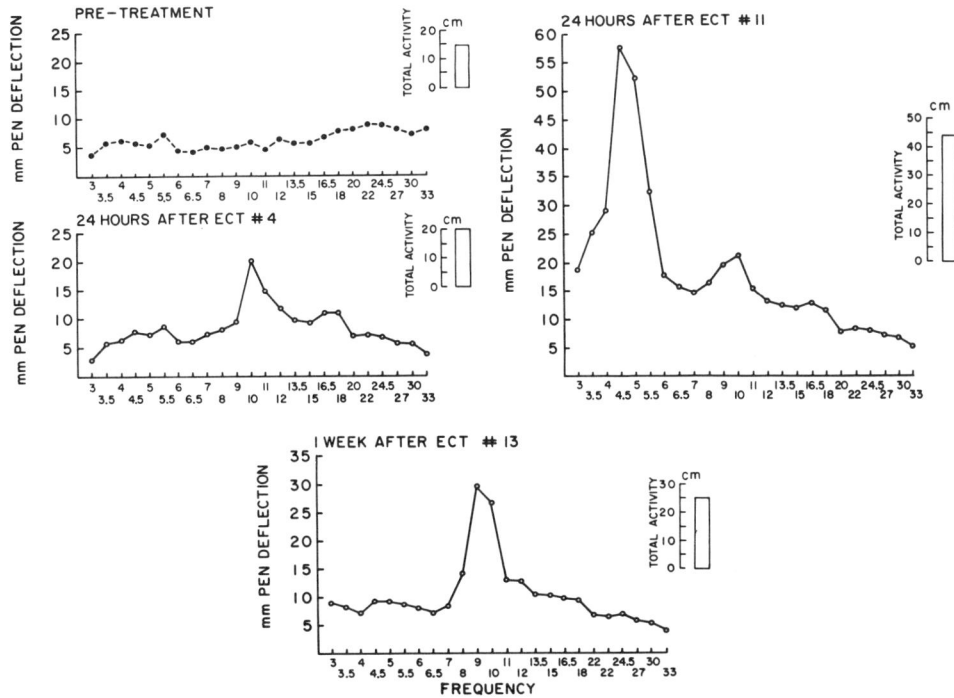

FIG. 8.4. EEG frequency analysis with ECT. Male, age 50, Left frontal, left occipital leads.

The degree of slowing is greater with alternating currents than after unidirectional and brief square wave stimuli. Although the differences are measurable, they are not significant. The principal difference is between seizure-producing and subconvulsive currents (Fig. 8.5). The degree of slowing is also greater after bilateral electrode placements than after unilateral placements and after pentylenetetrazol and flurothyl than after ECT (Chusid and Pacella, 1952; Liberson, 1953; Fink and Kahn, 1957; Fink and Green, 1958; Fink et al., 1958b; Abrams et al., 1973b; J. Small, 1974; Marjerrison et al., 1975). For example, in our comparison of the EEG slowing after flurothyl and after ECT, we found a somewhat higher percent time slow wave activity after flurothyl than after an equal number of ECT (Table 8.1).

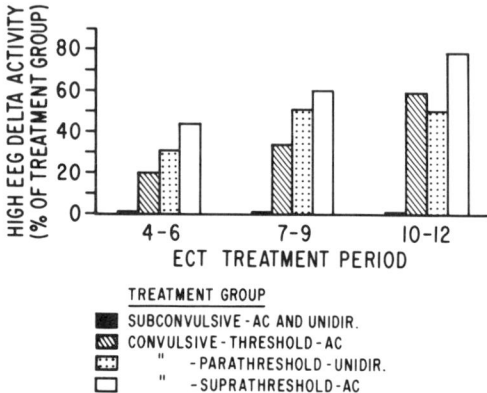

TREATMENT GROUP
■ SUBCONVULSIVE - AC AND UNIDIR.
▨ CONVULSIVE - THRESHOLD - AC
▥ " - PARATHRESHOLD - UNIDIR.
□ " - SUPRATHRESHOLD - AC

FIG. 8.5. Effect of ECT treatment type on EEG delta activity.

TABLE 8.1. Postconvulsive EEG slow waves[a]

	Average percent time				
		No. of treatments			
Treatment	Pretreatment	4–6	7–9	10–12	After 2 weeks
Flurothyl (15)	6.0	29.4	50.3	51.2	16.8
ECT (18)	4.0	29.8	39.2	47.5	18.0

[a] Data from Fink et al., 1961.

Some authors find the amount of slowing equivalent after bilateral and unilateral ECT when the findings are corrected for the shorter and incomplete seizures often seen in unilateral ECT (Sand-Strömgren and Juul-Jensen, 1975).

There is a great interindividual variability, however, in the amount, rate, and persistence of EEG slowing after ECT. In our studies, we noted a wide range in the degree of slowing which was only partly related to the induction features and number and frequency of seizures. What was surprising was the wide range in the degree of EEG slowing among patients with the same type of illness and age, who exhibited varying degrees of slowing with treatment (Figs. 8.6–8.8). Some of the variation is probably due to the difference in pretreatment EEG characteristics, and some of the differences are surely due to the induction methods, but features and differences still remain that reflect the psychopathology of the subject and factors in the EEG recording setting (Green, 1957, 1960).

The interseizure slow wave activity is usually symmetric, but there may be an accentuation of slowing over the dominant hemisphere after bilateral ECT (Volavka, 1972; Volavka et al., 1972; J. Small, 1974). In unilateral ECT, accentu-

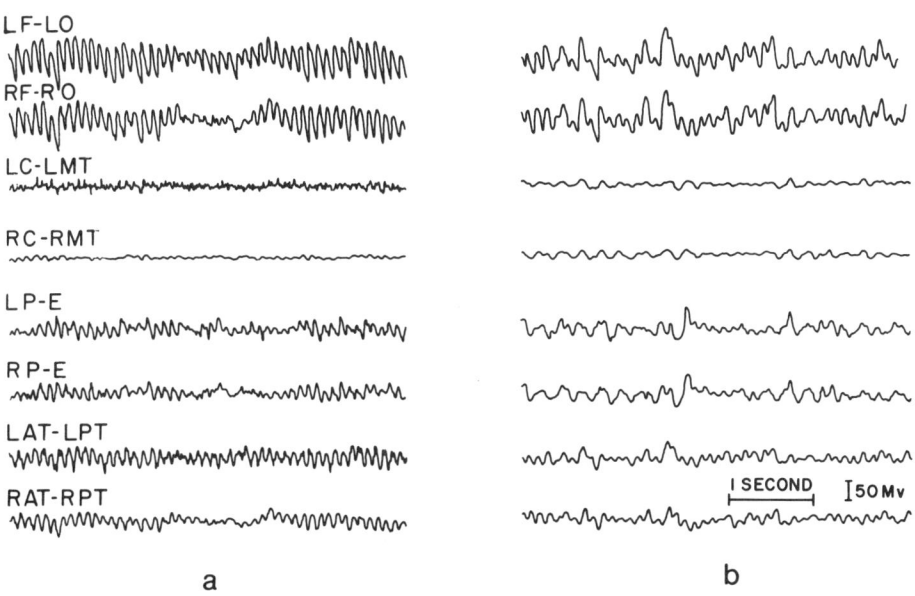

FIG. 8.6. Intermediate degree EEG slowing. (a) Pretreatment. (b) 24 hr after EST no. 10.

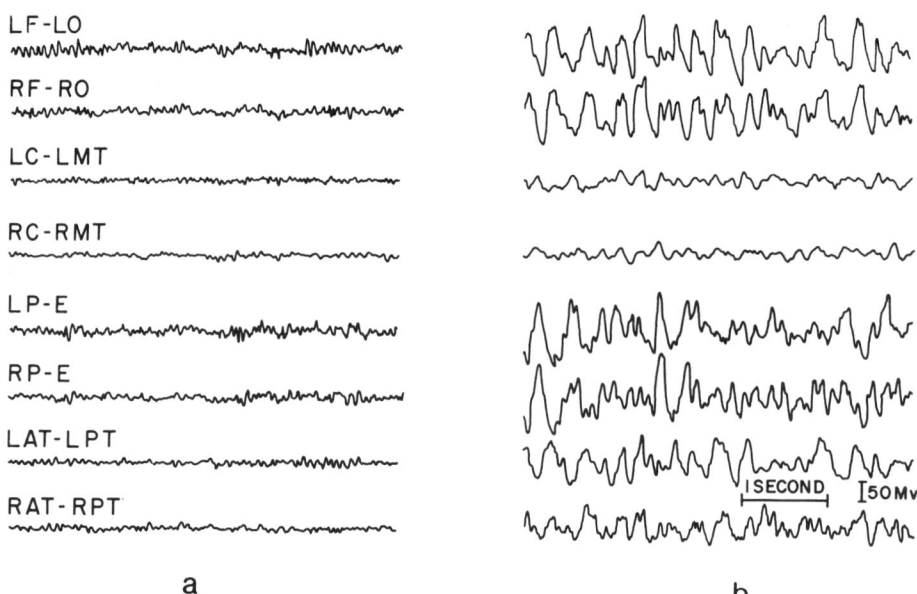

FIG. 8.7. High degree EEG slowing. (a) Pretreatment. (b) 24 hr after EST no. 11.

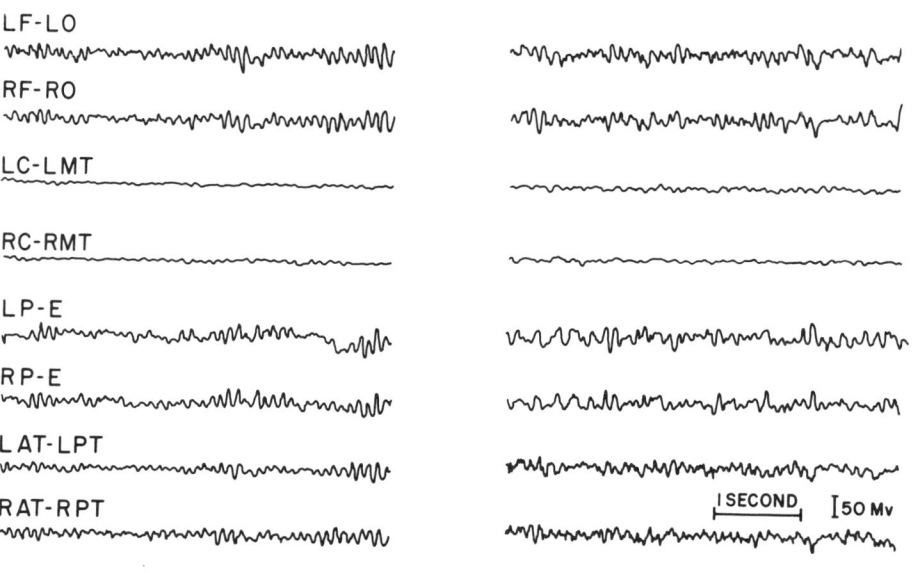

FIG. 8.8. Low degree EEG slowing. (a) Pretreatment. (b) 24 hr after EST no. 12.

ation of the interictal EEG with greater slowing over the treated hemisphere is usually found (Fig. 8.9) (Martin et al., 1965; Sutherland et al., 1969; d'Elia, 1970a; d'Elia and Perris, 1970, 1973; Abrams et al., 1970; Volavka et al., 1972; Small et al., 1973; J. Small, 1974; Marjerrison et al., 1975). After flurothyl, lateralization of the EEG was not observed (Small et al., 1973).

The asymmetry and focal accentuation, when it occurs, may be related to the anatomical asymmetry in brain structures seen in postmortem anatomical and *in vivo* computerized axial tomograms (LeMay, 1976; Galaburda et al., 1978).

When seizures are repeated rapidly within one sitting, as in multiple monitored ECT (MMECT), there is little increase in the amount of slowing over that which would have occurred in a single seizure of higher intensity (Blachly and Gowing, 1966; Abrams and Fink, 1972; Abrams et al., 1973b). We examined the EEG records in 18 patients who received multiple ECT (MECT) through either unilateral or bilateral electrode placements. EEG records were obtained in 160 of the seizures. The seizure activity was longer after bilateral MECT (61.9 ± 18.3 versus 51.5 ± 25.2 sec; $t = 1.98$, $p \leq 0.025$); and later seizures in a series were longer than the first seizure. Termination of the seizure was more precise for later seizures; in general, most seizures (43 of 57) ended in a precise fashion. Postseizure records after bilateral ECT were most often flat, whereas after unilateral ECT, the immediate postseizure record was frequently filled with mixed alpha and beta frequencies (Abrams et al., 1973b).

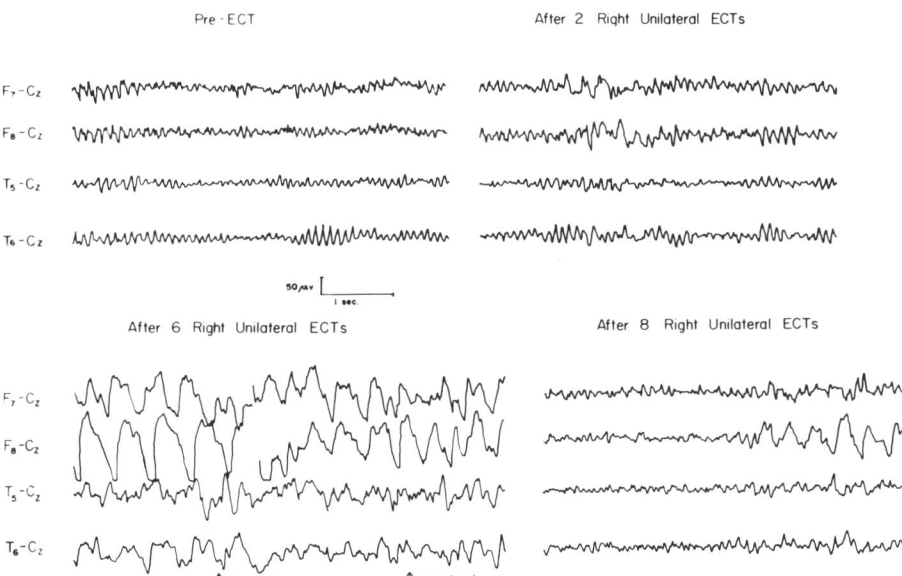

FIG. 8.9 Interseizure EEG with unilateral ECT.

The amount of slow waves is not maximal immediately after a seizure but increases in time, suggesting that the sustained EEG changes are correlated with developing biochemical events and not the seizure induction itself. In intensive electroshock in schizophrenic patients who received four seizures daily for 7 days, Callaway and Boucher (1950) found the slow waves to increase progressively during treatment and after the last treatment. The maximum EEG change occurred from 3 to 6 days after the last treatment.

The amount of slow wave activity in the interseizure and postseizure EEG varies with the setting. If patients are tense and anxious in the laboratory, the degree of slowing is reduced. With hyperventilation, drowsiness, or after the administration of barbiturates, the amount of slowing is enhanced (Roth, 1951).

Another effect of ECT is to modify the alpha-blocking response to photic stimulation. The duration of this response is longer in retarded depressed patients (Wilson and Wilson, 1961) and increases to average levels after ECT (Ulett et al., 1962; d'Elia et al., 1974) as after antidepressant drugs (Zung, 1969).

Various interpretations have been given to the EEG patterns during and after the seizure. The neurophysiologic basis for these features is ill defined, although most reporters ascribe the origin of bilaterally synchronous discharges seen in epilepsy and indistinguishable from those patterns found in ECT as originating in diencephalic structures having easy access to homologous areas of both hemispheres (Jasper, 1949; Roth, 1951). One view of the changing seizure EEG patterns proposed by Adrian (1936) attributes the electrical phenomena of the tonic, clonic, and postconvulsive phases of the convulsion to excessive firing and recruitment of cortical cells, afterdischarges, and exhaustion, respectively.

The Postseizure EEG

Following the last treatment, there is a progressive disappearance of slow wave activity. The mean frequency increases toward the normal alpha range within 2 to 6 weeks. In some patients, resolution may be slower, with abnormal frequencies persisting for months (Pacella et al., 1942; Levy et al., 1942; Cremerius and Jung, 1947; Fink and Kahn, 1957; Sutherland et al., 1969). The rate of resolution may be as rapid after intensive ECT as after conventional ECT, as noted by Callaway and Boucher (1950), who found slow waves to disappear within 9 to 21 days after a course of 28 treatments given in 7 days. Klotz (1955) examined the records of patients up to 6 months after treatment and observed that 81% had abnormal slow records at the end of treatment, 12% after 1 month, 5% after 2 months, and less than 2% after 3, 4, and 6 months.

In clinically responsive patients, the EEG records usually become filled with well-modulated alpha activity. The persistence of slow waves or the early reappearance of low voltage fast activity is considered a poor prognostic sign (Hoagland et al., 1946; Chusid and Pacella, 1952).

Other Physiological Measures

Few studies have examined changes in variables other than the alert, resting EEG following ECT. The few studies are reviewed by Mendels et al. (1974) and Small et al. (1978b). With respect to the averaged evoked response, they note that a recognizable visual evoked response is elicited in subjects with typical petit mal episodes in the EEG, suggesting that not all cortical neurons participate in seizure activity. In studies of the interictal EEG after bilateral and unilateral ECT, Small and Small (1971a) were unable to show significant differences in visual or auditory evoked responses. The evoked potential configurations were remarkably unchanged, despite obvious alterations in the resting EEG. The delayed recovery time in the somatosensory evoked response seen in depressed patients returned to a normal recovery time with behavioral improvement after ECT, in a manner similar to that seen after tricyclic antidepressants (Shagass, 1972).

Studies of the contingent negative variation have been equally unproductive, the changes associated with ECT being inconsistent (Small and Small, 1971a, b).

Interest in the effects of ECT on the sleep EEG arose from two observations: (a) the prominence of insomnia in depression and its value as a favorable predictor of outcome with ECT, and (b) the experimental study that REM-deprived cats given ECS did not experience a compensatory increase in REM sleep time. In a study of cats, Cohen and Dement (1966) and Cohen et al. (1967) reported that as few as four ECS reduced REM pressure. REM sleep time was reduced in cats by daily ECS, also without a rebound in compensatory REM time (Kaelbling et al., 1968). In depressed patients, disturbances in sleep EEG patterns include a shorter total sleep time (greater periods of wakefulness), longer sleep latency, more early morning awakening, less delta and REM sleep, and shorter REM latency (Kupfer and Foster, 1975; Coble et al., 1976; Gillin et al., 1978). Studies of the effects of ECT are variable and the results unclear, largely because of methodologic problems. The consensus finds that total sleep time and amount of time in stages 3, 4, and REM increase, with a decrease in REM latency. There is a reduction in spontaneous awakenings and, in general, sleep is less disturbed, longer, and closer to control values after ECT (Green and Stajduhar, 1966; Zarcone et al., 1967; Mendels et al., 1974).

The autonomic correlates of ECT were also examined; in general, the effects of ECT were minimal (Bassett and Ashby, 1954; Stern and Sila, 1959; Stern and Word, 1961; Stern et al., 1961; Noble and Lader, 1971; Dawson et al., 1977). Depressed patients tend to exhibit lower skin conductance levels, smaller phasic skin conductance responses with longer latencies, higher tonic heart rates, and smaller heart rate changes to stimuli than do nondepressed controls. Following ECT, there is little change in the electrodermal or heart rate responses. One group (Bassett and Ashby, 1954), however, related an increase in skin conductance response after ECT to clinical improvement.

SIGNIFICANCE OF EEG CHANGES

The EEG patterns during and after ECT are a consistent accompaniment of the process, and their significance has been studied extensively. Many questions have been asked, principally, the relationship of EEG changes to outcome and as evidence of brain damage and its persistence. Some authors have used EEG measures to monitor the treatment of the individual patient, and others have sought clues to the mechanism of the antidepressant effects of ECT.

EEG Measures as an Index of Brain Damage

In clinical neurology, the appearance of high voltage EEG slow waves of 2 to 6 Hz bursts in focal and asymmetric patterns is evidence of a pathologic process in the brain. The abnormalities are associated with seizure disorders, organic confusional toxic states, and cerebral impairment caused by trauma, mass lesion, and vascular deficiency. The time course, persistence, and distribution over the head are the usual guides to their clinical significance (Strauss et al., 1952; Hill and Parr, 1963; Kooi, 1971).

The induction of a seizure, as administered today, is a regular feature of convulsive therapy, and persistent EEG slow waves are a necessary part of the treatment. But the EEG changes do not persist beyond 2 to 4 weeks after the last treatment (Pacella et al., 1942; Levy et al., 1942; Fink and Kahn, 1957; Turek, 1972; J. Small, 1974). This is also true for multiple seizures, in which extensive alterations in brain functions are developed (Callaway and Boucher, 1950; Exner and Murillo, 1977). Slow wave activity disappears within 3 weeks, and records taken at follow-up after 1 year are indistinguishable from control subjects. In ECT, normalization of the EEG with an increase in the amount and regularity of alpha activity is a regular feature of responsive patients after ECT.

ECT has been compared to reversible head trauma, and it is likely that in the usual case, ECT does not result in persistent brain damage (Roth, 1952; Fink 1966, 1972c). A special case is raised by the reports of the persistence of spontaneous seizures. In such instances, it is probable that some brain damage did occur; as a result of the electric currents, vascular hyperemia, or cerebral hypertension, a focus of injury was created, which became the source for spontaneous seizures. Even such episodes are reported as reversible, although persistence for up to 3 years has been noted (Karliner, 1956; Assael et al., 1967). As such episodes are uncommon, we lack the EEG and neurologic studies to document such a focus.

Relationship of EEG Measures to Outcome

Two aspects of the problem have been studied: (a) the predictive value of the pretreatment EEG, and (b) of the interseizure or postcourse EEG. Some authors found that patients with a normal (alpha) EEG pretreatment had a better prognosis than patients with low voltage fast tracings (Turner et al., 1945; Weil and Brinegar, 1947; Kennard and Willner, 1948; Mosovich and Katzenelbogen, 1948; Fink and Kahn, 1957). Others failed to find such a relationship (Moriarty and Siemens, 1947; Chusid and Pacella, 1952). Hoagland et al. (1946) report a positive relationship between the amount of fast activity in the pretreatment EEG and clinical outcome with ECT in a group of involutional depressed women.

As with so many physiological measures, the post-ECT EEG was most clearly related to the pre-ECT EEG (Johnson et al., 1960b; Volavka et al., 1972; Turek, 1972). In the absence of any relationship between the resting EEG and clinical psychopathology, it is no surprise that the efficacy of the ECT therapeutic process, which is so closely related to clinical diagnosis, is not related to the resting EEG. Furthermore, in these studies, diagnostic classes were not well defined with populations made up of schizophrenic and depressed patients; also, seizures were not monitored. Thus neither the number nor duration of seizures was well defined.

Is there a relationship between the amount of slowing in the interictal EEG and clinical efficacy? Most studies, using visual descriptions of the EEG and global outcome statements, failed to find a relationship and concluded that slowing of the EEG occurs in all patients, independent of outcome (Cremerius and Jung, 1947; Weil and Brinegar, 1947; Moriarty and Siemens, 1947; Mosovich and Katzenelbogen, 1948; Blaurock et al., 1950; Chusid and Pacella, 1952). Nevertheless, there was a general impression that a relationship exists between the abnormality induced in the EEG and outcome. As expressed by Lewis (1945):

> Electroencephalographic changes occur during the course of treatment (electric shock) and correlate with amnesia as other evidence of impaired mental function. When there is no evidence of impaired mental function and no electroencephalographic alteration, clinical improvement does not occur.

In the same period, three observers, using quantitative measures for EEG and careful behavioral assessments, reported EEG-behavioral relationships with both theoretic and clinical significance.

EEG Predictors

Roth (1951, 1952) recorded the EEG changes in ECT after thiopental (Thiopentone, Pentothal) anesthesia. Patients were examined before ECT, within a few hours of treatment, and for a number of weeks after a course of ECT. He found that thiopental revealed latent changes in the EEG, usually most clearly after the third treatment when the resting EEG failed to show consistent changes. The typical response to thiopental consisted of rhythmic, frontally preponderant, bilaterally synchronous, paroxysmal high voltage delta discharges at 2 to 3

Hz, lasting 100 to 200 sec. The slow discharge was followed by a quiescent stage in which slow activity was absent from the record, even when it had been prominent in the resting EEG. Roth concluded that there was some relationship between EEG and clinical change, since an atypical thiopental response was associated with a poor therapeutic result. He was intrigued by the theoretic significance of the observations. As the site of action of thiopental was thought to be in deep midline structures, it was likely that ECT had its primary effects in the diencephalon, a structure with ready access to all cortical areas but with particular connections to the frontal lobes.

Using these observations as a base, Roth et al. (1957) applied the thiopental technique to 41 cases of psychotic depression. The patients received between 6 and 12 ECT, and thiopental activation records were obtained before the first treatment, within 4 hr after every treatment, and weekly after the last treatment for up to 2 months. Thiopentone (5%) was injected at a rate of 1 cc every 15 sec with a 5-sec pause (equal to 150 mg/min) until eye closure and regular deep respiration occurred. Total dose varied from 150 to 300 mg. A typical response was the development of high voltage slow activity, usually followed by a prolonged period of low voltage fast EEG. The slow wave burst activity was readily evoked during this period by sensory stimulation. With successive treatments, patients showed an increase in the amount of slow wave activity, usually peaking with the last treatment. Thereafter, slowing was rapidly reduced to less than one-half the peak amount by 3 weeks, and to less than pretreatment levels by the end of 2 months.

Roth and his co-workers failed to find a relationship between peak values in the percent time slowing and immediate outcome. When the records of relapsed cases were examined, however, a clear relationship was found between low peak values of slow waves (less than 40%) and the rate of relapse at both 3 and 6 months after discharge. The higher relapse rates were related to low peak delta values irrespective of the number of ECT, age, prior illness, or duration of symptoms before treatment. Roth et al. (1957) concluded that the relationship between recovery and EEG change was indirect, with the EEG changes tending to promote recovery

> ... by impeding in some way the physiological processes underlying the psychotic illness. But the EEG changes alone do not ensure success ...

They emphasized the nonspecific nature of the ECT process and considered that other psychopathologic features influenced the outcome, while the EEG changes

> ... may serve to indicate whether or not a quantitatively adequate physiological basis for recovery has been provided by treatment ... [p. 233].

As a practical matter, they suggested that thiopental activation was too cumbersome for routine use but that it may be helpful to determine the time to terminate a course of treatment. If a thiopental record taken a few hours after a treatment exhibited between 35 and 50% percent time delta activity, the treatment may be considered adequate, while lower values would be a basis for further treatment.

Our own studies were based on the concepts of Weinstein et al. (1952) that altered brain function provided the milieu for the expression of denial in ECT. Our studies encompassed different measures of brain function, including memory and perceptual tests, language, and EEG.

In our initial series, 24 patients referred for electroshock were studied (Fink and Kahn, 1957). EEG records were obtained prior to and at weekly intervals during and after bilateral ECT using a Reiter C-47 Electrostimulator. During treatment, records were taken 1 day after a treatment, usually 25 to 31 hr later. Records were examined and artifact-free samples identified from the resting and posthyperventilation periods. For each of three lead pairs (left fronto-parietal, anterior temporal-vertex, and parietal-ear lobe), various indices were determined: (a) percent time slow waves (7 Hz and slower) in the record and in each lead; (b) slowest frequency in the sample, (c) highest voltages, and (d) duration of longest burst. When records were ranked according to each of these criteria, the sample was divided into thirds, and records were classified as highest, middle, or lowest third of the total sample. In percent time, high degree delta records were characterized by at least 18% for an average delta index, 21% or more in one of the three measured leads, slowest frequency less than 3¾ Hz, amplitude at least 100 μV, and burst duration at least 2½ sec. Clinical response was determined by a combination of global assessment by staff, patients, and relatives during the 2 months of observation after the last treatment. In a second study, the EEG records of 54 consecutive, unselected patients referred for ECT were examined using similar quantitative EEG and behavioral criteria.

There was a well-defined relationship between the early appearance of high degree slow wave EEG records and global assessments of improvement (Table 8.2). Of the 11 patients rated as much improved, 80% of the EEG records were classed as high degree in the second and third weeks of treatment, whereas

TABLE 8.2. High degree slow wave EEG records[a]

Clinical rating	No. of treatments			
	1–3	4–6	7–9	10–12
Much improved (11)	25	80	91	88
Moderately improved (6)	0	16	50	40
Unimproved (7)	0	0	0	20

[a] Data from Fink and Kahn, 1957.

none of the records from the seven unimproved patients were so classified. The relationships were the same in the analyses of the individual indices of EEG slowing, as these were highly intercorrelated, with the correlations ranging from 0.47 to 0.98.

Believing that the rate of development and degree of EEG slowing was prognostic of outcome, we obtained resting EEG records during the second (ECT 4–6) and third (ECT 7–9) weeks of treatment and related these measures to the clinical global ratings in the next 54 patients referred for ECT (Table 8.3). Of the patients in whom high degrees of EEG slowing developed, 67% were rated as much improved; only 30% without high degrees of EEG slowing were so rated. We concluded that the early induction of slowing was an important feature of the ECT process (Fink and Kahn, 1957).

Another set of observations was provided by Ottosson (1960), who examined the significance of the EEG seizure discharge by using lidocaine to reduce the duration and amount of EEG seizure activity. Lidocaine shortened seizure activity and modified the seizure termination. Instead of abrupt terminations in electrical silence, lidocaine seizures transformed rapidly to postcentral alpha activity. Lidocaine-modified seizures were less effective than unmodified seizures in their antidepressant efficacy. Although Ottosson made no direct claim for a relationship between interseizure slowing and antidepressant efficacy, his studies demonstrated that there was less clinical efficacy when immediate postseizure slowing was reduced.

TABLE 8.3. *Patients with high degree slow wave EEG records during second and third weeks of treatment*[a]

	Clinical rating		
EEG slowing	Much improved	Moderately improved	Unimproved
Both high (18)	12 (67%)	4 (22%)	2 (11%)
One high (16)	4 (25%)	8 (50%)	4 (25%)
None high (20)	6 (30%)	7 (35%)	7 (35%)

[a] Data from Fink and Kahn, 1957.

Unilateral ECT

In a later study, we examined the EEG and behavioral effects of unilateral and bilateral ECT (Abrams et al., 1970, 1972; Volavka et al., 1972). From a sample of 103 patients, we were able to examine the relationship of EEG slowing to clinical outcome in 31 depressed patients who received unilateral nondominant ($N = 9$) and bilateral ($N = 22$) ECT and who had a full range of satisfactory EEG records (Volavka et al., 1972). The EEG data were reduced by period analysis using digital computer programs (Fink et al., 1968). The behavioral scores were derived from a modified Hamilton depression rating scale completed 1 day after the fifth or sixth treatment in the series.

The changes in average frequency and in percent time delta activity were found to be the principal features of the ECT response. These were related to changes in the adjusted depression scale score. While the expected relationship between EEG variables and the number of treatments was observed, no relationship was found between the degree of slowing and Hamilton scale change. In addition, EEG lateralization differences were found between the two electrode placements; here too, there was no relationship to the change in depression scale score.

In a reassessment of the relationship of EEG to clinical outcome, Volavka (1974) found the evidence to be limited and could not find any secure relationship. Kurland et al. (1976) also reexamined this relationship in a group of 19 depressed patients. They reported that the clinically improved patients had greater amounts of alpha activity and lesser amounts of slow waves than the unimproved patients, in direct contrast to our findings (Fink and Kahn, 1957).

What is to be made of these data? Despite some effort, no clear relationship has been defined between EEG slowing—the characteristic EEG response to seizure—and clinical outcome. In reexamining our studies (Fink and Kahn, 1957), it seems that our success was probably based on the mixed sample of depressed and schizophrenic patients that was recommended for ECT at that time. The correlation was derived from the responsivity in both EEG and behavior of the subset of depressed patients, and the delayed behavioral response and lesser degrees of EEG slowing in the schizophrenic subjects. Our failure to define a relationship in more recent studies may be attributable, in part, to our more homogeneous (depressive only) samples but also to the short-term assessment that we used. Roth et al. (1957) also failed to find a relationship between pentothal-induced slowing and short-term improvement but could define one for relapse rates.

Our studies highlight one interesting physiological observation. Depressed patients exhibit a greater sensitivity to neurophysiological changes after seizures than other (schizophrenic) patients, as evidenced by the more rapid evolution of EEG slowing both in the spontaneous interseizure EEG and in response to thiopental.

Slowing of the EEG after ECT is evidence that a cerebral seizure (or a series of cerebral seizures) has occurred. Such evidence is the best available index among our present techniques to assure us that the changes in brain function ordinarily necessary for a therapeutic response have occurred. Although EEG slowing is not directly related to antidepressant efficacy, its appearance seems necessary, although not sufficient, for the evolution of antidepressant activity. Perhaps improved methods of inducing ECT, or biochemical-pharmacological replacements, will be developed which will make the development of EEG slowing as irrelevant to antidepressant efficacy as is amnesia.

Effects of Drugs

The induction of seizures in patients under the influence of a barbiturate and succinylcholine (or curare) affects the efficacy of the treatments little, and presumably also affects the seizure parameters as little, although the seizure threshold rises. The administration of a barbiturate in the interictal period enhances the degree of EEG slowing, increasing the amplitude and amount of theta and delta activity (Fig. 8.10).

Following an observation that large doses of atropine could prevent EEG slowing following experimental seizures in the monkey, Ulett and Johnson (1957) examined the effects of atropine and scopolamine on the EEG after ECT. Seven schizophrenic patients received daily doses of intramuscular atropine (1 to 5 mg) and five received scopolamine (1 to 3 mg) during and for a few days following a course of ECT. The patients were maintained on the atropine regimen for 21 to 36 days and on scopolamine for 9 to 36 days. EEG records taken during

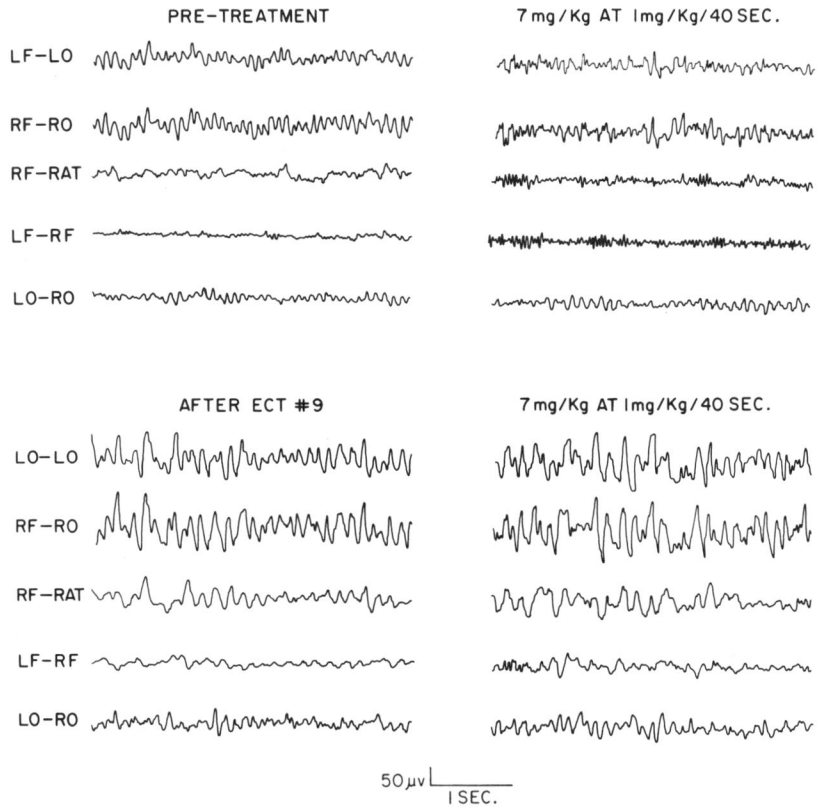

FIG. 8.10. Effect of intravenous amobarbital on EEG slowing pretreatment and postconvulsion. Female, age 25.

the treatment course (numbers of treatments not specified) did not exhibit the usual EEG slowing of ECT. When atropine was discontinued, slowing suddenly appeared, suggesting that the drugs suppressed the expression of the slow wave activity. Johnson et al. (1960a) attempted to replicate this study and found that difficulties in drug administration precluded an acceptable conclusion.

We also examined the effects of anticholinergic drugs on EEG activity, using a number of centrally active drugs, such as diethazine, benactyzine, and procyclidine, as well as the experimental compounds Ditran, JB-318, JB-336, and WIN-2299. The effects of the anticholinergic compound diethazine are shown in Fig. 8.11. In patients with EEG slowing and a reduction in their psychotic symptoms and mood disorder, the administration of the anticholinergic drug elicited restlessness, agitation, delusional thoughts, and a relapse in the mood disorder. These symptoms were associated with a reduction in slow wave activity and a desynchronization of frequencies. The language patterns of denial—use of third person, qualification, and displacement—which were associated with improvement with ECT also were reversed. As the effects of the anticholinergic drugs waned, the EEG slowing would return and with it an improvement in behavior and a return of the denial language patterns. These observations led to the

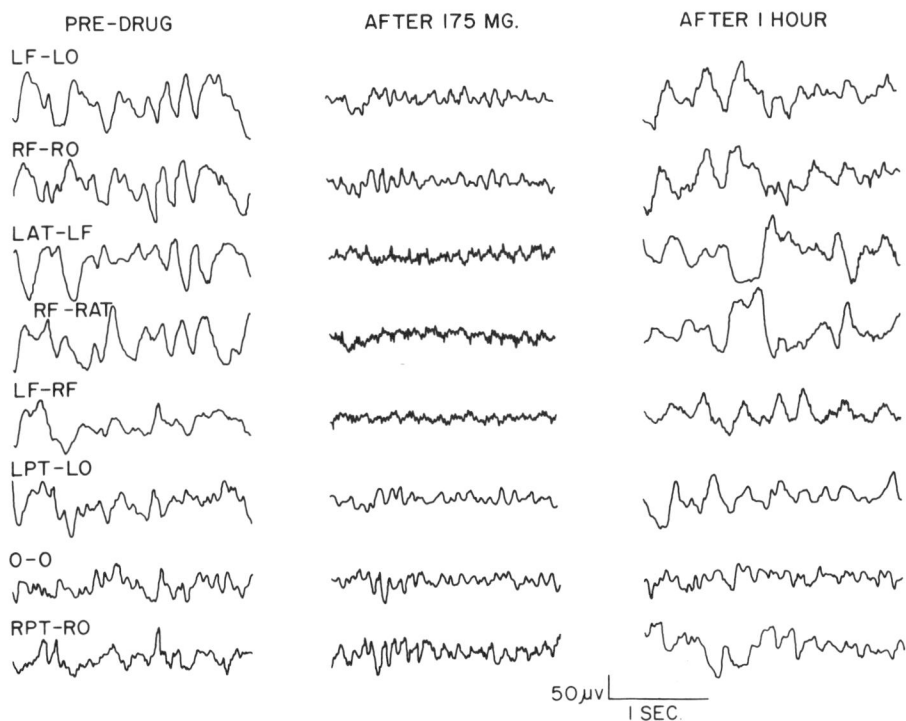

FIG. 8.11. Effect of diethazine on EEG delta. Female, age 34, 24 hr postconvulsion no. 12.

suggestion that an enhancement of cholinergic mechanisms was an important feature of the ECT process (Fink, 1958a, 1959a, 1960, 1966).

The interictal EEG slowing is also reduced by amphetamine (Lennox et al., 1951), mescaline (Merlis and Hunter, 1955; Denber, 1955), diphenhydramine (Diaz-Guerrero et al., 1956), and LSD-25 (Bente et al., 1958) (Fig. 8.12). The duration of the ECT seizure was reduced by lidocaine, with a sharp reduction in spike activity and without an elevation in the seizure threshold. Lidocaine shortened the postictal silence, with an early reappearance of alpha activity and eye opening (Ottosson, 1960).

The barbiturate reactivity of subjects is related to clinical outcome with ECT. In the sedation threshold, patients with low thresholds (requiring less amobarbital for a defined EEG effect) had better prognosis for ECT than patients with a high sedation threshold (Shagass and Jones, 1958; Perris and Brattemo, 1963). These observations are consistent with the better prognosis in ECT of patients who show language patterns of denial in response to intravenous amobarbital (Weinstein and Kahn, 1955; Kahn et al., 1956).

In retrospect, it is clear that further study of the interaction of drugs with different central neurohumoral effects would have contributed to our understanding of the ECT process. These analyses indicate that adrenergic, cholinergic,

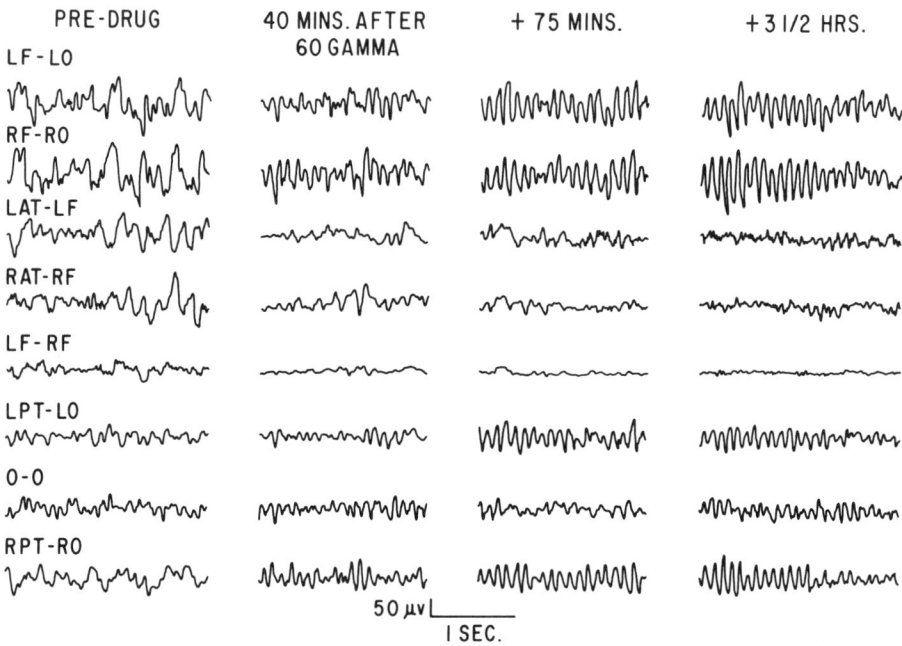

FIG. 8.12. Effect of intravenous LSD on EEG delta. Female, age 44, 24 hr postconvulsion no. 9.

and histaminic neurohumors are involved in the expression of the slow wave activity of the ECT process.

EEG Indices in Clinical Management

EEG measures have been used infrequently in clinical management. Blachly and Gowing (1966) recommended EEG monitoring of seizures to determine the time to repeat a seizure in MMECT. Monitoring also provided a measure of the type of seizure termination ("fit switch"). Difficulties with the successful application of unilateral ECT led other observers to examine the usefulness of seizure monitoring. d'Elia and Raotma (1975) found unilateral and bilateral ECT clinically equivalent in only one-half the published studies. d'Elia suggested that seizure induction with unilateral ECT was more difficult, with more inductions incomplete and aborted. This conclusion was made more likely by the prevalent use of modified ECT, in which objective measures of the duration and characteristics of the seizure are hidden by anesthesia and muscle paralysis. Missed seizures were considered the basis for the lesser efficacy of unilateral ECT by Sand-Strömgren and Juul-Jensen (1975), who were able to equate the clinical efficacy of the two treatments by adjusting for the short and incomplete inductions with unilateral ECT. Similar conclusions were presented by J. Small (1974). It is worthwhile to consider some procedure to monitor a seizure in order to reduce the number of treatments to a minimum. EEG monitoring provides an objective assessment of the termination of treatment in the individual patient and a measure of dosage in comparative ECT-pharmacotherapy assessments. Duration of seizure activity is a corollary to the plasma level measurements of antidepressant drugs.

EEG recordings are also useful in the management of the individual clinical case. When depressed, catatonic, or manic patients fail to respond to ECT within the anticipated period of treatment, a resting EEG recorded 24 to 72 hr after a seizure provides useful information. If the record does not show generalized, symmetric, high voltage EEG slow wave activity in bursts, it is likely that the subject has received an inadequate course of treatment, and further seizure inductions may be useful. If the record exhibits adequate amounts of such activity, however, then it is likely that further treatment will do little to enhance the therapeutic results. In the use of ECT in schizophrenic patients, the role of EEG changes is still unclear; in such instances, the clinical criteria are the best.

SUMMARY

A cerebral seizure is central to the antidepressant efficacy of convulsive therapy. EEG monitoring finds induced seizures to be similar to idiopathic grand mal seizures. EEG activity is similar, regardless of the mode of induction, exhibiting characteristic latency, tonic, clonic, and postictal patterns. The EEG changes are symmetric, with burst activity characteristic of centrencephalic epilepsy.

With successive seizures, thresholds rise, and duration of seizures falls. The interictal EEG exhibits progressive slowing of the mean frequency and an increase in the mean amplitudes. The degree of slowing is related to the number and frequency of seizures, to the psychopathology and age of the patient, and, to a lesser degree, to the type of currents and placement of electrodes.

The amount of slow waves is not linearly related to clinical outcome, but their early appearance and persistence is a necessary condition for improvement in the ECT process. EEG changes resolve after the last treatment, and thus they are no longer measurable after 2 to 6 weeks, except when the treatment is intensive.

EEG indices are useful in the successful management of patients, providing an objective index of adequacy of treatment under modern anesthetic conditions.

Chapter 9

Neuropsychology of ECT

Impairment of memory is the most known, most studied, and most pervasive consequence of induced seizures. It is the basis for the principal complaints of patients and their relatives. Despite much interest, the literature is complex and poorly controlled. The significance of amnesia for the therapeutic process is still debated. The arguments reflect differences in selection of subjects, tasks used for assessment, treatment parameters, and time of testing and retesting. The terms *memory, recall, forgetting,* and *learning* are imprecise, and in the testing, there is variability in the time of original exposure, in the measure of the intactness and the clarity of memory prior to ECT, in the modality tested (auditory, tactile, or visual), in the content (verbal or figural), and in the procedures used (recall, relearning, or recognition) (Cronholm and Ottosson, 1961a; Fox, 1961; Riddell, 1963; Inglis, 1969; Brunschwig et al., 1971; Dornbush, 1972; Squire, 1977). Despite these complexities, there is a commonality of experience that provides answers to some of the pressing questions about convulsive therapy:

Is amnesia essential to treatment outcome?
Are recent and remote events affected equally?
Does amnesia persist after treatment, and what is the rate of its recovery?
Can the severity of the amnesia be modified?

The data are distributed widely in the literature, but considerable help is afforded by the reviews by Cronholm and Ottosson (1961a), Miller (1970), Dornbush (1972), Foulon (1973), Dornbush and Williams (1974), Harper and Wiens (1975), and Squire (1977).

Seizures also affect other psychological processes, probably to an extent equal to their effects on memory. Many aspects have been examined, particularly visual-motor tests, reaction time, critical flicker fusion, tachistoscopic recognition, and tactile perception, but the data for any one aspect are limited and less well documented than the effects on memory.

EFFECTS ON MEMORY

Impairment in memory is so prominent with convulsive therapy that some investigators concluded that amnesia was central to its mode of action (Chapter 13). With improvements in induction, placement of electrodes, and electric currents, the therapeutic antidepressant effects of ECT were seen as distinct from the amnesic effects; thus elimination of amnesia should not interfere with therapeutic efficacy.

The amnesic effects were more marked when anoxia was accepted as a part of the therapeutic process. After Holmberg (1955, 1963) demonstrated that the clinical efficacy of seizures was not reduced when the inhalation of oxygen prevented anoxemia, the emphasis changed to a further reduction in amnesia by selective electrode placements, light anesthesia, oxygenation, and minimal currents to induce seizures (Chapter 15).

Estimates of the effects of seizures on memory vary with the modality (auditory, tactile, or visual) and the content (verbal and nonverbal) tested. The changes in current path resulting from varying electrode placements affect modality and content differently, indicating that the brain response is not unitary to a seizure but is quite varied (see below). There is a differential sensitivity in the memory process to seizures, with subjects finding recognition tasks the easiest to accomplish and least sensitive to impairment; recall, particularly after an interpolated delay (as with the learning of a nonsense task between learning and recall), is the most difficult and most sensitive to impairment with ECT.

Cronholm and his associates (Cronholm and Molander, 1957, 1961, 1964; Cronholm and Blomquist, 1959; Cronholm and Ottosson, 1960, 1961a, b, 1963a–c; Ottosson, 1960) examined the effects of ECT on various tests: a visual recognition test (20-figure tests), a paired associate verbal test (30-word-pair test), and a reproduction of verbal items accompanied by a visual stimulus (personal data test). For each test, the number of correct responses immediately after learning (immediate reproduction) and 3 hr later (delayed reproduction), and the difference between the scores (forgetting) were calculated. With ECT, both forgetting and delayed reproduction were impaired in the three tests. In one study (Cronholm and Ottosson, 1961a), changes in these tests were examined in relation to the severity of the depression and the response to ECT. Depressed patients displayed impaired learning (poorer scores in immediate and delayed reproduction) compared to controls, with the greatest difference in the personal data tests. The forgetting scores did not differ. With ECT, those patients who were clinically rated as improved or recovered exhibited an improvement in the immediate reproduction test but an increase in forgetting in the three tests. Delayed reproduction was impaired for the word-pair test and slightly improved on immediate reproduction. A similar relationship between the improvement in memory tests with improvement in depression was also observed by others (d'Elia, 1970a; Sand-Strömgren et al., 1976).

ECT affects the memory for events experienced before (retrograde amnesia) and after (anterograde amnesia) the seizure. Many factors are important in determining the severity and duration of the amnesia, including time, quality of the stimulus, and mental status at time of perception (learning) and at retest. The closer the event occurs to the seizure, the more its recollection is seriously impaired. However, events that cannot be recalled on testing immediately after the seizure may often be remembered later; there is an apparent "shrinkage" of retrograde amnesia with time.

Emotionally important, familiar, and easily assimilated events are recalled more easily than complex and unfamiliar events (Williams, 1950a, b, 1966). Studies of the symbolic meaning of memories led Janis (1948, 1950a–c) to suggest that ECT was effective because it led to the forgetting (repression) of painful memories.

Registration is essential for the recall of any event. Depressed patients have an impairment in learning (registration), which may selectively affect the recall of events of little personal meaning or those that were not clearly defined so that the individual failed to attend to the event for its registration and later recall. At the time of recall, familiarity, reminders, and other clues to the memory to be recalled may be necessary to elicit material that was registered. It is the complexity of these aspects of memory testing, as well as the selection of the modality, content, and delay factors, that make these analyses so difficult (Dornbush and Williams, 1974; Harper and Wiens, 1975).

Pattern of Amnesia

During each seizure, there is both retrograde and anterograde amnesia, which varies in extent. There is a subjective cloudy period before the anesthesia induction (or before the treatment in unmodified ECT) and a subjective period of confusion, lack of clarity in perception, and disorientation after the seizure. The period of confusion and amnesia is measured in minutes in unmodified ECT but may be considerably longer when anesthesia is used, as in modified ECT. The extent (severity) of the amnesia and its durability (persistence) is proportional to the number and frequency of seizures (Zubin, 1948; Korin et al. 1956; Zamora and Kaelbling, 1965; Miller, 1970; Dornbush et al., 1971; Fromholt et al., 1973). Age is negatively correlated with performance on memory tests, but the interaction of age and ECT is not well defined. Some studies find the impairment in performance with ECT to be greater in older patients (Fromholt et al., 1973); others find no such relationship (d'Elia and Raotma, 1977).

The degree of amnesia varies with the type of psychopathology. Amnesia is usually less in nondepressed patients, particularly in schizophrenic patients who may be resistant to the amnesic effects of seizures. Whether this is a reflection of their younger age or a difference in brain responsivity is unclear. A similar resistance to change may occur in the development of EEG slowing, response to amobarbital and pentothal in sedation threshold and sleep threshold studies, and psychomotor tests. Cronholm et al. (1973) found age-related differences in memory testing after ECT, which were the result of pretreatment, age-related differences in learning and retention but were not a direct effect of the seizures.

We also sought to relate the changes in recall and learning to improvement in ECT (Korin et al., 1956). Patients ($N = 40$) and controls ($N = 21$) learned lists of eight three-letter words, each word being exposed for 10 sec on flash cards. Recall was tested under two conditions: (a) immediately after an interpolated learning of a list of nonsense syllables, or (b) after a 10-min rest period during which a copy of a popular photonews magazine was read. Treatments were given three times weekly and testing was done twice weekly on nontreatment days. Controls were tested with the same tests and at the same frequency. As treatment progressed, the patients made more errors in learning the word lists; but when the frequency of treatments was reduced from three times to twice weekly, learning improved. After the last treatment, learning ability returned rapidly. Thus within 1 week the number of errors was less than pretreatment (Fig. 9.1). The controls showed a progressive improvement in learning. Interpolation of nonsense syllables impaired the recall of the learned word lists so that errors were already apparent during the first week of treatment (one to three treatments), while interpolation did not interfere with recall in the untreated controls (Fig. 9.2). Interpolation impaired performance on the test and increased its sensitivity as a measure of interference. We found no relationship in this study between the degree of clinical improvement and the interference in learning and recall tests.

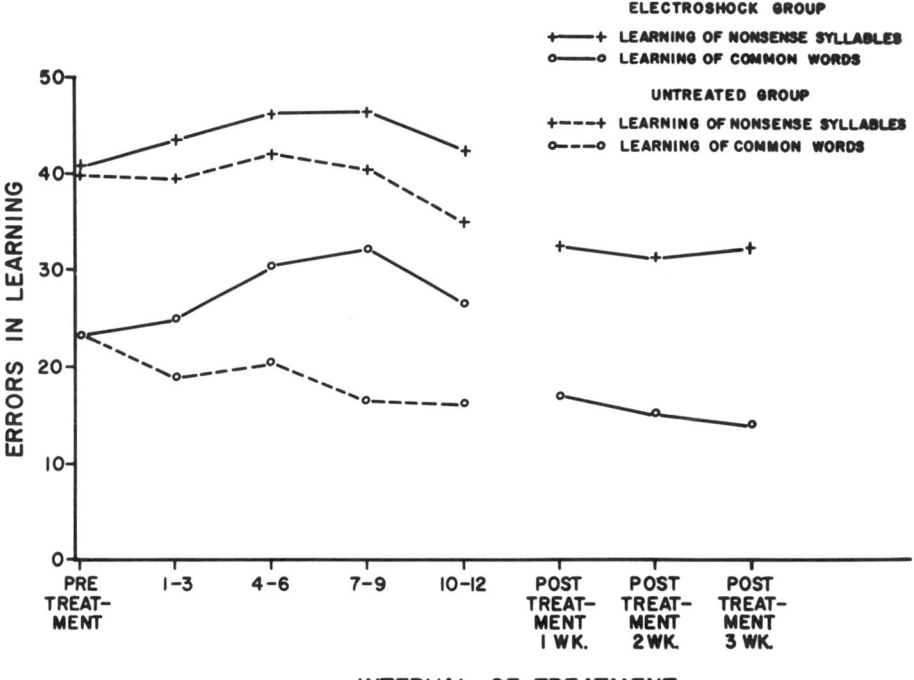

FIG. 9.1. Relationship of errors in learning to ECT. From Korin et al., 1956.

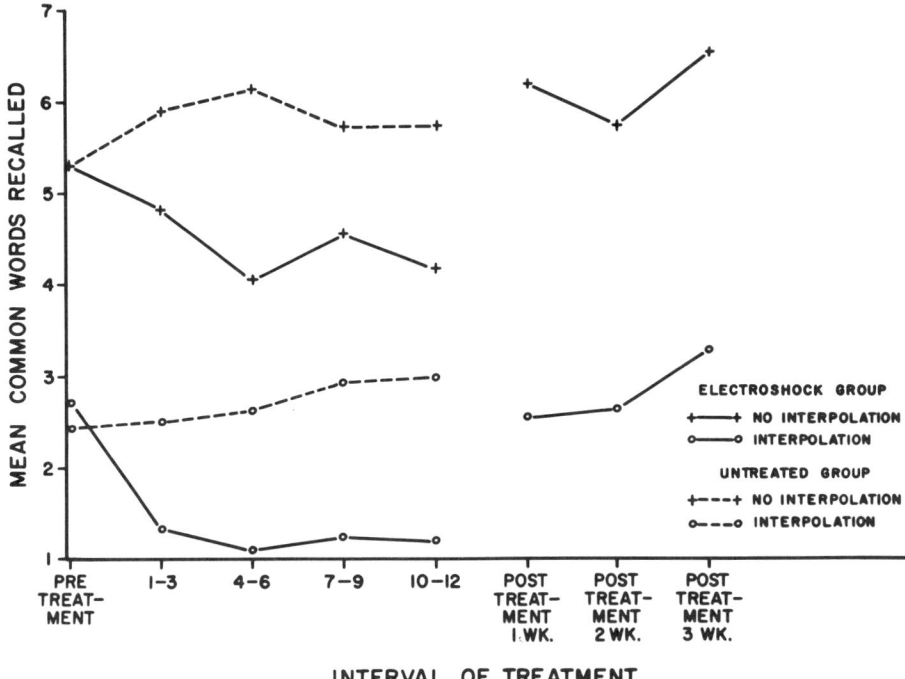

FIG. 9.2. Relationship of recall of common words to ECT. From Korin et al., 1956.

Patients' learning is impaired after each seizure. The pattern of recall of material learned from 30 min to 6 hr after a treatment and retested at various times thereafter is interpreted to indicate that the deficit is in the storage of the learned tasks rather than in the perception or learning (Cronholm and Ottosson 1963a, b; Hunt, 1965; Harper and Wiens, 1975; Squire et al., 1976b; Reichert et al., 1976a, b).

The effect of a "reminder" on the memory trace affected by ECT has also been examined. In animal studies, material may be forgotten if the animal is retested (reminded) just before ECS so that the trace is active at the time of ECS. Patients learned a 32-item recognition test 18 hr before ECT. Just before ECT, a reminder trial was given. After ECT, the material was retained as well or better in the reminded patients as in those not given the reminder, suggesting that amnesia is not specific to events fresh in storage at the time of treatment (Squire et al., 1976c; Squire, 1977).

Effect of Frequency and Number of Seizures

Performance on memory tasks decays with each successive seizure during the course of treatment. After the first seizure, impairment is measurable for a few hours; after four to six seizures, it is measurable for 48 hr and longer; and after eight to 10 seizures, it is measurable for 4 to 7 days and longer (Brengelmann, 1959; Goldman et al., 1972; Squire et al., 1975). Impairment is greatest proximal to the seizure and improves after each seizure, with progressive recovery of performance when seizures are terminated. Measures taken a few weeks after the last treatment usually show scores on memory tests to be equal to or better than the scores before ECT (Korin et al., 1956; Miller, 1967; Turek and Block, 1974). For many patients, memory functions reach preillness levels for the recall of life events within a few months of the last treatment (Squire and Miller, 1974; Squire and Chace, 1975; Squire and Slater, 1975; Squire et al., 1975). For others, however, memory deficits may last a year or longer (Levy et al., 1942; Brody, 1944).

The frequency of seizures affects the extent and rate of development of amnesia. When seizures are given at the conventional rate of three times weekly, the impairment in recall and learning is measurable in the second week; when the frequency is reduced to twice weekly, amnesia becomes more difficult to measure and may be apparent only with sensitive tests. When the frequency of treatment is increased to daily or multiple seizures in 1 day, the difficulties in memory become severe after a few days, often accompanied by disorientation, confabulation, and confusion (Kennedy and Anchel, 1948; Glueck et al., 1957). Patients who received extended courses of treatment at the increased frequency showed no greater impairment of memory on follow-up than did patients who received treatments at the conventional rate or who received drug therapy (Murillo and Exner, 1973a; Exner and Murillo, 1977).

An interesting modification in increasing the frequency of seizures was that of multiple ECT (MECT), in which the patient has three to eight seizures, one immediately after the other, with one anesthetic induction. Forced ventilation with oxygen is also a feature of this regimen (Blachly and Gowing, 1966). In the initial report, confusion and amnesia were estimated to be the same as one or two conventionally spaced ECT; these estimates were confirmed by others (White et al., 1968; Bidder and Strain, 1970; Bridenbaugh et al., 1972). An organic mental syndrome with a severe amnesia, however, did develop in some patients (Strain and Bidder, 1971; Abrams and Fink, 1972). In our study of MECT, we treated 38 patients with either unilateral or bilateral MECT-4 or MECT-6 (Chapter 15). While the anticipated rapid clinical response occurred in only one patient, and the remainder required additional conventionally spaced treatments, we also noted that four seizures at one sitting altered the recall to paired associate learning tests as little as a single ECT. Postictal sleep, however, was often prolonged, and drowsiness, disorientation, and confusion were greater than usually seen in conventional ECT.

In a study comparing two and four unilateral nondominant ECT treatments weekly in depressive patients, Sand-Strömgren et al. (1976) found no greater impairment with four treatments weekly. The two groups were equal in clinical efficacy and in memory tests, suggesting that the antidepressant effects balanced any amnesic effects of treatments given with increased frequency.

The severity of the amnesia after repeated seizures spaced hours apart in 1 day or when induced on a daily basis is in striking contrast to the relative lack of impairment when an equal number of seizures is given in one sitting. The amnestic effects of ECT are partly a result of the currents, but this factor is not as large as that due to the biochemical sequellae of the seizure. Although these sequellae are as yet ill defined, they are processes measurable in hours rather than in the moments required for the seizure itself or for some of the measured neurohumoral events (Chapter 11).

Effect of Current Path

Changing electrode placements alters the cerebral path of the electric currents, modifying the extent of the amnesia and the affected modalities. With unilateral electrode placements, memory is disrupted less than with bilateral placements. This is true whether the electrodes are placed over the dominant or the nondominant hemisphere. These differences have been examined extensively, and the data are well summarized (d'Elia, 1970a, 1974, 1976; Dornbush and Williams, 1974; Harper and Wiens, 1975; Squire, 1977).

The asymmetry of the localization of cerebral functions provides a basis for the differential effects of the location of the stimulating electrodes on modality and content of memory tests. Unilateral placement allows a greater effect of the current on the tissues under and between the electrodes. The effects on verbal tasks are greater when electrodes are placed over the dominant hemisphere and on nonverbal and visual tasks when the electrodes are placed over the nondominant hemisphere (Dornbush, 1972; Dornbush and Williams, 1974). A detailed study of these relationships is presented by Cohen et al. (1968), who randomly assigned depressed patients to one of three treatments: bilateral, unilateral nondominant, or unilateral dominant ECT. Performance on a paired associated learning test (verbal) and a recall of unfamiliar visual designs (nonverbal, visual) was tested at various times during the course of treatment. Patients treated with unilateral dominant ECT showed a greater impairment in the verbal task; those treated with unilateral nondominant ECT showed their greatest impairment on the nonverbal task; whereas patients treated with bilateral ECT showed an impairment in both. In a replication study, Berent et al. (1975) examined the effects of a single seizure with stimulation to either the dominant or the nondominant hemisphere and reported the same findings: greater effects on verbal tests when electrodes were placed over the dominant hemisphere and greater effects on nonverbal (forms) tests with placement over the nondominant hemisphere.

Similar findings are also reported by Kronfol et al. (1978) who compared dominant and nondominant ECT in depressed patients. Pretreatment they found impairment in performance tests, greater in tests of the functions of the nondominant hemisphere. With one ECT, the impairment in performance worsened. At the end of the course of 8 nondominant unilateral ECT, however, performance in the tests of nondominant hemisphere functions improved over pretreatment values. After dominant unilateral ECT, tests of dominant hemisphere functions showed persistent disruption.

In studies in our laboratories, we also found better performance on tests of auditory and visual short-term memory and on the paired associates learning test in patients treated with unilateral nondominant ECT than in patients treated with bilateral ECT (Figs. 9.3–9.5). When the retention interval from presentation

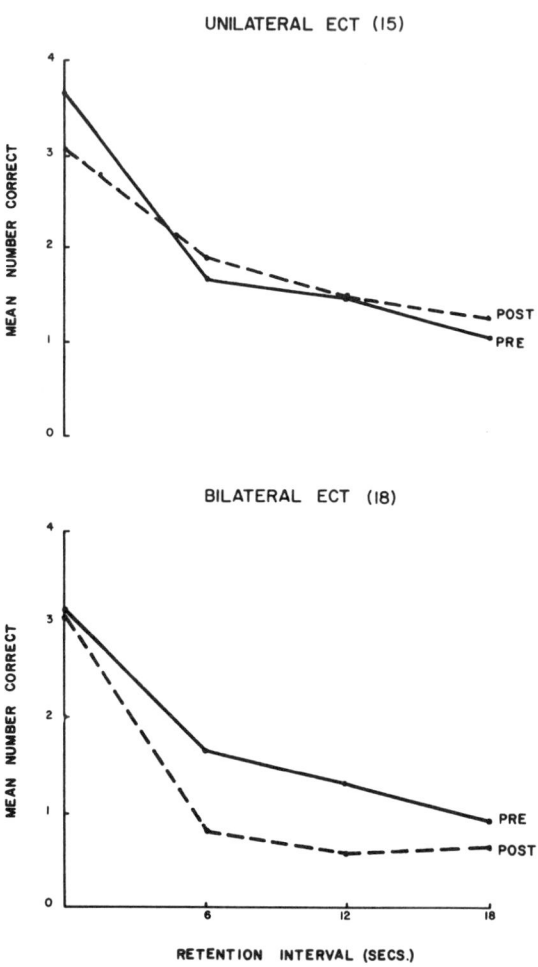

FIG. 9.3. Auditory short-term memory with unilateral and bilateral ECT. From Dornbush et al., 1971.

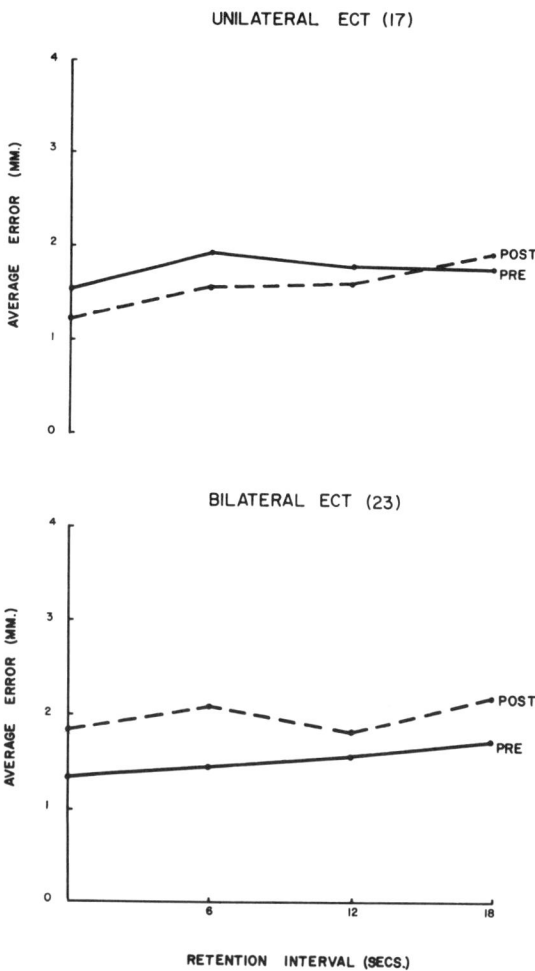

FIG. 9.4. Visual short-term memory with unilateral and bilateral ECT. From Dornbush et al., 1971.

to recall was lengthened (from 0 to 18 sec) the impairment was greater with the longer delay intervals (Dornbush et al., 1971). Similar findings were also reported by Stones (1973).

The disruption in performance on verbal memory and auditory tests is most severe with dominant unilateral electrode placements, next with bilateral, and least with nondominant unilateral placements. For nonverbal and visual tests, disruption is more severe with nondominant unilateral treatment, and least with dominant unilateral treatment (Zamora and Kaelbling, 1965; Gottlieb and Wilson, 1965; Wilson and Gottlieb, 1967; Halliday et al., 1968; Strain et al., 1968; Sutherland et al., 1969; Bidder et al., 1970; d'Elia, 1970a; Dornbush et al.,

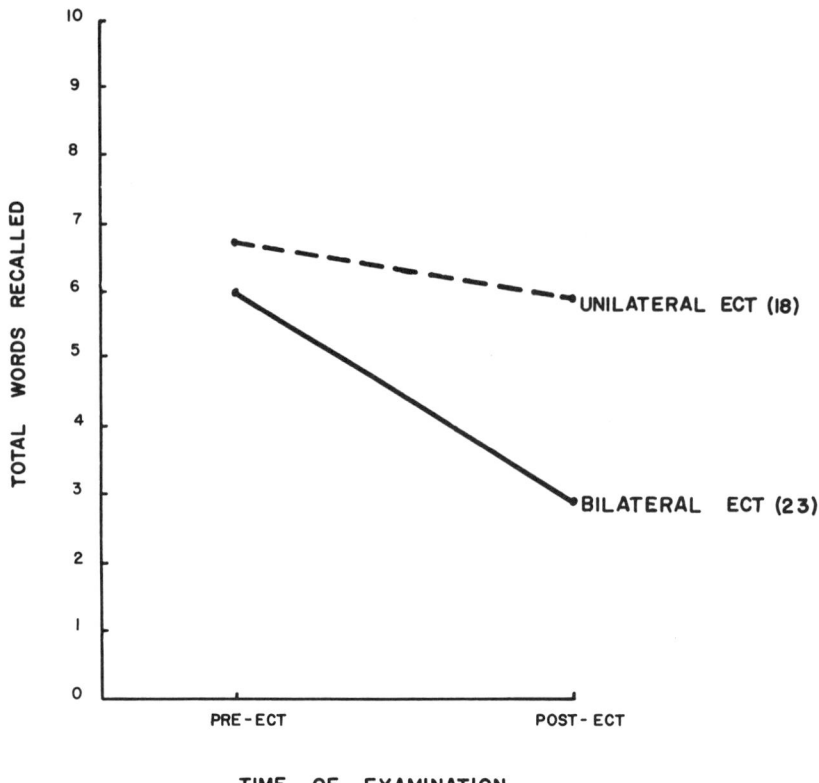

FIG. 9.5. Paired associate learning with unilateral and bilateral ECT. From Dornbush et al., 1971.

1971; Sand-Strömgren, 1973; Stones, 1973; Squire and Chace, 1975; d'Elia et al., 1976; Reichert et al., 1976a,b; Squire, 1977; Squire and Slater, 1978).

The symmetry is not defined in all studies, there being some differences occasioned perhaps by test design, test administration, or time in relation to treatment (Dornbush and Williams, 1974). The differences are clearly seen in performance on the various subtests of the Wechsler memory tests (where decreased performance is generally found with unilateral dominant and bilateral electrode placement, but an improved performance on retesting after nondominant unilateral treatment) (Martin et al., 1965; Zamora and Kaelbling, 1965; Levy, 1968; Halliday et al., 1968; Cohen et al., 1968; Sutherland et al., 1969; Fleminger et al., 1970; Dornbush et al., 1971; Abrams et al., 1972; Squire and Chace, 1975). In clinical tests of orientation, confusion, and in the simple repetition of learned items, observers uniformly find unilateral nondominant treatments least disruptive (Wilcox, 1956; Frost, 1957; Lancaster et al., 1958; Cannicott, 1962; Abrams, 1967; Cannicott and Waggoner, 1967; Zinkin and Birtchnell, 1968; Man and Bolin, 1969; d'Elia, 1970a).

Harper and Wiens (1975) assessed the many studies of unilateral and bilateral ECT as to whether they involved learning alone, learning and retention, or short- and long-term memories. On learning tests, there is a gain in the Wechsler memory test scores after ECT, a finding attributable to the relief from depression (Martin et al., 1965; Zamora and Kaelbling, 1965; Sutherland et al., 1969), and that learning is better after unilateral nondominant ECT than after unilateral dominant ECT (Cohen et al., 1968; Fleminger et al., 1970). In the learning and retention tests, nine studies are cited, and despite methodological faults, Harper and Wiens (1975) conclude that learning and retention are less affected by nondominant unilateral ECT than by bilateral ECT (Gottlieb and Wilson, 1965; Valentine et al., 1968; Halliday et al., 1968; Zinkin and Birtchnell, 1968; Costello et al., 1970; d'Elia, 1970a; Dornbush et al., 1971; Abrams et al., 1972; Fromholt et al., 1973). Six studies were cited as measures of the effects on long-term memory, and despite methodological difficulties, they again concluded that long-term memory is less affected by unilateral nondominant ECT than by bilateral ECT (Cannicott and Waggoner, 1967; Levy, 1968; Strain et al., 1968; Bidder et al., 1970; Cronin et al., 1970; Squire et al., 1975).

d'Elia and his co-workers have examined the effects of different placements of the electrodes in unilateral ECT—frontoparietal, frontofrontal, and temperoparietal—and found little difference in memory tests related to these locations (d'Elia and Widepalm, 1974; d'Elia, 1976; d'Elia et al., 1977a). The effects are more marked in comparisons of the nondominant and dominant placement. Abrams and Taylor (1973) examined the clinical and memory effects of anterior bifrontal placement and found that the clinical effects were intermediate between bilateral and unilateral electrode placements; on memory tests, however, they were unable to measure memory changes either clinically or on the Wechsler memory scale.

The decrease in the memory test disruption with unilateral electrode placement was interpreted as the result of less drastic or less traumatic inductions, but the dissection of the differences in performance on different memory tests (i.e., auditory and visual, verbal and nonverbal) suggests that the currents contribute directly to some of the amnesic effects. Since the therapeutic efficacy among the different electrode locations is virtually equal, the differences in memory tests among electrode locations suggest that the antidepressant activity of ECT is not based on amnesia. It is more likely that both the direct effects of the seizure and current characteristics, particularly the current path, contribute to the degree and type of amnesia but little to the antidepressant efficacy of ECT (Ottosson, 1960; Cronholm and Ottosson, 1963a, b; d'Elia, 1970a; Fink, 1972c, 1974c; Abrams et al., 1972; Sand-Strömgren, 1973).

Effect of Current Intensity

Changes in memory tests have frequently been used to measure the efficacy of different types of current (Chapter 15). Currents of high intensity disrupt memory the most. Observers have often been satisfied with a clinical assessment of the organic mental syndrome, reporting lesser effects after seizures induced by unidirectional and brief stimulus currents than after alternating current inductions (Bayles et al., 1950; Alexander, 1953; Liberson, 1953). In a parametric study, Kendall et al. (1956) found that the effects on memory were the same for unidirectional and alternating current inductions except for a test of new learning, in which the unidirectional current inductions showed better scores (less interference). Cronholm and Ottosson (1963b, c) found no difference on memory tests for treatments induced by unidirectional or ultra-short square wave currents. The question was reexamined by Weaver et al. (1974, 1977), who compared the clinical and amnesic effects of standard alternating current inductions with an experimental current which delivered 150 ultra-short square wave pulses of alternating polarity, with a low (16 joules) energy output but sufficient to induce a clinical seizure. They found no difference in tests of memory using measures from the Wechsler-Bellevue and the Halstead-Reitan tests.

Comparisons of ECT and Flurothyl

At one time, it was thought that the amnesic effects were largely due to the direct effects of the currents and of cerebral anoxia. When anoxemia was precluded by adequate ventilation with oxygen, the amnesia remained. Although the clinical experience with pentylenetetrazol seizures indicated that the amnesia was associated with the seizure and not the induction path, the introduction of flurothyl provided another opportunity to examine the role of the currents in the amnesic process.

Flurothyl seizures interfere with the consolidation of the memory trace and produce retrograde amnesia in mice (Alpern and Kimble, 1967) and chicks (Cherkin, 1974). Flurothyl seizures in humans elicit confusion, disorientation, and amnesia (both retrograde and anterograde), virtually the same as that elicited by ECT. The effects on memory tests are comparable, including the effects on the Wechsler memory scale, Cronholm-Molander test battery, Graham-Kendall memory for designs, the embedded figures, California F-scale, Bender Gestalt, and block design tests (Kurland et al., 1959; Fink et al., 1961; Spreche, 1964; Scanlon and Mathas, 1967; Small et al., 1968b; Kafi et al., 1969; Fieschi et al., 1970; Laurell, 1970). When differences are noted, the effects of flurothyl are somewhat less than those of ECT (Scanlon and Mathas, 1967; Small et al., 1968b; Kafi et al., 1969; Laurell, 1970).

In our studies, we found the effects of flurothyl and bilateral ECT on memory tests equal (Fink et al., 1961) (Figs. 9.6, 9.7). There were no differences on test performance prior to treatment among the 12 patients treated with ECT and the 15 treated with flurothyl (Table 9.1). Performance on some subtests of the Wechsler-Bellevue, an embedded figures test, and the California F-scale was equally impaired in the two groups at the fourth week of treatment and showed equivalent recovery 2 weeks after the last treatment. Postconvulsive EEG slow waves increased with the two treatments (see Table 8.1). When the

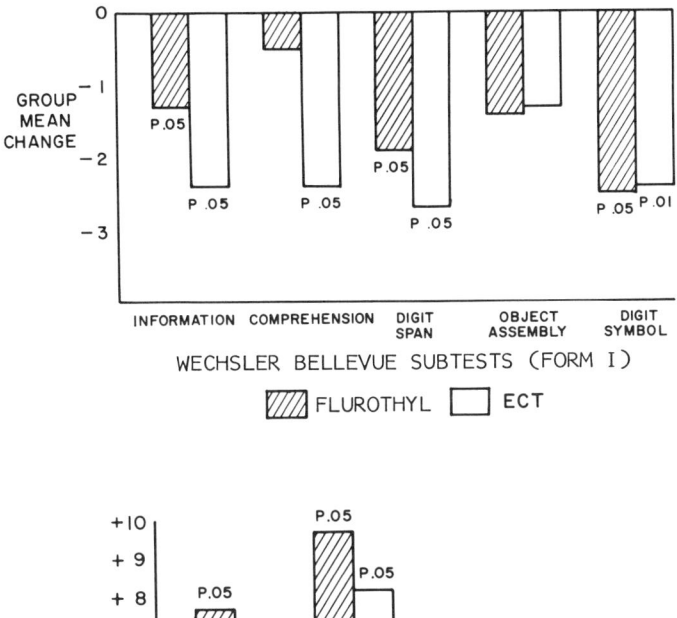
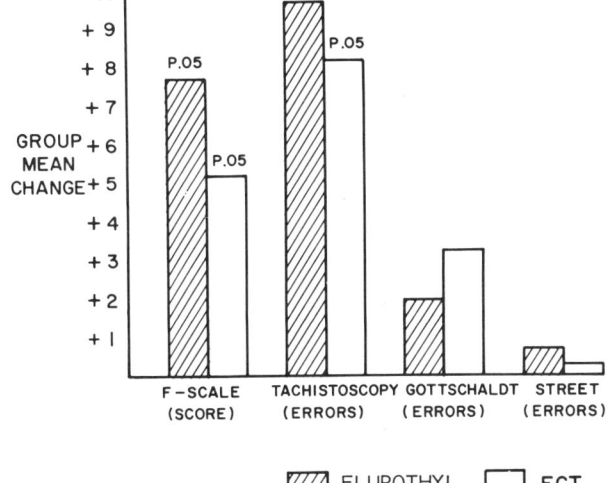

FIG. 9.6. Group mean change in test scores during convulsive treatment, Flurothyl and ECT. From Fink et al., 1961.

changes in memory test scores were correlated with the increase in EEG slow wave activity, there were significant relationships in the changes at the fourth week of treatment (Table 9.2).

The amnesic effects of the two treatments are found to be comparable. There is some indication that flurothyl seizures may be longer in duration (Karliner and Padula, 1962; Gander et al., 1967; Small and Small, 1968; Laurell, 1970), but the incidence of missed and incomplete seizures may also be higher (Laurell,

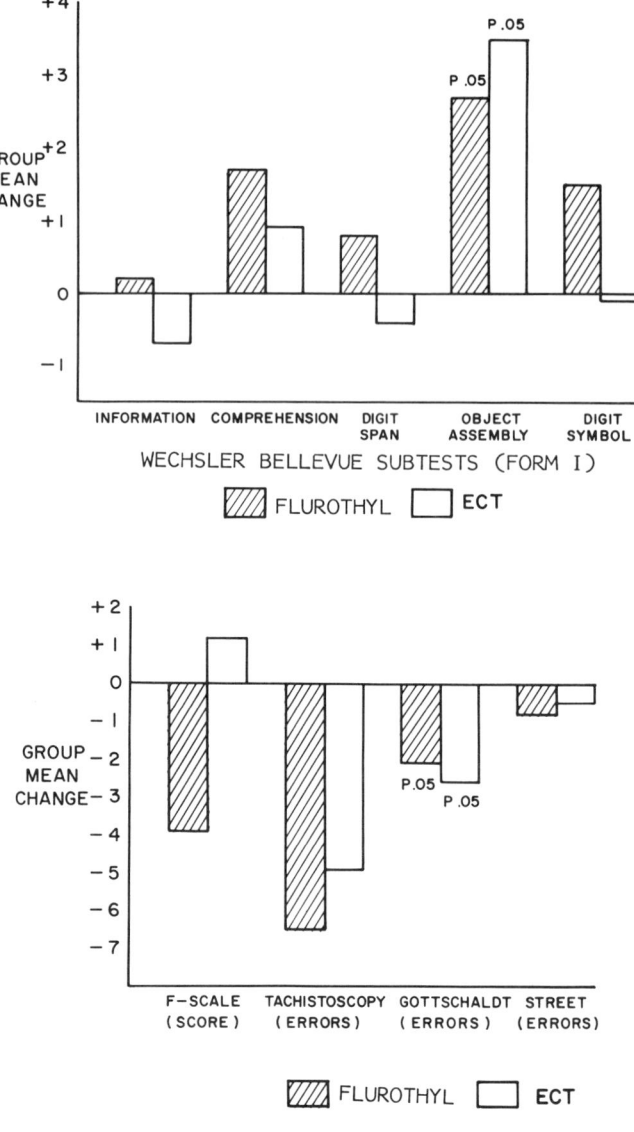

FIG. 9.7. Group mean change in test scores following convulsive treatment, Flurothyl and ECT. From Fink et al., 1961.

1970). Since reliable measures of the cerebral changes in induction are lacking in these studies, we are unable to judge whether the amnesic effects are truly comparable or whether there is a distinct component added by the passage of the currents. A satisfactory trial of flurothyl seizures at threshold doses with monitoring of the seizure activity and duration is yet to be done.

TABLE 9.1. Effect of flurothyl and ECT on psychologic test performances[a,b]

Test		Pretreatment and fourth week	Pre- and posttreatment	Fourth week and posttreatment
Wechsler-Bellevue (weighted subtest score)				
Information	Flu[c]	−1.3[d]	+0.2	+1.5[e]
	ECT	−2.4[e]	−0.7	+1.7[e]
Digit span	Flu	−1.9[d]	+0.8	+2.7[e]
	ECT	−2.7[d]	−0.4	+2.3[f]
Object assembly	Flu	−1.4	+2.7[d]	+4.1[d]
	ECT	−1.3	+3.5[e]	+4.8[f]
Digit symbol	Flu	−2.5[e]	+0.8	+3.3[f]
	ECT	−2.4[f]	−0.1	+2.3[f]
Tachistoscopy (errors)	Flu	+9.7[d]	−6.5	−16.2[f]
	ECT	+8.2[d]	−4.9	−13.1[f]
Embedded figures (errors)	Flu	+2.0	−2.1	−4.1[f]
	ECT	+3.3	−2.6[d]	−5.9[f]
F-scale	Flu	+7.7[e]	−3.9	−11.6[f]
	ECT	+5.2[e]	+1.2	−4.0[e]

[a] Data from Fink et al., 1961.
[b] Scores expressed as mean differences.
[c] Flu, Flurothyl.
Using Wilcoxon's T for paired replicates: [d] $p < 0.02$; [e] $p < 0.05$; [f] $p < 0.001$.

Comparison of Subjective and Objective Tests

There is generally an improvement in performance when test results obtained after a patient's recovery are compared to those taken during the illness and prior to ECT. Although part of the improvement in memory performance was thought to be due to the patient's familiarity with tests that were repeated, this explanation was deemed insufficient for the amount of improvement that occurs. Comparing the subjective reports with the results of objective tests of memory, Cronholm and Ottosson (1963a) found that the self-ratings of memory improved, while the retention scores showed the expected decrement (increase

TABLE 9.2. Change in task performance and degree of EEG slow wave activity (pretreatment versus fourth week; rank order correlations).

Treatment	Wechsler-Bellevue form 1				Tachis-toscopy	Embedded figures	F-scale
	Infor-mation	Digit span	Object assembly	Digit symbol			
Flurothyl	0.73[b]	0.54[c]	0.31	0.38	0.62[c]	0.13	0.12
ECT	0.28	0.72[c]	0.60[c]	0.34	0.80[b]	0.37	0.66[c]
Flurothyl and ECT	0.25	0.61[b]	0.46[c]	0.31	0.67[b]	0.43[c]	0.38[c]

[a] Data from Fink et al., 1961.
[b] $p < 0.01$; [c] $p < 0.05$.

in forgetting) in depressed patients who received up to four ECT. The depressive state improved with treatment, and the patients showed a positive correlation in self-assessments of their memory and their improvement in clinical symptoms. Cronholm and Ottosson concluded that clinically improved patients seldom complain of objective impairments since they judge their welfare in relation to their improved learning and perception rather than their impaired retention. Unimproved patients tend to complain more about memory dysfunction among other complaints (Cronholm and Ottosson, 1963a).

In comparisons of different inductions, I. Small (1974) and Squire and Chace (1975) found that subjective self-reports of impaired memory were greater on long-term follow-up after bilateral ECT than after unilateral ECT or flurothyl. In a 6- to 9-month follow-up, Squire and Chace (1975) reported that two-thirds of the patients treated with bilateral ECT complained of persistent impairment in memory compared to one-quarter of those treated with nondominant unilateral ECT.

In a follow-up study of schizophrenic patients treated with either flurothyl, bilateral ECT, or unilateral ECT, there were no differences among the groups on Wechsler test scores (I. Small, 1974). There was a trend for patients who received unilateral ECT to have better test results. The results with bilateral ECT were the poorest; with flurothyl, the results were in-between. Patients' subjective assessment 2 to 5 years after treatment found complaints of memory loss in 46% of those treated with bilateral ECT, 22% of those treated with flurothyl, and 9% of those treated with unilateral ECT.

In a recent study, Squire (1977) examined patient self-ratings of their memory performance 6 months after a course of ECT and found selective time periods for which the patients complained. Their greatest impairment was for events closely related to their illness and treatment. The complaints diminished by 6 months after treatment, but the self-ratings reflected awareness of some impairment, in contrast to the objective tests, which showed a recovery of performance.

These observations are confounded by reports that the depressive illness itself, in the absence of ECT or drug therapy, is associated with a measurable amnesia for the period of the illness (Sternberg and Jarvik, 1976). The amnesia improves when the illness subsides. It is probable that the deficit in the retention and recall of events during the illness parallels the withdrawal, introspection, preoccupation with obsessive thoughts, and the ruminations that often dominate the thinking of severely depressed patients. With relief of symptoms, there is an improvement in perception, retention, recall, objective test performance, and subjective assessments of memory. It is in the treatment failures that the dissociation between subjective complaints and objective tests occurs.

Extent of Retrograde Amnesia

Another concern has been the extent to which seizures may interfere with the recall of memories of events remote from the illness and treatment. The concern was reinforced by the depatterning and regressive EST (REST) treatments in which a severe organic mental syndrome develops, including impaired performance on memory tests (Chapter 15). In a recent study of the recovery of performance in memory and other tests after REST, Exner and Murillo (1977) compared the performance of schizophrenic patients successfully treated with REST ($N = 28$) to pharmacotherapy ($N = 16$) 11 months after discharge from the hospital. The REST patient had received an average of 26 treatments (range, 12 to 54). The authors found no difference between the groups in performance on the subtests of the WAIS, Bender Gestalt, embedded figures, object sorting, or memory quotient tests. They also obtained EEG records at follow-up and observed some differences in the records between the REST and the drug-treated samples, with the REST-treated patients showing less slow wave activity and a higher mean EEG frequency than those who were drug treated. The change in EEG was opposite to that which they expected if EEG slowing, a characteristic acute effect of REST, had persisted.

More elaborate studies of the effects of ECT on remote memory have been carried out by Squire and his associates (Squire, 1974, 1975, 1977; Squire and Miller, 1974; Squire et al., 1975, 1976a, b, c; Squire and Slater, 1975; Squire and Chace, 1975). In one test, patients were asked to recognize the name of television programs that were broadcast for a single season up to 17 years before the test sessions. The programs were selected for their equivalent exposures to the public and their appearance during a single year only. Tests were given before and 1 hr after the fifth ECT treatment. There was a temporal gradient of impairment in long-term memory in patients receiving bilateral ECT, with marked impairment of the recognition of programs broadcast 1 to 3 years before their treatment; programs broadcast 4 to 7 years previously were remembered as well after ECT as before. The memory loss largely recovered on retest 1 to 2 weeks after the last treatment. No deficits in the test were observed in patients who were treated with right unilateral ECT (Squire et al., 1975; Squire and Slater, 1975).

ECT produced a greater loss of temporal order information than of other tests of memory (Squire et al., 1976a). Following five bilateral ECT, the patients were unable to place the names of television programs broadcast from 1 to 16 years before in a proper temporal sequence. The impairment was worst for recent events, extending to programs that occurred 4 to 7 years before but not 8 to 16 years before. The deficit persisted up to 2 weeks after the last treatment. Squire (1977) summarized his studies by noting that information acquired 2 to 20 years prior to bilateral ECT was temporarily lost but fully recovered by 6 months retesting. Information acquired in the week prior to treatment may be permanently lost; that acquired from 1 week to 2 years prior to treatment appears to be recovered by 6 months retesting, but the data are insecure.

A second concern is the effects of ECT on autobiographical and personal events, the anxiety being that these may be selectively impaired. Janis

(1950a–c) examined the recollection of events related to early schooling, travel, job history, and other life experiences in 19 patients who were to receive ECT and in 12 control patients. Interviews were done before ECT, 4 weeks after the last ECT (average of 17 treatments), and, for five patients, again 3 to 5 months after treatment. On repeat interviews, the patients exhibited amnesia for some events that had been reported initially, and some deficits remained up to 5 months. While Janis did not specify the time period of the memories not recalled, Squire (1977) reassessed the Janis protocols and noted that the memories that were lost were primarily those related to the immediate hospitalization or the year preceding hospitalization rather than earlier biographical reports, which were spared. In their studies of the effects of unilateral and bilateral ECT on memory, Strain et al. (1968) included questions of personal memories and found no differences in their recall in a follow-up assessment 10 days after courses of unilateral or bilateral ECT.

Effects of Drug Treatment

The effects on memory of the interaction of ECT and drugs have been studied little. Ottosson (1960) found that treatments given after lidocaine (which reduced seizure time and the extent of EEG seizure changes) resulted in less effects on memory tests, particularly in the forgetting scores, than treatments given without lidocaine.

We examined the interaction of drugs and ECT, although we emphasized the effects on language and EEG more than the effects on tests of memory (Chapters 8 and 10). When drugs reduced the amount of EEG slow wave activity after ECT, as after anticholinergic and stimulant drugs, there was a decrease in the denial language scores and an increase in the variability of speech; conversely, when EEG slow wave activity was increased, as after barbiturates, there was an enhancement of denial language scores and a decrease in speech diversity. Presumably, these changes were associated with an improvement in performance tests after anticholinergic and stimulant drugs and a decrease after barbiturates (Fink 1958a, 1959a; Fink et al., 1960). Some studies assessed the influence of succinylcholine and barbiturates on the clinical efficacy of ECT and on tests of memory and found that the contribution was negligible (Brenglemann, 1959; Cronholm and Molander, 1957, 1961; Miller, 1970). A reduction in ECT-induced amnesia was reported with pemoline (Cylert) (Small et al., 1968a) but not for the peptide ACTH 4–10 (Small et al., 1977) or piracetam (Mindus et al., 1975). Although there was some thought that these compounds may have direct effects on the memory processes involved in ECT, the recent report that ECS-induced amnesia may be reduced by amphetamine suggests that the effect may be nonspecific, related to a general alerting effect of some drugs (Mah and Albert, 1975). ECT given to patients receiving maintenance lithium treatment increased the complications, particularly those referable to the CNS, including a greater impairment of memory (Small et al., *personal communication*).

More recently, d'Elia et al., (1978) examined the effects of *l*-tryptophan on memory in ECT. Depressed patients receiving ECT were assigned to two groups; one received 6 g of *l*-tryptophan daily, and the other received placebo capsules. On a number of tests, patients receiving ECT and *l*-tryptophan performed less well than the group receiving ECT alone, suggesting that *l*-tryptophan may have an amnesic effect. There were no advantages in clinical behavioral assessments in the *l*-tryptophan-treated group (d'Elia et al., 1977*b, c*).

PERFORMANCE TESTS

In addition to amnesia, seizures are associated with impairment in perception, a slowing in motor performance, and errors in psychomotor tasks. As with amnesia, the decrease in perceptual acuity and slowing in motor performance are proportional to the number and frequency of seizures. The decrements are ·maximal at the time of seizure and recover rapidly; thus performance is at pretreatment levels or improved within 2 weeks of the last seizure. The impairment in performance is reflected in simple and complex sensory tests, psychomotor tests, and tests requiring complex discriminations. Performance is less disrupted and recovers more rapidly on simple than on the more complex tests, particularly those tests in which the stimuli are presented near threshold, or where speed of performance and interpolated distractions are a feature of the test.

Some attention has been paid to the effects of ECT on the performance subtests of the Wechsler-Bellevue test: picture arrangement, picture completion, block design, object assembly, and digit symbol tests (Fisher, 1949; Fink et al., 1961; Strain et al., 1968). Such changes have also been reported for the critical flicker fusion frequency, where there was a significant drop in the fusion frequency during ECT which returned to pretreatment levels within 2 weeks of the last treatment (Landis et al., 1956). Landis et al. also found that the time to complete a choice reaction time task increased with treatment and returned to baseline or better within 2 weeks. The perception of the aftereffect to the Archimedes spiral was impaired (Robbins et al., 1959), as was the perception of random shapes (Ashton and Hess, 1976) and the Benton visual gestalt figures (Strain et al., 1968); and both tapping speed and speed on the maze and peg board tests decreased, while errors in the latter tests increased, with ECT (McAndrew et al., 1967).

We examined the effects of seizures on the perception of simultaneous tactile stimuli (Korin and Fink, 1957, 1959; Fink et al., 1959*a*), on the embedded figures test (Kahn and Fink, 1957; Kahn et al., 1960*a*), and the tachistoscopic presentation of embedded figures (Pollack et al., 1962). In the tactile perception tests, we first confirmed that psychiatric patients were likely not to correctly identify two stimuli simultaneously applied to different body areas when the stimuli are at threshold levels. The errors, described as errors of omission (extinction) or displacement, were observed when electrode pairs were placed 1 inch apart on both cheeks, dorsa of the hands, and calves of the legs and threshold stimuli applied in combinations, such as face-hand, face-leg, face-face (Korin and Fink, 1957; Fink et al., 1959a). In patients referred for convulsive therapy, the tests were repeated before treatment, after 10 to 12 treatments, and again 2 weeks after the course was completed. More errors of confabulation and displacement but not of extinction were made after ECT, with a return to pretreatment performance 2 weeks after ECT. In this study, the instructional set also influenced the results, with more errors made when the subject was asked, after each stimulus presentation, whether he had been stimulated "Anywhere else?" (Korin and Fink, 1959).

In the Gottschaldt embedded figures test, 53 patients referred for ECT attempted to identify a simple shape in a complex figure—a 25-item, time-limited, visual discrimination test of increasing complexity (Kahn et al., 1960a). An example is seen in Fig. 9.8. The figures begin with simple forms (a, b) and progress to more complex ones (c, d).

Of the patients, 29 received bilateral convulsive therapy and 24 subconvulsive currents. Treatments were given three times weekly and testing occurred 1 day after treatment. The errors declined in the subconvulsive group and increased in the convulsive group (Table 9.3). The changes in these scores were also

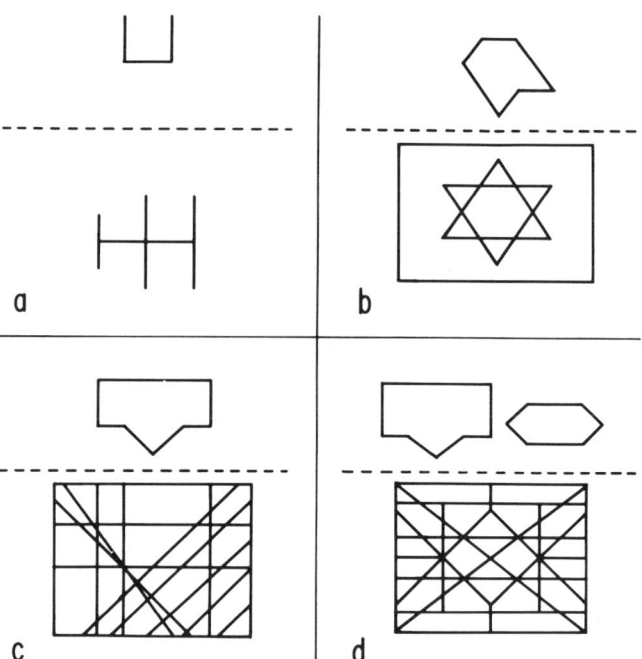

FIG. 9.8. Hidden figures test. **a, b:** Simple forms. **c, d:** More complex forms. From Kahn et al., 1960a.

TABLE 9.3. *Intragroup comparisons for number of errors in figure ground tests before and during ECT[a]*

Type of treatment	N	Before ECT	During ECT	Difference	p[b]
Subconvulsive	24	10.0	7.7	−2.3	< 0.02
Convulsive	43	9.5	11.8	+2.3	< 0.02

[a] Data from Kahn et al., 1960a.
[b] Intragroup analyses in this and in subsequent tables are based on Wilcoxon's method of paired replicates.

positively related to the increase in EEG slow wave activity and the increased manifestation of denial language after intravenous amobarbital, such that the patients who had the most changes in EEG and language also had the greatest decrement in performance on the complex figures test (Table 9.4). Two other relationships were of interest: the patients with the greatest decrement in the figures test exhibited the greatest change in behavior, as reflected in staff behavioral ratings; furthermore, the fewer the correct perceptions in the test before ECT, the greater the degree of EEG abnormality and the greater the number of positive amobarbital tests during the course of treatment.

Similar results were recorded in the perception of the tachistoscopic presentation of embedded numerals using the pseudoisochromatic plates for the perception of color-blindness (Pollack et al., 1962). In this study, 62 psychiatric patients were examined: 38 received ECT, 20 received phenothiazine drug therapy, and 10 control patients were not treated with either but received psychotherapy. Examinations were done before treatment, after 10 to 12 ECT or 4 weeks of phenothiazine therapy, and again 2 weeks after the last treatment for the ECT

TABLE 9.4. *Intragroup comparisons for number of errors in figure ground tests before and after ECT in relation to degree of physiologic change[a]*

Physiologic index	N	Mean difference in no. of errors during treatment	p
Amobarbital test			
None or one positive	13	−0.2	NS[b]
Two or three positive	28	+3.7	< 0.01
EEG			
None or one high delta	23	+1.7	NS
Two or three high delta	18	+3.3	< 0.05
Combined physiologic			
0–3	21	+1.0	NS
4–6	20	+3.9	< 0.01

[a] Data from Kahn et al., 1960a.
[b] NS, not significant.

TABLE 9.5. Error scores in tachistoscopic tests by group and treatment[a]

Group	N	Pre-treatment		Treatment		Post-treatment	
		Mean	SD	Mean	SD	Mean	SD
Convulsive	38	66.9	13.1	74.8	12.7	60.4	13.5
Drug	20	60.2	11.8	51.0	13.6	—	—
Control	10	57.8	13.7	49.3	15.3	—	—

	Significance of Intragroup Differences					
	Pretreatment vs treatment			Pretreatment vs posttreatment		
	MD	t	p	MD	t	p
Convulsive	+7.9	2.7	0.01	−6.5	2.1	0.05
Drug	−9.2	2.2	0.05	—	—	—
Control	−8.5	1.2	NS[b]	—	—	—

[a] Data from Pollack et al., 1962.
[b] NS, not significant.

group. The 12 figures were projected at nine preset durations from 50 to 5,000 msec. The figures were exposed at the fastest exposure time first, and then at progressively slower speeds until all the numbers were correctly perceived. The total errors, perseverations, and additions were scored. The number of errors increased with ECT, only to return to better than pretreatment levels by 2 weeks after the last treatment (Table 9.5). Phenothiazines also reduced the number of correct responses. In this test also, there was a correlation in the increase in errors and the amount of EEG slow wave activity (rho $= 0.67$; $p \gtreqless 0.01$).

In comparisons of the effects of flurothyl and ECT, the effects on performance tests failed to show differences between the two inductions (Kurland et al., 1959; Fink et al., 1961; Spreche, 1964; Scanlon and Mathas, 1967; Small et al., 1968b). Some of our data are seen in Figs. 9.6 and 9.7 and in Tables 9.1 and 9.2. In tests designed to examine the performance related to each cerebral hemisphere in unilateral ECT, McAndrew et al. (1967) failed to relate differences in performance to the side of electrode placement in tapping speed and maze and pegboard time and error scores.

CONCLUSION

These data provide the basis for answers to some of the questions frequently asked about the effects of ECT on memory and performance. Amnesia is a feature of depression and is most severe for the events that transpire when the illness is at its worst. With ECT, there is an additional impairment in memory, with a greater effect on forgetting than on learning, a slowing in motor activity, and an impairment in sensory discrimination. The impairment in memory and performance is directly related to the frequency and number of seizures, the mode of induction (particularly the location of electrodes and the strength of currents), and the time between a seizure and the testing of memory functions. Deficits are maximal immediately after each seizure and recover rapidly, so that most tests of memory or performance fail to show deficits 2 weeks after a series of treatments.

Memory and recall of events prior to the illness recover completely, while memory for events that occurred during the treatment or related to the immediate pretreatment (hospitalization) period may be permanently lost.

The severity of deficits in memory and performance may be modified by maximum spacing of treatments and by the judicious selection of electrode placement and current characteristics. Since there is little reason to believe that amnesia is necessary for the therapeutic process, in most cases the technique that reduces these deficits should be employed, including forced ventilation with oxygen, minimal currents for induction, unilateral nondominant placement of electrodes, minimal barbiturate anesthesia, and as wide a spacing of treatments as therapeutically feasible.

Chapter 10

Behavior, Language and Attitude

Seizures affect brain functions and elicit a variety of neurological and behavioral syndromes. The type and degree of the behavioral change depends on (a) the initial psychopathology and the personality of the patient, (b) the parameters of seizure induction, such as the frequency and number of seizures, electrode location, and currents, (c) the expectations of the patient and the observer, and (d) the stresses of the setting for the interaction. Many adaptations follow seizures, reflecting the behaviors that patients bring to the treatment.

Seizure induction is accompanied, in unmodified treatments, by the motor, reflex, and systemic changes characteristic of convulsions. Patients exhibit the classic tonic and clonic phases of a convulsion, with changes in cardiovascular and respiratory systems. The duration of the convulsion varies, and there is some suggestion that longer seizures are associated with better clinical results.

Tendon reflexes may be absent or may increase in strength during the convulsion. Pupils do not react during and usually dilate immediately after the seizure, returning to normal functioning within a few minutes. Corneal reflexes are absent during a convulsion and also return promptly. Abnormal reflexes are commonly seen for hours afterward (Kino and Thorpe, 1942; Kino, 1943, 1944; Savitsky and Karliner, 1948).

A more prominent neurological sequel to seizures is the change in mental state and the development of an organic mental syndrome. Although there is a relationship between the number and frequency of seizures and the change in sensorium, an organic psychosis may occur with few treatments (Kalinowsky and Worthing, 1943; Kalinowsky, 1945; Weinstein et al., 1952; Elmore and Sugerman, 1975). The syndrome may include disorientation, amnesia, agnosia, confabulation, aphasia, apraxia, and delirium, the latter being seen principally as the postseizure emergence delirium (Glueck, 1942; Juba, 1948; Gallinek, 1952b). As is reported in patients with aphasia, a patient reverted to the use of her native language (French) for 2 weeks after a course of ECT for depression (Lipsius, 1975). These syndromes occur with regressive ECT (Kennedy and Anchel, 1948; Glueck et al., 1957; Murillo and Exner, 1973a); and are occasionally seen in patients who receive four to six seizures in a single session, as in multiple ECT (Strain and Bidder, 1971; Abrams and Fink, 1972).

In an unusual study of the effects of ECS on behavior, monkeys reared in isolation were studied and their response to ECS was compared to the response of monkeys reared with their mothers during the first few months of life. The isolated monkeys exhibited a range of abnormal behaviors defined as self-disturbing, submissiveness, decreased sociability, and decreased environmental interaction. When control monkeys received sham ECS, they became less active and exhibited less social interaction, effects that became more definite and persistent after ECS. In the experimental monkeys, sham ECS had no effect, and ECS elicited an increase in activity level with less submissive behavior, increased aggressivity, and increased environmental activity (Lewis and McKinney, 1976). Although this initial and limited sample study did not provide a clear idea as to the mode of action of ECT, it did show that social behavior was alterable in experimental animals by ECS, providing a means for more detailed study.[1]

These manifestations of brain dysfunction, when seen in humans, are relatively infrequent and generally transient. More enduring in convulsive therapy are the changes in mental performance and interactive behavior, including mood, language, attitude, thought processes, and judgment. The range of possible adaptations is broad, but the range of syndromes seen in patients referred for ECT is restricted (Fink and Kahn, 1961; Fink, 1974a).

MODES OF ADAPTATION

In our studies, we described four frequent adaptations in our patients: (a) *euphoric-hypomanic,* (b) *somatization,* (c) *paranoid-withdrawal,* and (d) *panic modes* (Fink and Kahn, 1961). The variety of adaptations that we observed in our sample of 73 patients resulted from the variety of patients referred for convulsive therapy at the time of the study: depressive psychoses of manic-depressive, involutional and reactive varieties, and schizophrenic psychoses of paranoid, mixed catatonic and pseudoneurotic types. Patients were randomly assigned to modified treatments with either convulsive or subconvulsive currents, and two assessments were made: (a) behavioral change, without value judgment as to the advantages for the patient, and (b) clinical improvement, including value judgment (Table 10.1).

The *euphoric-hypomanic* adaptation was seen in depressed and retarded patients who increased their motor activity and rate of speech. They became more tractable and compliant, with elevated mood and feelings of well being, denial and minimization of symptoms, and an inhibition in the expression of delusional and paranoid ideation, even on direct inquiry. In such patients, tests of memory, calculation, orientation, and performance were either intact or impaired. In agitated depressed patients, the response was the same, except that agitation decreased and motor behavior became less restless and active. The *euphoric-hypomanic* adaptation developed in half the patients, who were generally rated as much improved or recovered.

---

[1] Another model for an animal study of the effects of ECS on behavior is provided by the development of rats with serotonin and norepinephrine depletion after the administration of selective monoamine neurotoxins. The animals with norepinephrine depletion are inactive, have hunger deficits, and are models of depression, whereas animals with serotonin depletion are hyperactive, frightened in novel situations, and models of anxiety (Ellison, 1977).

TABLE 10.1. Adaptive mode and clinical improvement[a]

Mode	N	Improvement rating			
		Recovered	Much improved	Improved	Unimproved; worse
Euphoric-hypomanic	36	11	14	10	1
Somatization	10	0	1	5	4
Paranoid-withdrawal	7	0	0	2	5
Panic	7	0	0	2	5
No change[b]	13	0	0	1	12

[a] Data from Fink and Kahn, 1961.
[b] Included subconvulsive treated subjects without a second course of ECT.

Patients in whom the *somatization mode* developed complained increasingly of their bodily symptoms and loss of memory, demanded reassurance, and were preoccupied with feelings of unreality and confusion. They remained unkempt and, when such adaptations occurred early in treatment, refused further treatment. Their speech was principally in the present tense and first person, with minimal use of third person speech, cliches, denial, or qualifications. At the end of treatment, the symptoms for which they were referred for convulsive therapy were no longer present. Although complaints were prominent, their relationship to the treatment and their transient nature were so generally accepted by the staff and the patients that the results were often evaluated as beneficial.

In some patients, paranoid ideation, suspiciousness, hostility, ideas of reference, and delusions became more marked. These patients, who exhibited the *paranoid-withdrawal mode* of adaptation, failed to care for themselves and remained unkempt. Speech was sparse and not spontaneous. They were hostile and uncooperative in interviews, denied illness, and minimized the symptoms that led to their hospitalization. They were uncooperative for testing, insisted on leaving the institution, and refused further treatment.

A fourth adaptation was exhibited by some patients who became increasingly anxious, agitated, restless, sleepless, and refused to eat. The adaptation was labeled the *panic mode,* for the patients feared treatment and hid on treatment days. They demanded to see their therapists and were fearful of damage to their mind. Ideation was generally unchanged, and the patients became increasingly uncooperative, continuing with other treatments only if reassured that they would no longer be given ECT. Such patients usually have low scores on the California F-scale, are generally younger, have high scores on anxiety scales, and have few of the vegetative features of endogenous depression (Pollack and Fink, 1961). Gordon (1946) also found that patients who object to treatment were refractory.

The last two adaptations were infrequent and were seen in patients who would no longer be considered suitable for convulsive therapy, being classified as the pseudoneurotic or mixed types of schizophrenia, or depressive psychoses of the reactive type.[2]

The adaptations that interested us were those described as *euphoric-hypomanic* and *somatization*. It was among these patients that the most favorable clinical improvement was seen. For the most part, these patients had been suffering from a depressive psychosis, although patients with syndromes of mania and schizophrenia occasionally exhibited the adaptations. At the time, two aspects of their behavior were of interest: (a) the changes in language and attitude that accompanied the behavioral changes, and (b) the personality characteristics that could predict the type of adaptation that developed. Our studies were based on concepts that the changes in brain functions, as induced by convulsive therapy, barbiturates, or other psychoactive drugs, elicited different behaviors, depending on the characteristic modes of adaptation of the subject. Such concepts of the dependence of psychological mechanisms on the integrity of brain functions were derived from the studies of Head (1926), Jackson (1932), Schilder (1932), Goldstein (1939), and Gerstmann (1942). More recently, Bender (1952) and Weinstein and Kahn (1955) examined the sensory and linguistic aspects of changes in brain function and emphasized the significance of instructional set and premorbid adaptation in the responses of subjects. Weinstein and Kahn focused particularly on the adaptation of denial of illness; in a seminal report, they suggested that the denial adaptation was the basis for improvement in convulsive therapy (Weinstein et al., 1952). They defined denial in behavioral (as in withdrawal and ludic behavior) and linguistic (as in explicit verbal denial, minimization, displacement, third person reference) terms.

LANGUAGE CHANGES

Patients tend to become more repetitive in their speech, to decrease their speech time, to become more hesitant, and to show less discrimination with ECT. These changes are seen in both content and form analyses of speech. For the most part, the content analyses examine denial of symptoms and illness (Kahn et al., 1955, 1956; Kahn and Fink, 1958, 1959; Jaffe et al., 1961; Fink, 1974a), whereas the form analyses examine the changes in rate, number, and variety of words occasioned by ECT (Jaffe, 1957, 1958; Fink et al., 1960; Jaffe et al., 1960). Some changes in language are reflected in attitudinal measures [as in the California F-scale (Fink et al., 1959b; Kahn et al., 1960b)] and the confabulation responses in perceptual studies [as in the tachistoscopic perception

---

[2] Similar studies of the typology of patients treated with imipramine and phenothiazines at the time of these studies found parallel changes in adaptation. In patients referred for imipramine therapy, we described six patterns of response: *mood elevation, explicit verbal denial, and manic* modes, occurring chiefly in depressive patients; and *reduction in episodic anxiety, agitated disorganization, and anhedonic socialization* seen in patients with other diagnoses (Klein and Fink, 1962a). With phenothiazines, eight principal adaptive modes were described: *suppressive denial, reduction in anger, affective stability, autistic compliance, decreased agitated depression, somatization, episodic agitation, and episodic anxiety.* The relationship to diagnosis was less secure for these adaptive responses (Klein and Fink, 1962b).

of embedded figures (Pollack et al., 1962) and perception of simultaneous tactile stimuli (Korin and Fink, 1957, 1959; Pollack and Fink, 1962)].

The language effects of ECT are usually subtle and observable in the usual patient only when the series of treatments has been completed or after special testing. In examining patients with minimal brain lesions, Weinstein and his associates demonstrated that doses of amobarbital sufficient to induce nystagmus and slurred speech exaggerated the language changes so that they became more prominent and were easily quantified. They described the procedure as the amobarbital test (Weinstein and Kahn, 1955) (Fig. 10.1). In principle, this application is similar to the elaboration of EEG slow waves after pentothal reported by Roth (1951) and Roth et al. (1957).

To questions of orientation and awareness of illness, the normal individual responds both before and after amobarbital with referential responses; they are not altered after amobarbital. Psychiatric patients may show transient changes of disorientation, denial, withdrawal, and ludic behavior, but their transient nature and fluctuating pattern distinguish them from patients with organic brain disease (Kahn et al., 1955). We examined the changes in syntactic language in 65 patients who received modified bilateral ECT three times weekly for 10 to 15 treatments (Kahn and Fink, 1958). The amobarbital test was done before ECT and on a day after four to six and seven to nine seizures. The amobarbital inquiry was presented before amobarbital and again after the injection of 0.05 g/min and nystagmus, slurred speech, drowsiness, and errors in counting backward had been recorded. While the answers to the full test were recorded, the analysis found the principal effects in the answers to the questions: "What is your main trouble?," "Why did you come to this place?," and "If you could have one wish, what would you wish for?"

Among the patterns found during treatment and prior to amobarbital were changes in the syntactic use of person (third person referent instead of first person), evasion (answer a question with a question), explicit verbal denial, increased use of qualifiers, change in tense (past instead of present), displacement, and exaggerated use of cliches and stereotyped expressions. After amobarbital, the number of these responses increased and appeared earlier in the course of treatment. In addition, patients exhibited cryptic responses (a personalized reference without obvious relevance to the question) and withdrawal reactions (incomplete sentences, incoherence, perseveration, use of a foreign language, blocked speech). The relationship of each response to clinical improvement is pictured in Fig. 10.2.

The language changes, which were interpreted as adaptations of denial in the milieu of altered brain function, persisted for up to 3 weeks after the last treatment. Patients who showed more language changes during the second and third weeks of treatment were evaluated as more improved than patients who failed to show these language changes or showed them only after amobarbital. The number of changes was also related to the percent time EEG delta activity (Kahn et al., 1956; Kahn and Fink, 1958).

FIG. 10.1. Amobarbital test.

	Before	After
What is your main trouble?		
Why did you come here?		
What do you call this place?		
What kind of a place is this?		
Where is this place located?		
How far from here do you live?		
Have you ever been in any other hospital of this name?		
Where were you last night?		
What is today's date?		
What month is this?		
What year is this?		
What time is it now?		
What part of the day is it?		
Who am I?		
Have you seen me before?		
**********		
* If you had one wish, what would you wish for?		
* Can you think of a joke?		

Adapted from Kahn et al. 1955; and Weinstein and Kahn, 1955.

Amobarbital is given intravenously in a solution of 0.5 g in 10 cc distilled water at a rate of 0.05 g (lcc)/min. As the drug is administered, the patient is asked to count backwards from 100; the injection is continued until the patient shows rapid nystagmus on lateral gaze, slurred speech, errors in counting, and drowsiness. (The usual amount is 0.2 to 0.5 g.) Immediately after, the questions are asked again. For each error, the question is repeated, and only persistent errors are counted.

The following changes, when persistent, are called positive and are indicative of cerebral dysfunction.
1. Denial of illness.
2. Denial of major aspect of illness, such as attributing entry into the hospital to a trivial or prior illness.
3. Misnaming the hospital, either its proper name or by a euphemism, such as "rest home."
4. Displacement of the location of the hospital, such as to another city.
5. Confabulated journey.
6. Reduplication of the hospital.
7. Disorientation for time of day, confusion of day and night.
8. Misidentification of the interviewer, as entertainer, lawyer.
9. Disorientation for year.

* These questions are added for psychiatric patients, to explore changes in symbolic expression.

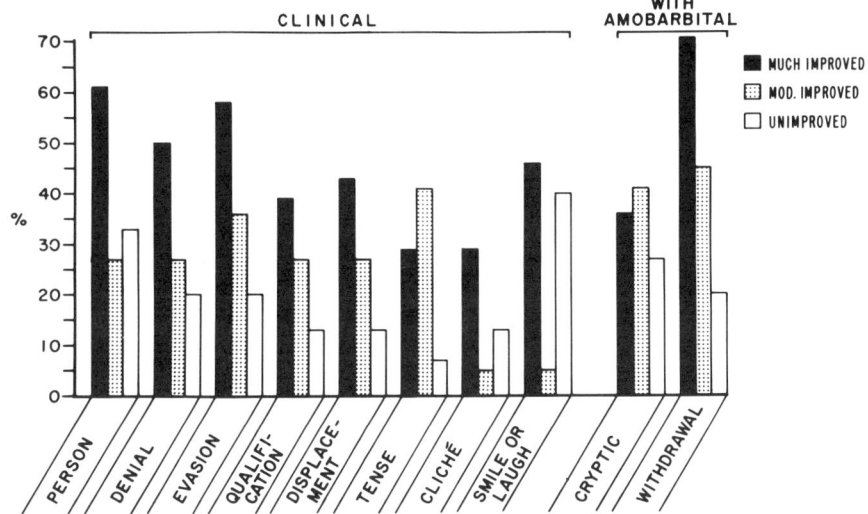

FIG. 10.2. Percentage showing each language pattern according to response to treatment. From Kahn and Fink, 1958.

We also examined the effects of ECT on formal language measures in unstructured clinical interviews. Measures of the variability and repetitiveness of speech, known as the type-token ratio (TTR), were calculated for successive 25-word samples in the first 500 words of an informal interview between the patients and a single interviewer. The dyadic TTR (the measure of redundancy in the combined speech patterns of patient and examiner) showed a significant decrease in the mean and an increase in the variability (standard deviation) in the subjects receiving ECT but no difference in patients receiving subconvulsive therapy under double-blind conditions. The degree of change in the dyadic scores was related to the degree of induced EEG slow wave activity. In patients in whom high degrees of interseizure EEG delta activity developed, the mean TTR decreased significantly; there was no relationship for the patients in whom high degrees of EEG slowing failed to develop (Table 10.2). Dyadic scores also

TABLE 10.2. Dyadic TTR and EEG delta activity

Delta group	N	Mean differences		
		Mean	SD	CV
High	7	−2.36	+2.24[b]	+3.11[a]
Low	6	−1.68	+0.32	+0.62
None	10	−0.84	−0.52	−0.58
Delta difference				
High–low		0.68	1.92[a]	2.49
High–none		1.52	2.76[c]	3.69[c]
Low–none delta		0.84	0.84	1.20

[a] $p < 0.05$; [b] $p < 0.02$; [c] $p < 0.002$.

changed in structured interviews based on the amobarbital interview protocols (Fink et al., 1960; Jaffe et al., 1960). These language changes, both those that are described as characteristic of denial and those in TTR, are manifestations of altered brain function, which, like amnesia and EEG slow wave activity, bears some (indirect) relationship to clinical outcome with ECT.

Not only does the language of the patient change with treatment, but also that of the staff. Jaffe (1958) examined the effects of altered brain function on the language and attitude of the *dyad;* a change in behavior in one affects the behavior of the other as well. The changes in language on the part of the staff are seen in the alteration in the reports and the attitudes of therapists as patients were treated, first with subconvulsive stimulation, which failed to alter brain function, and later by convulsive therapy, which altered both brain function and behavior, with resulting change in behavior and language of the therapist (Jaffe et al., 1961) (Fig. 10.3).

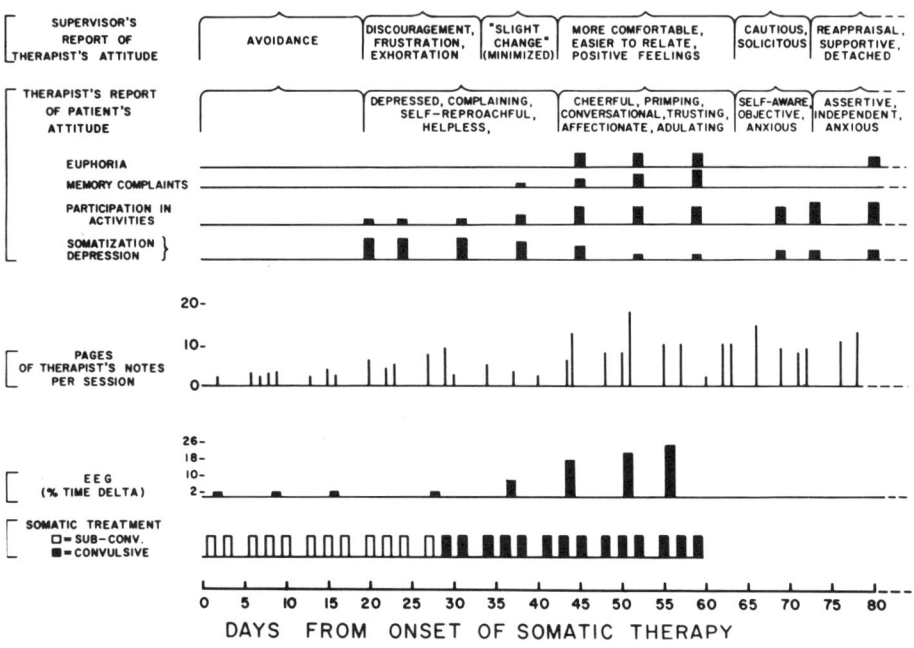

FIG. 10.3. Effect of changing brain function on psychotherapy. From Jaffe et al., 1961.

Effects on Attitude

ECT induces changes in attitude as well as language. Patients become more compliant and acquiescent with treatment. This is reflected in a number of measures, especially the California F-scale (Kahn et al., 1960b). The scale was designed to measure prejudice and authoritarianism, but the changes have been interpreted as reflecting the psychological aspects of rigidity and stereotypy (perseveration and lack of flexibility in response) and conventionalism. We noted that the F-scale was a prognostic scale, with patients who scored high on the scale before treatment having better outcome ratings than patients who scored low (Chapter 6).

The F-scale was also repeated on the day after the twelfth treatment and again 2 weeks after the last ECT. There were 59 patients who received a minimum of 12 bilateral ECT and a control group of 10 patients who received an equal number of subconvulsive stimulations only. With ECT, the mean F-score increased, while the score remained unchanged in the control group (Table 10.3).

TABLE 10.3. Effect of convulsive treatment on F-score[a]

| | | Mean F-score | | | |
Group	N	Pre-treatment	During treatment	Mean difference	t
Convulsive	59	45.3	51.0	+5.7	2.02[a]
Control	10	48.7	49.2	+0.5	0.02

[a] Significance at 0.05 level.

Of the control group, seven continued in treatment and received 12 convulsive treatments. Their F-score, which had been unchanged (+0.1) after subconvulsive treatments, increased significantly (+9.1).

EEG records taken the day after the twelfth ECT were scored for the degree of delta activity (Fink and Kahn, 1957), and the 54 records were divided in half: a high (>40%) and a low delta index (Table 10.4). The greatest change in F-score was associated with the greatest increase in EEG delta activity. When F-scores were obtained 2 weeks after the last treatment, the scores had returned to pretreatment levels, as had the increase in EEG slow wave activity.

These observations, as well as our experience with the reverse F-scale in which patients who scored high on the conventional scale (agreed with the statement) also scored high on the reverse scale, suggested that ECT alters the patient's attitude toward one of more compliance and less discrimination. This change in attitude is also reflected in two recent reports (Hillard and Folger, 1977; Spencer, 1977). Hillard and Folger (1977) found that patients reported they improved more and had fewer side-effects when they were on a treatment unit where more patients were receiving ECT than when they were among few ECT patients. In the study by Spencer (1977), 50 patients who

TABLE 10.4. Change in F-score and degree of induced cerebral dysfunction[a]

Degree of slow wave activity	N	During treatment			
		Pre-treatment	During treatment	Mean difference	t
High delta index	27	43.9	52.5	+8.6	2.3[b]
Low delta index	27	45.6	49.0	+3.4	0.8

Degree of slow wave activity	N	After treatment			
		Pre-treatment	Post-treatment	Mean difference	t
High delta index	21	42.2	40.6	−1.6	0.4
Low delta index	16	42.6	42.1	−0.5	0.1

[a] From Kahn et al., 1960b.
[b] Significance at 0.05 level.

were to receive ECT were given a set of general statements about ECT and were asked to give the extent to which they liked or dreaded an aspect of the treatment. More than half the patients liked or did not mind ECT or many of its more frightening aspects; only a few patients dreaded the treatment.

Confabulation

Another change in behavior that may often occur is confabulation—replacing a lost memory by an incorrect and imaginary response that has the quality of completing the answer and satisfying the inquiry. Confabulations were seen frequently in the study of the tachistoscopic presentation of complex figures (Pollack et al., 1962) and the perception of threshold simultaneous tactile stimuli (Korin and Fink, 1959). In both studies, the prominent errors were not omissions or extinctions but the completion of poorly perceived partial figures or mislocations and displacement of the sensory stimuli. These responses also have a quality of acquiescence and may reflect the same attitudinal change as seen in the F-scale.

ECT AND PSYCHOTHERAPY

Many authors have examined the relationship between the somatic therapies and psychotherapy, seeking a rational basis for the combined use of these modalities. The concerns were more marked in the initial years of study when the treatments were seen by some as facilitating and by others as competitive and antagonistic (Schilder, 1939; Grinker and MacLean, 1940; Weigert, 1940; Levy and Grinker, 1943; Moriarty and Weil, 1943; Linn and Rosen, 1950; Freeman and Cameron, 1953; Hill and Patton, 1956). A review of the early reports finds authors combining the modalities (Linn and Rosen; 1950), seeing:

> . . . The goal of ECT is securing and maintaining the psychotherapeutic accessibility of the patient. The final goal should be the psychotherapeutic restitution of the patient.

Some authors suggest an exploratory type of psychotherapy, claiming that ECT releases dynamically significant conflicts (Grinker and MacLean, 1940). Other authors, however, find that the same ECT results are achieved whether or not the patient sits through therapy sessions; indeed, the results are said to be better in the absence of psychotherapy (Kalinowsky and Hoch, 1952).

We also sought to integrate ECT with psychotherapy. We had observed a variety of responses to ECT but focused our attention on those patients in whom the pattern of euphoric-denial developed (or in whom we thought it would develop). As such patients were minimizing and denying their difficulties, displacing their feelings, and showing acquiescence, confabulation, and redundancy in speech, it seemed unlikely that the interpretive, exploratory, and referential type of psychotherapy would be useful or adaptive. In this view, we were encouraged by reports of the experience with intensive psychotherapy in depressive cases (Cohen et al., 1954). Based on our linguistic experience, we sought to modify the psychotherapeutic relationship by encouraging denial and repression and by discouraging exploration of repressed material by a directive attitude on the part of the therapist (Esecover et al., 1958; Jaffe et al., 1961). At one time in the treatment, the patient was receiving subconvulsive electrostimulation only, and the psychotherapy approach was unrewarding. When the treatments changed to ECT, however, the attitude of both the patient and the therapist changed with encouraging results (Fig. 10.3). For many patients receiving ECT, however, we did find that the psychotherapy sessions were *pro forma* with the patients' behavior changing independent of the therapy sessions.

A detailed examination of the interaction of psychotherapy and ECT is reported by Freeman and Cameron (1953), who found that severe anxiety developed in a number of patients after ECT—an anxiety not related to the treatment procedures but to life events and unconscious conflicts. They found psychotherapy helpful, particularly those procedures that encouraged patients to identify with supportive and authoritative figures in their acquaintance.

Our present views of the mode of action of ECT suggest that the efficacy of the treatment is independent of specific psychotherapy; and in combined therapy, the interpretations of the psychotherapist are largely irrelevant to the patient's improvement. To the extent that there is some benefit, it may be to encourage denial and repression of instinctual conflicts and to help the patient understand the limitations imposed by his illness and by the neurologic effects of the treatment.

Chapter 11

Biochemical Effects of Induced Seizures

Biochemical changes after induced seizures have been measured in many body fluids and structures, including blood, urine, gastric secretions, saliva, cerebrospinal fluid (CSF), and brain tissues. Considering our present views of the ECT process, the significant biochemical changes must be those occurring in the central nervous system (CNS). The therapeutic efficacy of repeated seizures is related to the occurrence of seizures in the brain and not to aspects of the motor convulsion, the psychological consequences of the treatments, or the mode of induction of the seizure (Fink, 1966, 1972c, 1974b, c, 1977b; Ottosson, 1960, 1968, 1974). Although the changes in blood, urine, and other nonneurogenic fluids have been studied extensively, the findings have limited clinical or theoretic interest. The changes in cerebral and cerebrospinal fluid measures are emphasized in assessing the effects of ECT in this chapter.

Some biochemical changes are short-lived and are probably directly related to the events of the seizure and the stress of the convulsion; others are of longer duration and may reflect effects with a greater therapeutic relevance. A biochemical change is more likely to be pertinent if it has a similar time course to the clinical or behavioral effects, if the biochemical change is fairly specific and not one of a large number of changes that could be attributed to overactivity, anoxia, or their sequellae, and if the change is compatible with other evidence arrived at independently from a different point of view (Kety, 1974). Considering these caveats, many of the measures cited by Ashby (1949), Fleming (1956), Holmberg (1963), Ottosson (1974), and Ilaria and Prange (1975) probably reflect events that are only indirectly related to the antidepressant efficacy of ECT. Furthermore, most of the changes in the blood, urine, CSF, and brain tissues that have been studied are probably consequences of the neurochemical changes underlying the therapeutic effect or coincidental, parallel phenomena of little interest to the therapeutic process; only a few may be considered central to the therapeutic process or to defined side-effects (Ottosson, 1974).

Another problem in relating biochemical measures to the mode of action of the convulsive therapies is that many studies are done in healthy animals rather than in depressed humans. Lacking an acceptable pathogenesis and pathophysiology of depression, it is questionable whether studies in normal animals are relevant for disease states (Ilaria and Prange, 1975).

HYPOXIA AND ENERGY METABOLISM

Cerebral oxygen consumption increases during each seizure. If oxygen saturation is maintained and muscle activity is restricted, lactate and carbon dioxide levels do not rise, glucose levels do not fall, and cerebral blood flow does not increase. With hypoxemia and inadequate muscle paralysis, however, lactate and carbon dioxide levels rise, glucose levels fall, and cerebral blood flow increases (Plum et al., 1968; Beresford et al., 1969; Szirmai et al., 1975). As Ottosson (1974) notes, however, clinical ECT is rarely given under controlled experimental conditions, and some degree of hypoxia and hypoxemia usually occurs. Nevertheless, hypoxia and its associated changes in energy metabolism are not factors in the therapeutic process, although they may be a factor in the development of memory changes. This is seen in the failure of nitrous oxide or carbon dioxide inhalations to have antidepressant activity.

Connections have also been sought between the effects of ECS and changes in glucose, adenosine triphosphate (ATP), oxygen, carbon dioxide, cyclic AMP, nucleotides, lactate, creatine, and creatinine in brain tissues with ECS (Essman, 1973). Few of the studies controlled oxygenation and/or anesthesia, and no consistent picture of the role of these changes in the therapeutic process has emerged. A significant increase in the urinary excretion of cyclic AMP was reported in 12 of 13 patients who received ECT, while four controls who received all aspects of the treatment, except the convulsive current and the seizure, showed a fall in urinary cyclic AMP (Hamadah et al., 1972). This observation was confirmed by Moyes (1972), who concluded that the increase in cyclic AMP in brain tissue was the basis for the antidepressant efficacy of ECT. Another report (Choi et al., 1977) found that red cell membrane sodium, potassium, and calcium ATPase levels are significantly lower in patients with endogenous depression than in controls, and that ECT increased the amount of these substances to control levels. Another study (Post et al., 1977) assessing the cyclic AMP levels in CSF of manic and depressed patients failed to find any increase in response to imipramine, amitriptyline, lithium, tryptophan, or ECT.

MINERAL METABOLISM

Since the introduction of lithium, mineral metabolism has been a focus of the study of depression. Coppen and Shaw (1963) reported that depression was accompanied by an increase in intracellular sodium and water. With ECT, diuresis occurs (Russell, 1960; Gibbons, 1960), and exchangeable sodium decreases in patients who improve (Gibbons, 1960). Potassium levels usually remain stable (Gibbons, 1960; Platman et al., 1970) or rise with lithium and ECT treatment (Coppen and Shaw, 1963; Coppen et al., 1966). CSF pressure increases transiently with each seizure (Deshaies and Renard, 1948), and its conductivity is increased, in part because of an increase in potassium and phosphate ions, which remain elevated for up to 3 days (Spiegel and Spiegel-Adolf, 1941).

The urinary excretion of calcium decreases with ECT in depressed patients; this decrease persists after the treatment course. While plasma calcium levels are within normal levels, there is a decrease in the levels with treatment. There is a shift to a positive calcium balance; this change was assumed to have therapeutic significance (Flach, 1964; Faragalla and Flach, 1970). These findings were recently confirmed (Carman et al., 1977), accompanied by a fall in calcium levels in the CSF. The hypocalcemia did not appear with the first few ECT but developed after three to five seizures, coincident with an acceleration of the antidepressant effects of the treatment. Carman and Wyatt (1977) carry the hypothesis further:

> That the observed decrease in CSF Ca [calcium] is specific to the function of ECT as an AD [antidepressant] is supported by similar findings with other AD modalities, and by the observations that schizophrenic or epileptic patients undergoing variously induced seizures exhibit no significant effects on CSF Ca [Katzenelbogen et al., 1939; Ueno et al., 1961; Eiduson et al., 1960]. The only previous study of changes in CSF Ca during AD response to ECT found Ca unchanged, although phosphate was increased [Björum et al., 1972].

Plasma magnesium levels are lower in depressed patients, and after ECT the levels are comparable to those of controls (Frizel et al., 1969; Carney et al., 1973). Cade (1964), however, reported higher plasma magnesium concentrations in depressed patients before and after recovery.

In a review of the significance of changes in mineral metabolism, Ottosson (1974) concluded that the changes were secondary to the recovery and were not a direct effect of the ECT process (type 2 effects).

BLOOD-BRAIN BARRIER PERMEABILITY

ECT elicits an increase in cerebrovascular permeability, which may persist for several days after a treatment (Spiegel and Spiegel-Adolf, 1941; Aird and Strait, 1945; Bjerner et al., 1944; Aird, 1958; Lee and Olszewski, 1961; Brown et al., 1963; Angel et al., 1965; Arneson and Ourso, 1965). Permeability to norepinephrine (Rosenblatt et al., 1970) and to tricyclic antidepressant drugs (Angel and Roberts, 1966) is also increased. Angel et al. (1965) found an increase in cerebrovascular permeability to cocaine 6 hr after the last ECS in rats subjected to one ECS per day for 12 days. Permeability measures returned to basal levels in 24 hr but when the frequency of ECS was increased to 12 ECS in 48 hr., the permeability to cocaine persisted for 6 days. Pretreatment with trypan red (a molecule of large molecular weight with a capacity to block "spaces" in the blood-brain barrier) decreased the cerebrovascular permeability to cocaine and also prevented the usual ECS disruption of a previously learned response.

The entry of radioactive sodium (^{24}NA) and isotopic water (tritium) from the blood to the CSF was examined in psychiatric patients before and after ECT (Coppen, 1960). The passage of both radioactive sodium and tritium was normal in schizophrenic patients but only half normal in depressed patients. With recovery after ECT, the rate of entry was normal, whereas the patients who failed to improve with ECT continued to show low rates of entry.

Recently, Bolwig and his associates (1977a, b) used radioactive isotope dilution methods to reexamine the blood-brain barrier permeability in clinical and experimental studies. Seizures increased cerebral blood flow both during and for up to 6 min after the seizure, allowing greater penetration of some intravascular substances in the brain. They postulated that endothelial cells stretched and new capillaries opened during the seizure. They found similar changes in permeability with hypercapnia, however, and indicated that the change in permeability was not the result of the seizure per se but resulted from an increase in cerebral blood flow.

This increased permeability may be reduced by the administration of dexamethasone. In an experimental study in rats, Suzuki et al. (1976) found that the ECS-increased penetration to the brain of Evans blue was blocked by the intraperitoneal administration of 2 mg/kg dexamethasone.

The change in cell membrane permeability has also been cited as a cause of the convulsion (Spiegel and Spiegel-Adolf, 1941; Cicardo, 1945). Others suggest that the increase in vascular permeability may result from the release of catecholamines that follows the hypoxia and hypercapnia that characterize each seizure (Clemedson et al., 1958). The cerebrovascular changes may be relevant for the antidepressant effect of ECT, since these changes persist after treatments and similar changes are induced with antidepressant drugs (Ottosson, 1974).

Another evidence of changes in permeability is a persistent elevation of some enzymes in the CSF after ECT, reflecting the increased vascular transfer of high molecular weight substances. CSF transaminase was elevated 12 hr after ECT and returned to normal by 48 hr (Mann et al., 1960). The rapid resolution of bromide intoxication after ECT was claimed to result from increased cellular permeability allowing an accelerated elimination of bromides (Gibson, 1975).

PROTEIN SYNTHESIS

With memory loss a prominent finding in ECT, the effects on protein synthesis were of interest. Spiegel and Spiegel-Adolf (1941) reported that CSF protein levels did not increase with ECT, but the activity of proteolytic enzymes, nuclease and desaminase, did increase. They interpreted the increases to be derived from the brain and not from the blood and concluded that the effects of ECT on brain enzymes were important to the ECT process.

ECS was found to interfere in the incorporation of radioactive labeled leucine into cerebral proteins (Dunn et al., 1971). This finding was corroborated by Essman (1973, 1974), who also noted a fall in cellular RNA concentrations, and by Dunn in later studies (Dunn et al., 1974). These authors suggest that the interference with protein metabolism was related to the passage of the electric currents and not to the convulsion itself; but the design of the studies cannot clearly separate these effects.

Body weight decreased but brain weight increased with ECS in rats (Pryor and Otis, 1969; Pryor et al., 1972a, b; Pryor, 1974). Monoamine oxidase (MAO) and acetylcholinesterase activity per milligram protein in the brain increased without detectable changes in the total protein concentration. The findings with

MAO were consistent; those with acetylcholinesterase were variable. There were no changes in succinate hydrogenase, catechol-O-methyl transferase, or cholinesterase in the same samples. The changes in MAO developed slowly and differentially with daily ECS and dissipated slowly and differentially after the last ECS.

An additional factor in these studies is the effects of ECT on hemoconcentration and increased permeability of the blood-brain barrier. A fall in plasma protein levels and hemoconcentration after ECT was described (Altschule et al., 1948*a, b*).

NEUROENDOCRINE EFFECTS

Many early studies focused on the effects of ECT on the adrenal and pituitary glands, reflecting an interest in the adaptive mechanisms of the body to stress (Hemphill et al., 1942; Mikkelsen and Hutchens, 1948; Hoagland and Pincus, 1950). Convulsions in the rat induced a fall in adrenal cholesterol, similar to the effect of other severe generalized stresses, including the stress of a unilateral adrenalectomy. In patients, ECT produced a brisk outpouring of adrenal cortical steroids during the first few days of treatment, only to return to pretreatment levels with further treatment (Ashby, 1949, 1953; Kallio and Tala, 1959; Ferguson et al., 1964; Clower and Migeon, 1967; Elithorn et al., 1968). Blood levels of 17-hydroxycorticosteroids rose in ECT, an elevation related to the seizure and not to the quality of the electrical stimulus. The rise in corticosteroids was equivalent to the administration of 1.0 U corticotrophin. When the grand mal convulsion was blocked by diphenylhydantoin and other procedures, and only a psychomotor or aborted seizure occurred, the increase in corticosteroid levels was the same (Bliss et al., 1954):

> . . . suggesting that the major factors responsible for steroid elevations following electroshock were the cortical dysrhythmia and the central nervous system discharge.

That the adrenals are not essential to the therapeutic process was demonstrated by the successful treatment of a depressed patient by ECT in the absence of both adrenals (Guze et al., 1956). The administration of cortisone, however, improved the clinical response to ECT of a patient with Addison's disease (Cumming and Kort, 1956).

The weight of the adrenals increased in rats treated with multiple convulsions (Royce and Rosvold, 1953). They interpreted this functional hypertrophy as a sign of pituitary hyperfunction and suggested that the pituitary response could be the result of three mechanisms: (a) increased stimulation by epinephrine, (b) a metabolic effect, and (c) direct hypothalamic stimulation. They cited the evidence of Lorimer et al. (1949) that the electric currents of ECT directly affect the brainstem with the currents flowing along established pathways, and concluded:

That the hypothalamus is involved in electroshock is indicated by various experiments. The changes noted in temperature control and activity [Hoyt and Rosvold, 1951], appetite and body weight [Jensen and Stainbrook, 1949], and autonomic activity [Kessler and Gellhorn, 1941; Gellhorn and Safford, 1948] all implicate various hypothalamic nuclei. In addition, the fact that pituitary stimulation is not marked when electroshock is preceded by barbiturate medication [Graham and Cleghorn, 1951; Rosvold et al., 1952], the latter having a known depressant effect on the hypothalamus [Leitner and Grinker, 1934; Masserman, 1937] is another suggestive clue. The work reported here with animals bearing adrenal transplants and those receiving multiple electroshocks during one convulsion would also tend to emphasize the hypothalamic mechanism, since the results suggest that neither the sympathetic nor the metabolic pathways may be essential.

Beuret and Swanson (1969) reviewed many studies of the endocrines and ECT and found the treatments to produce signs of pituitary stimulation and heightened autonomic activity. They concluded that these changes were more parsimoniously explained by increased activity of the hypothalamus rather than as direct effects on specific endocrine glands.

The possibility that ECT is effective to the extent that it stimulated the secretion of ACTH was tested by direct ACTH administration, but the results were disappointing. Altschule et al. (1949, 1950) treated three patients with melancholia and found no improvement. The patients responded to ECT. Similar results were reported by Hemphill and Reiss (1942), Cleghorn et al. (1950), and Smith (1950). ECT has also reversed a iatrogenic induced hypofunction of the hypothalamus of the CRF-ACTH type (Pitts and Patterson, in press).

The plasma ACTH increased 10 min after ECT and returned to normal levels in 1 hr (Berson and Yalow, 1968; Yalow et al., 1969; Delitala et al., 1977). A similar increase occurred in cortisol, the increase varying inversely with initial levels (Stokes, 1972). The diurnal periodicity of cortisol hypersecretion is lost in depressed patients and returns to normal with ECT (Sachar et al., 1973b). Dexamethasone suppression of cortisol is well defined after ECT (Stokes, 1972).

ACTH also increased after multiple ECT (Allen et al., 1974). The elevation during the stimulation fell rapidly after the treatment, returning to baseline within 2 hr. Changes in cortisol followed the same course.

Other evidence of changes in pituitary function is seen in the increase in prolactin levels in depressed patients receiving ECT, whereas anesthesia alone failed to elicit the same elevation (Öhman et al., 1976; O'Dea et al., 1978). These studies in depressed patients find a plasma prolactin increase within five minutes of a seizure and a return to baseline by 24 hours. A similar study in schizophrenic patients finds the same sharp increase in prolactin levels immediately following a seizure and a rapid return to baseline, within two hours (Meco et al, 1978). Baseline prolactin levels did not rise, although the return to baseline was more rapid, with successive treatments. These observations indicate that the involvement of dopaminergic pathways reflected in the modulation of prolactin is a consequence of central neurochemical changes accompanying a seizure, and not a link in the therapeutic process (Chapter 14).

In males, urinary gonadotropins increase with ECT, as do serum levels of follicle-stimulating hormone (FSH) and luteinizing hormone (LH) (Ettigi and Brown, 1977; van Praag, 1977; Delitala et al., 1977). In some studies, thyroid-stimulating hormone (TSH) and growth hormone (GH) levels did not increase with ECT (Ryan et al., 1970; Thorell and Adielsson, 1973); while Delitala et al. (1977) reported an increase in serum GH but not in TSH. Others, however, found serum GH and glucose levels to increase 30 min after each ECT (Vigas et al., 1975, 1976). In another study, increased ACTH and cortisol production was not accompanied by changes in serum FSH, LH, TSH, HGH, or cyclic AMP (Ylikorkala et al., 1976). It is common for female patients to cease menstruation, either during depression or as a result of ECT (Michael, 1956). And, antidiuretic hormone levels rose immediately after ECT and were elevated one week after a course of therapy in schizophrenic patients (Narang et al., 1973). Similar increases in ADH were found after chlorpromazine therapy (Shah et al., 1973).

NEUROHUMORAL EFFECTS

The role of the neurohumors — epinephrine, norepinephrine, serotonin, dopamine, and acetylcholine—in depression and their response to antidepressant therapies have been studied extensively (Schildkraut, 1965; Kety, 1966; Kopin, 1972; Weil-Malherbe and Szara, 1971; Mandell, 1973; Baldessarini, 1975a, b; Mendels, 1975; van Praag, 1977). Few studies, however, directly assess the role of biogenic amines in ECT, and the few do not provide a clear picture of the influences of these neurohumors in the ECT process.

The effects of ECT on autonomic functions were first examined by measuring the blood pressure response to intravenous epinephrine and subcutaneous methacholine (Mecholyl) (Funkenstein et al., 1948; Gellhorn, 1953). Reduced responsivity to both agents was seen in depressed patients who later had a good response to ECT. Weil-Malherbe (1955) found that ECT elevated plasma levels of epinephrine and norepinephrine and that the elevation was suppressed by barbiturate premedication. Havens et al. (1959) confirmed these findings. Heightened sympathetic activity accompanied seizures but was not essential to the treatment course, since the barbiturate reduction in amine levels did not reduce clinical efficacy.

Increases in the turnover and synthesis rates of serotonin, norepinephrine, and epinephrine have been observed with ECS and ECT, but the findings have been interpreted to result from the stress of the procedures and not to be specific for the antidepressant activity of ECT (Garattini et al., 1960; Kety et al., 1967; Ladisch et al., 1969; Schildkraut and Draskoczy, 1974; Valzelli and Garattini, 1974; Baldessarini, 1975a, b; Grahame-Smith, 1976; van Praag, 1977; Editor, 1977a). Some authors infer that the efficacy of ECT is attributable to the increased turnover of norepinephrine (Dysken et al., 1976). Others, however, fail to find increased rates of catecholamine turnover in ECS (Papeschi et al., 1974).

After a series of ECS, both norepinephrine and serotonin levels are normal or increased. Levels of tyrosine hydroxylase are elevated, as are levels of MAO. These levels may remain elevated for up to 6 weeks, presenting one of the more persistent biochemical changes after ECS (Pryor, 1974). Dopamine levels also increase after ECS (Ilaria and Prange, 1975). Ebert et al. (1973) reported that 5-HT, 5-HIAA, and tryptophan increase for a few days after a series of ECS, indicating an increase in turnover of 5-HT. Modigh (1975, 1976) found a sustained increase in noradrenergic neuron activity but not dopaminergic or 5-HT activity after daily ECS; while daily ECS produced increased postsynaptic monoamine receptor sensitivity to 5-HT and dopamine (Evans et al., 1976; Green et al., 1977; Grahame-Smith et al., 1978; Costain et al., *in press*). These latter workers have carried out extensive studies to document their thesis that the efficacy of ECT is related to the brain changes that make the brain sensitive to agents that mimic the actions of brain monoamines. They emphasize that the changes are most likely in the postsynaptic neurons. Most recently, Green (1978) found that the effects of flurothyl were the same as those with repeated ECS.

Human studies are less secure. In our studies and in those of Ottosson, we failed to find an increase in CSF 5-HIAA or HVA with ECT (Nordin et al., 1971; Abrams et al., 1976); while Jori et al. (1975) reported CSF elevations of HVA and 5-HIAA after ECT in probenecid-treated patients. van Praag (1977) noted increased 5-HIAA and HVA levels in CSF after ECT in probenecid-treated patients, although the changes were not related to the clinical effects. In patients with reduced CSF levels of 5-HIAA and HVA, van Praag observed a normal response after successful ECT. He concluded that the turnover of 5-HT and dopamine probably increases in response to ECT.

Another approach was taken by d'Elia et al. (1977*b, c,*) who compared the clinical efficacy of ECT with and without *l*-tryptophan in patients with endogenous depression. The oral administration of 6 g/day did not enhance the antidepressant efficacy of ECT, nor was there an alteration in *l*-tryptophan levels associated with the number of treatments or the clinical response.

Summarizing the various neurohumoral studies, Baldessarini (1975*a)* noted that:

> The metabolic effects of ECT suggest that seizures can release catecholamines and serotonin acutely, but that effects of repeated seizures are likely to be nonspecific in the case of serotonin, and small and of short duration in the case of norepinephrine.

From these data, it is probable that ECS increases central monoamine activity, a finding that is neither at variance with nor supportive of the monoamine hypothesis of depression (van Praag, 1977).

In our studies, we have focused on the role of acetylcholine. In 1966, impressed with the rapid reversal by anticholinergic drugs of the interseizure EEG slow wave activity which followed ECT, I reviewed the available data concerning the role of acetylcholine in seizures, head trauma, behavior, and EEG (Fink, 1966). CSF acetylcholine levels increase after spontaneous seizures and after ECT (Sachs, 1957). The increases are accompanied by increased choline and cholinesterase levels; and the increase in specific cholinesterase is associated with behavioral improvement. The interseizure EEG, which becomes materially slower in rhythm and higher in amplitude with ECT, shows a sharp desynchronization with a loss of amplitudes and an increase in the mean frequency after anticholinergic drugs. This change was seen with atropine, experimental anticholinergic drugs (e.g., Ditran), and antiparkinson drugs (e.g., procyclidine). Prior to ECT, the effect of anticholinergic drugs is to decrease both the mean amplitude and the percent time EEG alpha activity. This is seen in patients with high and low pretreatment percent time alpha activity (Figs. 11.1, 11.2). With procy-

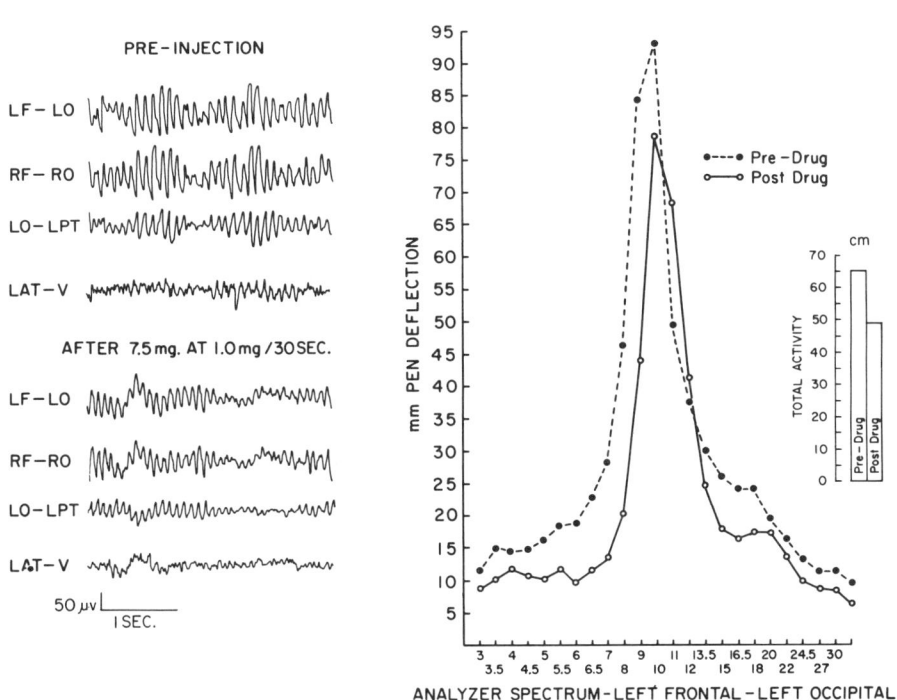

FIG. 11.1 Effect of intravenous procyclidine.

clidine, there is a sharp drop in the induced slow waves (Fig. 11.3; see also Fig. 8.11). This reversal in EEG measures is accompanied by behavioral worsening (Fink, 1958a, 1960; Itil and Fink, 1966; Bradley and Fink, 1968).

The chronic administration of atropine and scopolamine reduced the amount of EEG slowing and the clinical efficacy of ECT. In a controlled clinical study, Ulett and Johnson (1957) reported that marked clinical improvement occurred in four of six patients who received ECT but no anticholinergic drugs, compared to two of seven who received ECT and daily atropine treatment and one of five who received ECT and daily scopolamine treatment. In a replication study, however, these authors were unsuccessful (Johnson et al., 1960a).

Considering the paucity and the technical difficulties of studies of acetylcholine metabolism, it is unclear what role, if any, acetylcholine may play in the ECT process. It is possible that it may affect the release of hypothalamic hormones in a fashion similar to other biogenic amines from acetylcholine-sensitive receptor cells.

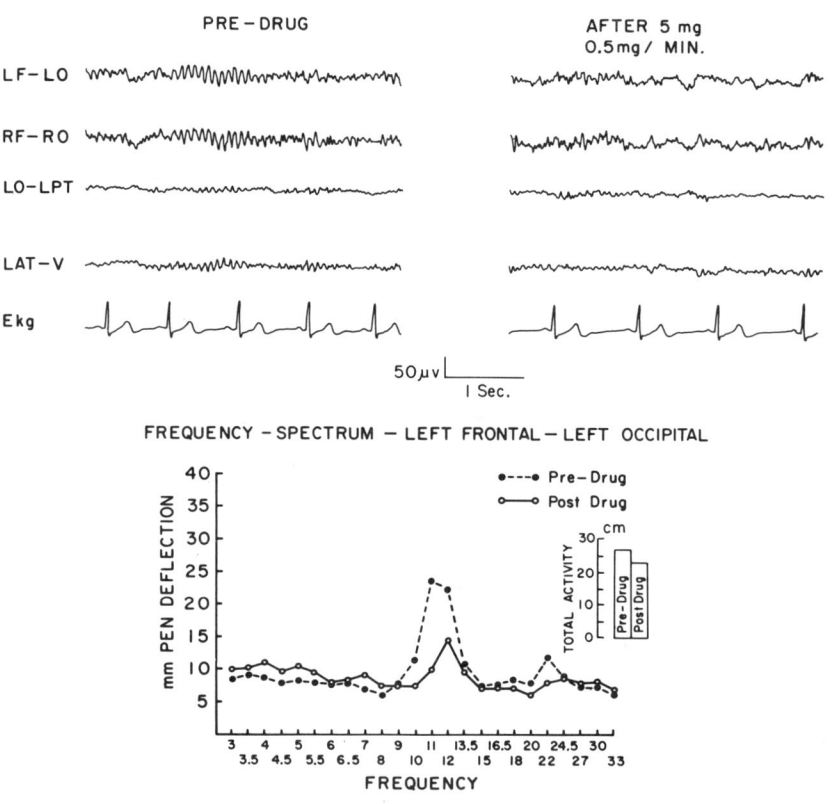

FIG. 11.2. Effect of intravenous procyclidine.

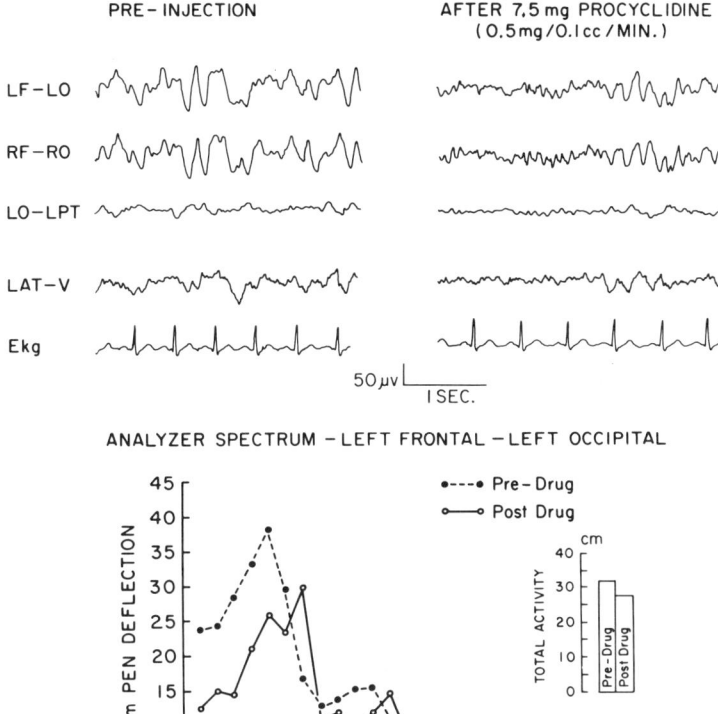

FIG. 11.3. Effect of intravenous procyclidine on post-ECT slowing. Male, age 20, 24 hr post-ECT no. 15.

Chapter 12

Vascular Effects: Cardiac and Cerebral

Seizures affect the vascular system, and extensive measurements have been made of both the cardiovascular (Perrin, 1961) and cerebrovascular systems. The chief changes in the cardiovascular system are the result of the activation of the autonomic nervous system and a Valsalva effect (the increase in heart rate and bimodal effect on blood pressure which results from forced respiratory straining against closed air passages); but anoxia, the accumulation of metabolites, and muscular activity also exert some influence.

During the seizure, heart rate increases to 120 to 180 beats/min and falls rapidly immediately thereafter so that it may be at or lower than pretreatment levels in 4 to 6 min. The effects are similar in modified and unmodified ECT. If atropine is not used, heart rate may fall with the passage of the current and rise during the seizure. In modified ECT, neither muscular activity nor the Valsalva effect is probably active, the principal changes resulting from an autonomic discharge and, to a lesser extent, from anoxia (Perrin, 1961).

Blood pressure also increases, with systolic measurements rising to 200 to 250 mm Hg and diastolic measurements to 110 to 150 mm Hg. A transient hypotension may follow a seizure, and the blood pressure effects are usually gone in 4 to 6 min (Deshaies and Renard, 1948). The changes in blood pressure are less in modified ECT and after atropine. Succinylcholine also reduces the extent of the blood pressure changes (Altschule, 1950; Brown et al., 1953a; Holmberg, 1953a, b; Holmberg et al., 1954; Perrin, 1961).

Pulse pressure changes little. Venous pressure rises with the same time course as for heart rate, and the effect is clearly reduced in modified ECT. Cardiac output increases, as do cerebral and peripheral blood flow measurements (Perrin, 1961).

Electrocardiographic measures have not been reported during the seizure, but in the immediate postseizure period, there is an increase in the amplitude of the P wave, especially in leads II and III, changes in the shape of the QRS wave, and reduction and inversion of the T segments. These changes have not been considered significant, except in rare instances (Perrin, 1961; Deliyiannis et al., 1962; Cropper and Hughes, 1964; Hussar and Pachter, 1968; Woodruff et al., 1969; Malik, 1972).

Cardiac Arrhythmia

Arrhythmias are frequent, occurring during and after the seizure; and both sinus bradycardia and auricular tachycardia have been reported. Many authors report these effects to be reduced by atropine, succinylcholine, and anesthesia, concluding that the vagal influences are affecting the rhythms (Altschule, 1950; Nowill et al., 1954; Lewis et al., 1955; Lewis, 1956; McKenna et al., 1970; Ward, 1974). Other observers indicate that ganglionic blocking agents can also reduce cardiac arrhythmia (Tewfik and Wells, 1957; Richardson et al., 1957; Anton et al., 1977).

While the changes have been described principally in man, parallel studies find the same changes in dogs and monkeys (Brown et al., 1953*a, b;* Colville et al., 1960; Plum et al., 1968; Anton et al., 1977). The changes are the same in seizures induced electrically and after pentylenetetrazol, with blood pressure rising an average of 72 mm Hg and cerebral blood flow increasing by 264% (Plum et al., 1968). These authors noted that cerebral oxygen consumption increased by 60% during a seizure, but the cerebral blood flow was so great that the oxygen tension rose during and after each seizure, reflecting the ability of the brain to adjust its vascular bed and systemic blood pressure to meet metabolic needs. As long as the adverse effects of the convulsion on respiration and skeletal musculature were eliminated, the cerebral oxygen tension was maintained to meet oxygen demands.

Similar effects of ECT on cerebral blood flow are described using the techniques of computerized cerebral impedance plethysmography (Doust et al., 1974; Doust and Raschka, 1975). The seizure induced a surging increase in cerebral blood flow, which persisted for at least 2 hr after the seizure. The increase was still present at 26 hr in some patients. The response of depressed and schizophrenic patients differed, with greater changes occurring in the depressed patients who showed clinical improvement.

The significance of autonomic effects in the cardiovascular response to ECS is emphasized in recent studies in dogs by Anton et al. (1977). They noted that the increased levels of circulating catecholamines were responsible for the hypertensive response to ECS, since the pressor response could be blocked by preventing the release of catecholamines by high spinal anesthesia or by inhibiting alpha-adrenergic receptors with phenoxybenzamine. Anton et al. suggested that the adrenal medulla was the source of the circulating neurohumors, and that asystole and arrhythmia were cholinergic effects since they were blocked by atropine.

There are also well-defined changes in blood constituents. ECT is followed by hemoconcentration, leukocytosis and lymphocytosis, and hyperglycemia, which are maximal 15 to 30 min after the seizure and which return to pretreatment levels in 1 to 3 hr (Ewald and Haddenbrock, 1942; Delay, 1946; Carse and Slater, 1946; Stern et al., 1949; Salomon and Gabrio, 1949; Parsons et al., 1949; Michael and Brown, 1951). Hemodilution, relative leukopenia and lymphopenia, and a reduction in eosinophiles are seen in later phases of the ECT-related changes (Parsons et al., 1949; Shattock and Micklem, 1952; Reichlin and O'Neal, 1962). An increase in the erythrocyte sedimentation rate and a lowering of the coagulation time have also been reported (Parsons et al., 1949).

These changes are related to the alterations in body economy caused by stress, altered oxygenation, motor activity, and disturbed food and fluid intake accompanying induced seizures, and are not related to the therapeutic elements in the process.

Cerebral Effects

ECT also has a profound effect on the cerebral vasculature. Increased arterial pressure and cardiac rate raise the cerebral blood flow and open the intravascular-cerebral spaces, allowing the passage of substances, including proteins, which are usually contained within the vascular bed (Aird et al., 1956a, b; Clark and Sarkaria, 1958). These observations have recently been confirmed by more elegant means (Hirano et al., 1970; Suzuki et al., 1976; Petito et al., 1976; Bolwig et al., 1977a, b).

Cerebral vessels contract during ECT, and the contraction may persist into the recovery period (Alexander and Lowenbach, 1944; Matakas et al., 1977). Parallel changes in the capillary system of the nail-bed have also been observed for up to 10 min (Davis et al., 1955).

In postmortem studies, cerebral hemorrhagic changes were occasionally reported in patients who died in ECT (Alpers and Hughes, 1942). In experimental studies, however, there were no vascular or tissue changes after ECS using light microscopy (Barrera et al., 1942; Heilbrunn and Weil, 1942; Neubuerger et al., 1942; Globus et al., 1943; Alexander and Lowenbach, 1944; Ferraro et al., 1946; Siekert et al., 1950). In more recent studies, there was astroglial swelling in the cerebral cortex of rats after pentylenetetrazol-induced seizures (De Robertis, 1969). Other studies found no decrease in neuron concentration after extended ECS (Colon and Notermans, 1975). Considering the transient nature of the changes that have been observed in the cerebral vasculature after ECS, it is not surprising that there are no measurable neuronal or glial changes in the brain; and it is unlikely that such transient changes result in long-lasting or demonstrable structural changes, even in electron microscopic examination (Garcia and Cervos-Navarro, 1978).

Cardiac arrest, arrhythmia, and coronary insufficiency represent the principal risks of ECT, being the most usual cause of death (Perrin, 1961; Arneson and Butler, 1961; Cropper and Hughes, 1964; Hussar and Pachter, 1968; Malik, 1972). The data from the cardiovascular studies indicate that the effects of seizures on blood pressure, heart rate, and cardiac rhythms are significantly reduced by modified ECT (succinylcholine and anesthesia) and by atropine. These data are the most compelling reasons for the use of modified ECT in practice.

THEORIES OF CONVULSIVE THERAPY

The resolution of the men who introduced convulsive therapy is astonishing. The treatment is so different and its manifestations so frightening that many have sought to explain its unanticipated success. Our concepts of the efficacy of a treatment arise from our views of etiology and pathogenesis; thus the theories of ECT reflect the kaleidoscopic history of modern psychiatric thought. A review of the theories and the studies undertaken to assess their validity (Chapter 13) provides the basis for another formulation (Chapter 14) that recognizes the dependence of the ECT process on psychopathology. The proposed formulation is based on the neurophysiologic and neuroendocrine consequences of repeated seizures.

Chapter 13
Review of Theories

> . . . the progress of science . . . [is] . . . not wholly unlike a pack of hounds, which, in the long-run, perhaps catches its game, but where, nevertheless, when at fault, each individual goes his own way, by scent, not by sight, some running back and some forward; where the louder-voiced bring many to follow them, nearly as often in a wrong path as in a right one; where the entire pack even has been known to move off bodily on a false scent.
>
> S. P. Langley, quoted by E. Anderson (1969)

Seizures have been induced in the severely mentally ill for more than 40 years, and yet no satisfactory explanation of how they elicit improvement in a patient's behavior has been accepted. Convulsive treatments lie outside the common experience of psychiatrists accustomed to verbal suasion, interpretation, and rational discourse. The development of this heroic treatment is not rooted in a long history, and the experience upon which a theoretic view can be erected is limited. We also lack a single, cogent view of the etiology of mental illness.

It is fashionable to say that the mechanism for the seizure therapies is unknown, that

> . . . there is no theory as to the nature of the shock treatments sufficiently comprehensible to be taken very seriously [Kalinowsky and Hippius, 1972].

There are no good general theories to explain the action of coma or, as they are often called, 'shock therapies' " [Redlich and Freedman, 1966].

In a recent critique of controversial issues in psychiatry, Clare (1976) writes:

> The most widely expressed criticism of electrical treatment is that nobody knows how it works. Not surprisingly, such ignorance worries many people.

Many theories have been proposed, and many are based on important aspects of the convulsive therapy process. The data and theories of ECT have been extensively reviewed in the continuing effort to extract the essential elements of this complex process. In addition to the descriptions in the texts by Sargant and Slater (1963) and Kalinowsky and Hippius (1972), the following are helpful for aspects of biochemistry: Ashby (1953), Spiegel and Spiegel-Adolf (1953), Fleming (1956), Ottosson (1960, 1974), Holmberg (1963), Beuret and Swanson (1969), Essman (1973), and Ilaria and Prange (1975). For behavioral aspects, Fleming (1956), Ottosson (1960), Riddell (1963), Miller (1967), Hurwitz (1974), and Turek and Hanlon (1977) are useful. The list of theories compiled by Gordon (1948) is of historic interest.

STRUCTURAL THEORIES

The first concepts of the mode of action of the shock therapies were based on cerebral pathology. The success of insulin coma was explained by inferring that nerve cells in dementia praecox were hypersensitive to external stimuli. Coma protected these abnormal cells from outside stimulation, and during the period of forced rest, the storage of glucagon increased and the abnormal functions of the affected cells were reduced (Sakel, 1956) or the abnormal cells were destroyed by repeated hypoglycemic insults (Arnold, 1959). Others thought the diseased cells were destroyed by the localized hypoxia resulting from spasms in brain capillaries (Stief and Tokay, 1932).

The seizures that occur spontaneously during insulin coma were thought to be hazards to be avoided (Sakel, 1938, 1956). The concepts of seizures as therapeutic agents were derived from a number of sources. One was the data regarding the differences in concentration in cerebral glial cells among patients with schizophrenia and epilepsy, with epileptic patients having higher concentrations than normal, and schizophrenic patients having lower concentrations than normal. In surveys in different mental institutions in Hungary, Steiner and Strausz had found that only 20 of 6,000 patients with schizophrenia had ever had an epileptic convulsion. Other scientists in Hungary had noted that in schizophrenic patients in whom epilepsy developed, the epilepsy rapidly disappeared; and in those epileptic patients in whom schizophrenia developed, the epileptic attacks had become infrequent at the beginning of the disease and had later disappeared. These observations encouraged the belief that these two clinical syndromes were biologically incompatible and did not coexist in the same patients; this led Meduna (1935, 1956) to undertake trials to increase gliosis in schizophrenic patients by inducing seizures experimentally. Within a few years, the concept of the incompatibility of schizophrenia and epilepsy was found to be erroneous, and the gliosis theory of seizure therapy was discarded.

Some authors thought a psychosis resulted from the accumulation of toxic substances in the brain; and seizures increased blood-brain barrier permeability, enhancing the removal of these substances (Danziger and Kindwall, 1946). Cerletti (1956) postulated the production of antipsychotic substances by a brain under extreme stress—substances that he termed "agonines." He believed he could develop agonines in the spinal fluid of pigs subjected to repeated electroconvulsive seizures and used such fluids to treat the mentally ill. The effort was unsuccessful.

Some clinicians sought the site of action of convulsions in the diencephalon, based on the belief that hypofunction of the diencephalon was a cause for schizophrenia. Sakel (1956) claimed that his interest in insulin was based on its actions in the hypothalamus. Ewald (1939) described the action of insulin coma as a stimulation of diencephalic centers, and Ewald and Haddenbrock

(1942) extended this explanation to ECT. Hemphill and Walter (1941), in a particularly broad report of their experiences with ECT in 75 mentally ill patients, noted the special responsivity of cases of agitated involutional melancholia and suggested:

> ... it is tempting to assume that alterations in the blood supply or perhaps direct stimulation have had a physical effect on the pituitary or the frontal and neighboring regions of the brain.

The focus on the diencephalon is also seen in the studies of the autonomic responses in ECT by Delay (1946), Delmas-Marsalet (1946), von Baeyer (1951), Ashby (1953), and Piette (1955).

The role of brainstem centers, particularly the hypothalamus, in the ECT process was recently reconsidered by Carney and Sheffield (1973, 1974) and Abrams and Taylor (1974, 1976b). Carney and Sheffield (1973, 1974) examined the effects of brief stimulus, low dose pulse ECT in cases of endogenous and neurotic depression and found that the efficacy of these minimal currents was significantly better in patients with endogenous depression. They thought that their observations supported the suggestion of Roth (1951) that the diencephalon mediated the therapeutic response. Abrams and Taylor (1974, 1976b) explained the differences in the response of depressed patients to seizures induced through unilateral, anterior frontal, and bilateral electrode placements by a direct therapeutic role for currents passing through brainstem centers.

The autonomic nervous system was also implicated. The responsivity of schizophrenic patients to sympathetic stimulants was found to be deficient or reduced, and central sympathetic reactivity was found to increase with ECT and direct stimulation of the hypothalamus. ECT was seen as redressing an imbalance in sympathomimetic and parasympathomimetic influences, particularly in the brainstem (Abely et al., 1948; Gellhorn, 1953; Fukuda and Matsuda, 1969).

Some sought the mechanism for ECT in changes in membrane permeability, noting that the blood-brain barrier is more permeable after ECS and ECT to both the release of substances from the brain and the introduction of substances into it (Spiegel and Spiegel-Adolf, 1941; Aird and Strait, 1945; Brown et al., 1963; Bolwig et al., 1977a,b) (Chapter 11).

Gordon (1948) identified other theories focused on enzyme and metabolic dysfunctions. These concepts, like some described in the preceding paragraphs, are more suitably applied to insulin coma therapy. Their juxtaposition with ECT reflects a failure to discriminate between insulin coma and ECT, a common error in the early decades of the use of the "shock therapies."

PSYCHOLOGICAL THEORIES

Gordon (1948) divided theories of ECT into two groups: 27 different somatogenic and 23 psychogenic theories. The latter sought explanations in concepts of inactivation of phylogenetic experiences, the reactivation of ontogenetic influences, desensitization of the psyche to conflicts and traumata, and the allaying of libidinal surges and unconscious conflicts. Amnesia was usually central to these views. The psychological theories of the mode of action of ECT were explicated by many, including Schilder (1939), Weigert (1940), Abse (1944), Frosch and Impastato (1948), Janis (1950a–c), and Weinstein, et al. (1952), and were recently summarized by Miller (1967, 1968).

The principal psychological consequence of seizures is an increase in repression, with a loss of recall of recent and remote events, particularly those with significance for the illness (Schilder, 1939; Abse, 1944; Miller, 1968). Repression is enhanced by each seizure, which the patient views as a threat of impending death (Schilder, 1939). Each induction of a seizure is a stress that elicits primal anxiety to which the organism has only one effective defense—repression of the threat (Abse, 1944; Sandison, 1950). The physiologic events of the seizure are equivalent to the stress responses to rage, fear, and other strong emotions. Under such stress the changes in behavior represent a regression to a more primitive, more infantile form of adaptation, thereby relieving the patient of the need to deal with the immediate problems of the illness (Abse, 1944). But the theoretic jump from a description of fear during the treatment to a psychological therapeutic mechanism is a large one and is not substantiated by direct observation (Miller, 1967). This view has become less tenable since the introduction of anesthesia for the convulsive therapies. Panic and fear have been curtailed without reducing the therapeutic efficacy of ECT.

Theory of Punishment

Others view ECT as a punishment, which assuages the feelings of guilt that are the basis for the patient's disturbances in affect (Schilder, 1939; Silbermann, 1940; Millet and Mosse, 1945). Schilder (1939) saw each recovery from a convulsion as a rebirth and a renewal of relationships with the significant persons in the patient's life. The joy of rebirth was the basis for the hypomanic elation often seen during recovery. Millet and Mosse (1945) considered the willingness of patients to undergo treatments as punishment for past sins at the hands of a trusted father-figure. This hypothesis is consistent with one facet of the ECT process, its greater efficacy in patients with endogenous depression, patients in whom guilt and preoccupation with suicide have been documented. Although this hypothesis has some attraction, it has not been verified (Miller, 1968).

Another analytic construct is suggested by Weigert (1940):

> The panic provoked by convulsion or shock destroyed on the one hand delusions of grandeur, intimidated overbearing aggressions, and on the other hand the threat to life mobilized a powerful erotization and turned the patient's interests from autistic fixations to the object of outside reality. Male patients showed a greater resistance and less favorable results from this overpowering treatment than female patients . . . the cruelty of the superego is replaced by a sadistic attack on the part of reality . . . this attack . . . mobilizes restitutive forces, an impulse towards instinct fusion, neutralization of libidinal and destructive instincts. Taking over the suicidal, self-destructive urge from the inward conflicts, reality becomes suddenly again the object of libidinal cathexes. The spectacular change in behavior turns introversion into extraversion.

These views of the effects of loss of consciousness on ego functions elaborate those of Kardiner (1932) and Schilder (1939).

Adaptations other than repression were also considered. Frosch and Impastato (1948) described two responses to seizures: (a) those that occur in all patients, such as memory defects and confusion, and (b) those that may be seen as an individual response to the illness and the defects following each treatment. The organic mental changes with difficulties with memory, disruption of body image and of ego boundaries, and disturbances in reality testing are threats to the individual ego. The subjects attempt to reintegrate their psychological functions at the highest level possible, using adaptations of repression; and if repression fails, they are further assaulted by the welling up of repressed emotions that must be dealt with, either by further repression or by another defense mechanism, such as displacement, regression, or denial.

Denial Theory

Following a similar reasoning, Weinstein et al. (1952) suggested that ECT elicits changes in brain function that allow more primitive adaptations to be expressed, particularly the explicit and implicit forms of denial of illness or anosognosia. This syndrome is augmented or elicited when absent in some patients by the administrations of intravenous amobarbital (Weinstein and Kahn, 1955). The neurologic sequellae of ECT were seen as a form of modified head trauma, which augmented a syndrome of anosognosia. In the verbal sphere, anosognosia was manifested by the language patterns of explicit denial, disorientation for place and time, reduplicative paramnesia (reduplication), confabulation, and paraphasia. The patient's feelings about his illness were also expressed by such nonverbal aspects of behavior as selective inattention, withdrawal, mutism, euphoria, mania, and altered sexual behavior. Weinstein and Kahn proposed that denial, both explicit and implicit, is the defense that achieves the greatest prominence in patients successfully treated by ECT. As support for their theory, they noted the experimental enhancement of the organic mental syndrome by the administration of amobarbital, which elicits denial in patients in whom the defense was either implicit or hardly discerned (Kahn et al., 1956). Studies in these laboratories found that the more successful results were seen in patients whose pretreatment or premorbid personality structure could be defined as denial-prone (Fink et al., 1959b; Kahn and Fink, 1959).

Amnesia Theories

Some emphasize amnesia as the therapeutic agent (Myerson, 1943; Stainbrook, 1946; Janis, 1950a–c; Cameron, 1960; Cannicott, 1968). A retrograde amnesia develops, usually for recent events during the period of the illness—events that may have an etiologic role in the development of the psychosis. Janis (1950a–c) suggests that the amnesia is a learned defense that allows the patient to repress painful experiences occurring subsequent to the treatments. He interviewed patients and controls before and after ECT and found that the amnesia of patients was greater for recent, emotion-ridden memories than for older, less stressful memories.

Cronholm and Ottosson (1960, 1963a–c; Ottosson, 1960, 1962b, 1968) studied the relationship among amnesia, neurophysiologic events, and clinical antidepressant ratings. The antidepressant efficacy of seizures was related to the amount of EEG slowing and only partially to the degree of memory impairment. Both retrograde and anterograde memory changes were tied to the induction of the seizure and, to a lesser extent, to a direct effect of the electric currents. They concluded that the antidepressant effects and memory disturbances varied independently of each other and were unrelated.

With the development of unilateral ECT, it was possible to further separate the antidepressant from the amnesic effects of ECT. While nondominant unilateral ECT is almost as therapeutically successful as bilateral ECT, it is not accompanied by measurable verbal memory loss, suggesting that the efficacy of ECT is not dependent on amnesia (Cannicott, 1962; Cannicott and Waggoner, 1967; Cohen et al., 1968; d'Elia, 1970a,b, 1974; d'Elia and Raotma, 1975; Sand-Strömgren, 1975; Squire, 1977).

If amnesia is the effective agent in the treatment process, perhaps clinical efficacy could be enhanced by treatments that exaggerate the memory deficits. A depatterning or regressive treatment was developed, in which the patient was treated more than once daily until he exhibited a severe organic mental syndrome and was unable to physically care for himself. When the treatments ceased, a reintegration of neurophysiologic functions and psychological processes occurred, with an amnesia for the traumatic events of the illness period, particularly the time just prior to and during the period of intensive ECT (Tyler and Lowenbach, 1947; Kennedy and Anchel, 1948; Cameron, 1960). Although the results seemed better for this treatment than for standard treatment regimens for schizophrenic patients, there is no evidence that this therapy was particularly useful or necessary for patients with depressive psychosis. Definitive studies of the relationships between memory functions and improvement in regressive therapy are yet to be done, although the recent studies by Exner and Murillo (1977) in schizophrenic patients are relevant.

In a study of the effects of ECS on conditioned responses in rats, Kessler and Gellhorn (1943) reported that both ECS and pentylenetetrazol seizures elicited a recovery of a conditioned response which had been inhibited by lack of reinforcement. They interpreted their unique observation as a reflection of the stimulatory effect of ECS on the hypothalamus.

ELECTROPHYSIOLOGIC THEORIES

The science of electroencephalography was showing rapid strides of discovery as the efficacy of ECT became known. Both developments shared a common interest in brain electrical activity and similar instrumentation. The discovery that epileptic patients exhibited characteristic disturbances in brain electrical activity provided another stimulus for a close association between the two techniques. As the electroencephalograph became commonplace in mental hospitals, it was used to study all aspects of mental illnesses, including their treatment. The events during insulin coma, seizure treatments, and the interseizure period were described in detail (Golla et al., 1940; Kalinowsky et al., 1942; Proctor and Goodwin, 1943; Hoagland et al., 1946; Polatin et al., 1940). ECT-induced seizures exhibited the same patterns of EEG high voltage spike and wave activity as did spontaneous epileptic seizures. The interseizure records showed a progressive increase in the amplitudes and a progressive slowing of the frequencies, so that after four to six seizures, the records were filled with high voltage theta and delta activity.

Many authors sought to relate changes in the EEG to clinical outcome, but the relationships, when found, were so indirect as to provide only an associative relationship to the ECT process (Hoagland et al., 1946; Roth, 1951; Roth et al., 1957). ECT was seen to affect the brainstem, with the EEG changes as a sign that an important brain change had occurred. Roth suggested that the psychoses represented recently acquired behavior patterns, which were more easily disrupted by any process that disorganized cerebral electrical activity, such as ECT or leucotomy. Since the EEG slow wave activity was symmetrical and diffuse over the whole scalp, it was seen as arising from deep central cerebral structures, most probably the diencephalon. ECT was believed to disrupt the thalamocortical pathways, which modulated emotional and ideational processes, particularly on recently acquired behaviors, such as the psychosis, leaving long-established personality traits intact.

Neurophysiologic-Adaptive Theory

Following our observation that patients who improved after ECT exhibited high degrees of EEG slow wave activity, my associates and I (Fink and Kahn, 1957; Fink, 1958a, 1960, 1962) saw the development of EEG slow wave activity as evidence that a persistent change in brain chemistry had occurred, which was necessary but not sufficient for clinical improvement. This hypothesis of ECT action was termed the neurophysiologic-adaptive hypothesis and was the basis for an extensive series of studies. In this theory, the increase in EEG slow waves indicated that the cerebral biochemistry was altered, thereby allowing physiologic and psychological adaptive processes to modify the expression of the psychoses. Denial of illness was emphasized as a prominent adaptation that favored improvement after ECT (Kahn et al., 1956). When EEG slow wave activity was reduced by anticholinergic drugs, the patient's clinical condition was found to worsen, leading to the suggestion that the EEG slow waves after seizures resulted from increased cholinergic activity in centrencephalic structures (Fink, 1958a, 1960, 1966). A similar relationship between EEG seizure activity and antidepressant activity was reported by Ottosson (1960, 1962b), who showed that the reduction in seizure activity by intravenous lidocaine was associated with a decrease in therapeutic efficacy.

Prolonged EEG slow wave activity was also considered a favorable prognostic sign in patients receiving insulin coma (Revitch, 1954). Persistent EEG slowing occurred in some patients, particularly after a prolonged coma, and Revitch (1954) ascribed a therapeutic benefit to the EEG changes.

Aird (1958) noted that an increase in permeability to metabolic substances resulted from seizures and was not a feature of the passage of currents alone. He concluded that the increase in permeability provided a mechanism for the prolonged neurophysiologic effects, which were the basis for the clinical activity of ECT.

At one time, REM sleep was compared to the desynchronized EEG seen in states of excitement and after hallucinogenic drugs. In sleep studies, various authors observed that the REM deprivation resulted in a rebound of REM sleep time during recovery, and that with ECS and ECT, the rebound in REM sleep was prevented. These observations led two groups to suggest that the efficacy of ECT was related to the effects on the sleep process (Cohen et al., 1967; Kaelbling et al., 1968).

BIOCHEMICAL THEORIES

From the beginning of the use of the convulsive therapies, it was apparent that electric currents or other convulsants provide a massive stimulation and discharge not only in the brain but also in the autonomic nervous system, the body musculature, and from the endocrine glands. Few systems of the body escape changes in their economy. The chemical homeostasis of the organism is profoundly disturbed, and biochemical measurements related to any of these body systems are likely to show large effects. As there is no dearth of biochemical effects associated with ECT, the difficulty lies in selecting those that are central to the therapeutic process (Ashby, 1949, 1953; Spiegel and Spiegel-Adolf, 1953; Fleming, 1956; Holmberg, 1963; Fink, 1966; Essman, 1973; Dunn and Bondy, 1974; Kety, 1974; Ottosson, 1974; Ilaria and Prange, 1975; van Praag, 1977).

The efficacy of ECT was related to its effects on the hypothalamopituitary-adrenal system by some observers (Altschule, 1949; Ashby, 1949, 1953; Hoagland et al., 1950; Taylor et al., 1951). These authors emphasized the increase in ACTH and adrenal corticoids reflected in diminished eosinophile counts, increased urinary 17-ketosteroid excretion, and fall in adrenal cholesterol. Others (Gellhorn, 1953; Weil-Malherbe, 1955) described increased activity of the adrenal medulla. The significance of these findings waned when ACTH administration was not clinically successful in patients who subsequently improved with ECT (Altschule et al., 1949, 1950).

Spiegel and Spiegel-Adolf (1953) observed an increase in CSF enzyme activity, particularly the enzymes related to nucleic acid metabolism, and suggested that increased enzyme activity was a factor in the efficacy of ECT. Changes in membrane permeability occurring with ECT were thought to allow the diffusion of these substances into the brain from the blood and the release of toxins from the brain into the blood (Cerletti, 1950; Spiegel and Spiegel-Adolf, 1953).

Hypoxia usually accompanies ECT. Hypoxemia and cerebral hypoxia were accepted as part of treatment and believed to be an aspect of the therapeutic process prior to the general use of anesthesia, muscle relaxants, forced ventilation, and oxygenation (Gellhorn, 1938; Gellhorn and Ballin, 1950). This view was encouraged by beliefs that ECT and insulin coma were similar in their effects. Weil-Malherbe (1955) and Holmberg (1963), however, found that oxygenation did not reduce the efficacy of the treatment.

Neurohumoral Theories

With increasing interest in neurohumors as mediators of mood and affect, changes in the level and activity of a number of substances were implicated in the ECT process. The activity of cholinergic and adrenergic systems was altered by the administration of methacholine and epinephrine, with the blood pressure response as the measured index. Increased responsivity of blood pressure was associated with a greater ECT response (Funkenstein et al., 1950, 1952). Others implicated serotonin (Lapin and Oxenkrug, 1969; Ebert, et al., 1973), dopamine (Ilaria and Prange, 1975), increased postsynaptic sensitivity to both (Evans et al., 1976), increased norepinephrine synthesis (Dysken et al., 1976), and an increase in noradrenergic but not dopaminergic neuronal activity (Modigh, 1975, 1976) as significant features of ECT.

In a detailed analysis of the role of acetylcholine in ECT, I noted that the cerebrospinal levels of acetylcholine increase, usually at the time when the patient shows clinical improvement. Choline and cholinesterase levels also increase in both blood and spinal fluid, and these changes were related to improvement after ECT. Anticholinergic drugs blocked the improvement in ECT; and if these drugs were given at a time when patients were improved, there was a reversal in behavior with a recurrence of the symptoms and language of the illness, again implicating acetylcholine in the therapeutic process.

Interest in protein metabolism led Essman (1973, 1974) and Dunn and his co-workers (1971, 1974) to find that ECS interfered with the incorporation of radioactive leucine into cerebral proteins and a fall in cellular RNA, implicating these processes in the amnesic effect of ECS.

Recent reviews of biochemical theories fail to define changes of significance to the ECT process, although they indicate those changes that probably bear little relation to outcome (Essman, 1973; Dunn and Bondy, 1974; Kety, 1974; Ottosson, 1974; van Praag, 1977). The latest contemporary survey based the antidepressant action of ECT on the enhancement of the postsynaptic responses mediated by serotonin and dopamine, with some contributions from an enhanced receptor sensitivity to norepinephrine rather than to any change in synthesis, concentration, or uptake of serotonin (Grahame-Smith et al., 1978). Their findings are consistent with the reports that ECS increases the concentration and disposition of brain serotonin, while not significantly affecting the disposition of other brain monoamines (Essman, 1973, 1978).

Chapter 14

A Theory of Convulsive Therapy

> Only in men's imagination does every truth find an effective and undeniable existence. Imagination, not invention, is the supreme master of the art of life.
>
> Joseph Conrad, 1912

A theory of convulsive therapy must account for the significance of the seizure but disregard the mode of induction, the direct actions of currents, and the distinctions caused by various electrode placements. It must consider the difference in response among patients with diverse psychopathologies and the time, measured in days, needed for a favorable outcome. Biochemical explanations must relate to changes in the brain rather than in the blood, urine, or other tissues. Psychological, personality, and linguistic considerations may affect the behavioral response and should be considered, but these are probably not central to the antidepressant efficacy of induced convulsions.

For a biochemical understanding, we may apply the postulates suggested by Ottosson (1974) and Kety (1974) (Table 14.1). A theory should encompass the release of hypothalamic hormones and changes in calcium metabolism. Increased levels and turnover of biogenic amines may also be important. Cerebral hypoxia and the changes in protein synthesis are probably related to the neurologic and amnesic sequellae that accompany the present technics of the administration of ECT but are not essential for the antidepressant efficacy. The relief of depressive affect is accompanied by many other biochemical changes, including altered diencephalic functions, increased responsivity of the adrenals and other endocrine glands, increased cerebrovascular permeability, changes in mineral and water metabolism, and elevated monoamine oxidases (MAO) and other enzymes. These are probably consequences of the processes and not central to the antidepressant efficacy of induced seizures.

The convulsive therapy process, although superficially similar in depression, schizophrenia, mania, and other disorders, probably cannot be subsumed by a single hypothesis and needs to be viewed differently for different clinical populations. This seems true at least for explanations and observations in the endogenous depressive psychoses and the acute schizophrenias, in which differences in dosage and efficacy are so great as to warrant such distinctions. Whether the response of manic and catatonic patients can be subsumed in either of these explanations or whether additional mechanisms will need to be elaborated is unclear at this time. In this regard, our understanding of the convulsive therapies today is similar to that of psychoactive drugs in the 1950s, when

TABLE 14.1. *Relevance for theory of ECT*

	Ottosson[a]	This chapter[a]
Release of hypothalamic hormones	—	1a
Norepinephrine (turnover and synthesis)	1a	1a
Serotonin (5-HT) (turnover and synthesis)	1a	1a
Acetylcholine increase	—	1a
Calcium metabolism	—	1a
Cerebral hypoxia	1b	1b
Protein synthesis	—	1b
Cerebrovascular permeability	1a	2
MAO in CSF	2	2
Diencephalic influence (weight, appetite, libido)	2	2
Mineral and water metabolism	2	2
Hormones (thyroid, sex, pituitary)	—	2
Adrenal medullary response		
Responsivity of adrenals	2	2
Epinephrine, norepinephrine activity	3	3
Adrenal cortical response (ACTH)	3	3

[a] Criteria of Ottosson (1974): 1a, direct link in process; 1b, link in side-effect; 2, consequence of central neurochemical effect; 3, coincidental phenomenon.

distinctions among the psychoactive drugs were best made by their effects in different clinical populations rather than by their individual chemical structure or pharmacology. Even today, after many decades of study, the clinical actions of psychopharmacologic agents remain diverse and do not allow a unitary theory of their mode of action.

DEPRESSIVE PSYCHOSES

Patients with primary depressive psychosis with endogenous features respond best to convulsive therapy, particularly if the vegetative signs of anorexia, insomnia, weight loss, decreased libido, diurnal variation, and inhibition of both motor activity and secretions are prominent. These symptoms, like depressive affect and suicidal preoccupation, respond rapidly, and their early relief is a favorable prognostic sign. Our present knowledge suggests that these functions are regulated by the hypothalamic-pituitary axis. A common pathway for the expression of the syndrome of endogenous depression is probably dysfunction of the hypothalamic centers serving these vital functions. The aspects of the ECT process that either augment or reduce the efficacy of seizure—methods of induction, electrode placement, and persistence of postseizure centrencephalic dysrhythmia—also point to the central brainstem region as critical to the success of the ECT process.

Modern biochemical theories of the pathogenesis of endogenous depression emphasize deficits in central aminergic activity. These theories are supported by the pharmacology of antidepressant drugs, both those with a tricyclic structure and the MAO inhibitors, which elicit an increase in the functional levels of monoamines at brain sites. ECT is a procedure that elevates both the levels and turnover rates of monoamines in the brain, and to the extent that these theories are relevant for our understanding of depression, they are supportive of the efficacy of ECT.

Hypothalamic dysfunction is a core process in endogenous depressive psychosis.
Convulsive therapy alters hypothalamic activity both by direct stimulation of hypothalamic cells and by increasing the functional neurotransmitter activity in the brain, thereby releasing substances, probably peptide hormones, that alter the vegetative functions of the body and the endocrine glands. Specific substances are released that modify mood and the behaviors associated with mood disturbances. The biochemical events that precede and accompany the seizure are the trigger for increased neurohumoral activity. In ECT, the direct stimulation of electric currents augment but are not necessary for the effects on hypothalamic functions.

This formulation extends the neurophysiologic-adaptive hypothesis of the mode of action of ECT. In the original formulation, psychological aspects were emphasized with the CNS changes as a trigger to achieve the adaptive response. The changes in brain function resulted in an impairment of critical perceptual and emotional discriminations, encouraging such psychological defenses as denial, repression, and displacement. EEG slow wave activity was evidence that cerebral functions had changed, and its persistence allowed new adaptations to develop. The present theory focuses attention on the hypothalamus and other brainstem structures and suggests that the increased release of peptide hormones of the hypothalamus is the basis for the relief of the depressive syndrome. The electrophysiologic measures (the persistence of EEG slow wave activity) provide an index that the neurochemical changes in the brain necessary for the therapeutic process have occurred, but their expression is not necessary for the clinical response.

The psychological events, which were central to the relief of symptoms in earlier theories, are now seen as supportive mechanisms, as changes in verbal and interpersonal relationships that encourage behavioral adaptations necessary for successful human intercourse.

This formulation is supported by a variety of observations derived from electrophysiology, biochemistry, anatomy, psychopathology, and experimental psychology.

Electrophysiologic Data

After ECT (or equally after chemical inductions, such as pentylenetetrazol or flurothyl), bilateral EEG slow wave activity occurring in burst patterns progressively dominates the interseizure record. Such EEG activity is characteristic of disturbances of midline brain structures, particularly the thalamus and hypothalamus; when spontaneous, such rhythms define a type of clinical epilepsy classified as centrencephalic. Seizures that result in bilateral and equal manifestations must have some mechanism for integration that has access to both hemispheres with the same facility.

Electrical stimulation of the intralaminar nuclei of the thalamus modifies the spontaneous activity of both hemispheres and stimulates rhythmic EEG activity in both cortices, with the rhythmic activity persisting beyond the period of stimulation (Morison and Dempsey, 1942). With increasing stimulation of these nuclei, symmetric convulsions are elicited (Hunter and Jasper, 1949). These observations led to the concept of a diffuse projection system connecting central structures, such as the thalamus, with the cerebral cortices. This system was later shown to be under the control of even more subcortical systems, e.g., the reticular system (Moruzzi and Magoun, 1949; Magoun, 1958).

EEG activity after ECT is reduced by lidocaine and anticholinergic drugs or enhanced by pentothal. Parallel changes in clinical behavior are seen when these EEG changes are observed. A reduction in EEG slow wave activity is accompanied by a recurrence of morbid symptoms and a regression to illness, whereas an enhancement of EEG slow waves is accompanied by euphoria, feelings of well-being, and clinical improvement.[1]

The electrophysiologic data, particularly EEG interseizure activity, are equivalent for seizures induced by photoconvulsive, pentylenetetrazol, electrical, or flurothyl means, and among the electrical inductions, they are virtually equivalent for different stimulation currents, such as alternating, unidirectional, or brief square wave stimuli. The differences in therapeutic efficacy among the various induction methods are much less than their similarities. In the number and frequency of the seizures needed for a therapeutic result in depressive psychosis, the various inductions are virtually equivalent, the difference at most being an average of 1 to 1.5 seizures for a course—clearly similar to the differences in dosages and times necessary for a therapeutic response among other treatments in psychiatry.

In ECT, however, there may be an added clinical component from the direct action of the currents. The principal current density is between the electrodes (Hayes, 1950; Weaver et al., 1976), although Lorimer et al. (1949) make a compelling argument for its passage along neuronal pathways, significantly affecting the brainstem. When electrodes are unilateral, the electric currents affect the brainstem less (Abrams and Taylor, 1976b; Weaver et al., 1976). Following bilateral ECT, the EEG exhibits greater slowing than after unilateral electrode placement; and in the latter, slow waves are asymmetric with accentuation of the slow waves on the side of the electrode placement.

Clinical efficacy varies with electrode placement. While the data are unclear, bilateral ECT may elicit clinical improvement more rapidly than unilateral ECT, although at the end of a clinical course the efficacy is equal. Although decreased

---

[1] These observations are consistent with the electrophysiologic classification of psychoactive drugs, in which the behavioral and clinical effects of drugs are directly related to their effects on EEG frequency, amplitude, and pattern (Fink, 1963, 1969, 1974e; Itil, 1961, 1964, 1974).

efficacy may result from missed seizures, it is also possible that electric currents passing through deep, midline structures may have a direct therapeutic component (Ottosson, 1974; Abrams and Taylor, 1976*b*). Thus placing electrodes far anteriorly should reduce the direct effects of currents in the brainstem and reduce their therapeutic efficacy, as observed by Abrams and Taylor (1973).

Biochemical Data

Functions of the pituitary and hypothalamus are altered during depression and return to normal after ECT.[2] For example, growth hormone (GH) normally rises in response to hypoglycemia; this response is reduced in depressed patients (Sachar et al., 1971*a, b,* 1973*b;* Sachar, 1976; Langer et al., 1976; Gregoire et al., 1977; Kendler and Davis, 1977). The GH response to *l*-dopa and the thyroid-stimulating hormone (TSH) response to thyrotropin-releasing hormone (TRH) are also reduced in depression (Gold, 1977). The return to an adequate response of TSH ($>$ 2.0 μU/ml at 20 and 60 min) after a challenge dose of TRH (200 μg) was seen in depressed patients who sustained the improvement of their depression after treatment with either ECT or tricyclic antidepressants but not in those patients who relapsed (Kirkegaard et al., 1975, 1978). Depressed patients also exhibit a deranged anterior pituitary responsiveness to hypothalamic releasing hormones, secreting abnormal amounts of GH, FSH and LH to an intravenous challenge of TRH, and abnormal amounts of GH to injections of LH-RH (Brambilla et al., 1978).

Depressed patients hypersecrete cortisol, and the administration of dexamethasone fails to suppress the hypersecretion (Stokes, 1972; Carroll and Mendels, 1976; Carroll et al., 1976*a–c*). CSF levels of cortisol were elevated in depressed patients; these levels fell with treatment and recovery. The CSF results paralleled the plasma total cortisol levels and the urinary excretion of free cortisol (Carroll 1976*d*). The corticosteroid response to methylamphetamine is lower (Checkley and Crammer, 1977), as is the TSH response to TRH (Loosen et al., 1976, 1977, 1978). Furthermore, cortisol excretion, which is usually phasic with a maximum during sleep, is not secreted in bursts in depressed patients and reverts to a normal phasic rhythm after treatment (Sachar, 1976; Ettigi and Brown, 1977).

It is through the monoaminergic regulation of the release of hypothalamic hormones that connections can be made among the biochemical theories of depression, treatment by antidepressant drugs, and the mode of action of ECT.

---

[2] Functions of the hypothalamus and the hypothalamopituitary axis, although poorly understood, are under intensive study, and new data and concepts appear with startling frequency. Present views include concepts of neurosecretory neurons producing transducers that change electrical signals into hormone release. There are complex interactions between brain structures and effector organs, and complex feedback mechanisms that so modify the levels of the substances measured and the activity of the endocrine glands that measurement of responses may be interpreted as a direct effect by one observer and a feedback effect by another. It is probably rash to summarize the present plethora of findings. As the views change, the indulgence of the reader is requested as he makes the necessary adjustments in the interpretation of the changes cited in these paragraphs.

The release of the hypothalamic hormones TRH, luteinizing hormone-releasing factor (LHRF), and GH release-inhibiting factor (GHRIF, somatostatin) is controlled by biogenic amines (Ettigi and Brown, 1977). Three input systems have been postulated: (a) noradrenergic-releasing fibers from medulla and pons, (b) serotoninergic inputs from raphe and median forebrain bundle, and (c) dopaminergic inputs from the nigrostriatum and the limbic and tuberoinfundibular systems. Increased serotonin or acetylcholine activity increases ACTH production, while increasing dopamine results in a fall in ACTH. GH secretion is increased by alpha-adrenergic or dopamine stimulation and decreased by beta-adrenergic stimulation. After ECS, norepinephrine, serotonin, and dopamine levels increase, as do tyrosine hydroxylase and MAO levels, reflecting increased monoamine activity (Ebert et al., 1973; Essman, 1973; Pryor, 1974; Baldessarini, 1975a, b; Ilaria and Prange, 1975; van Praag, 1977). Similar increased activity may be assumed for acetylcholine (Fink, 1966). Some authors have reported a reduction in parkinsonism in depressed patients treated with ECT, indicating that ECT has released increased amounts of dopamine in central brain regions (Brown, 1975; Lebensohn and Jenkins, 1975; Asnis, 1977).

From these observations, it seems probable that important functions of the brainstem and diencephalon, which subserve autonomic and homeostatic mechanisms, are partially regulated by neurons that synthesize and secrete monoamine neurotransmitters. The diffuse and widespread distribution of terminals arising from serotonin- and norepinephrine-containing neurons suggests that they serve functions having a long time course, for example, levels of arousal or consciousness, affect, and the tonic control of autonomic functions and their phasic responses to stress. They also regulate muscular tone and posture through the extrapyramidal motor system. Monoaminergic systems of the CNS represent a homolog of the peripheral autonomic nervous system, with the end-organ being the CNS itself. Monoaminergic systems are probably not involved in very precise, rapidly changing functions subserving sensation or control of the contraction of skeletal muscles; but they may be involved in disturbances of mood, drive, initiative, sleep and diurnal rhythmicity, sexual and feeding behavior, and hypothalamic-adrenal functions characteristic of the major affective disorders (Baldessarini, 1975a, b).

Calcium metabolism is an essential component of the release of hypothalamic and hypophyseal hormones. ECT shifts calcium metabolism to a positive balance, with an increase in intracellular calcium and a fall in plasma, CSF, and urinary calcium levels (Flach et al., 1960; Flach, 1964; Faragalla and Flach, 1970; Carman et al., 1977). Hypothalamic-releasing hormones alter the electrical characteristics of the plasma membrane of adenohypophyseal cells, facilitating the discharge of hormones; calcium ions are essential for this action. Changes in sodium and potassium ions play little role in this release process (Kraicer, 1974).

The behavioral effects of hypothalamic regulatory hormones are the least substantiated (and least studied) part of the theory. The demonstrations of the widespread nature of the effects of hypothalamic hormones compel their consideration as probable core substances in the alleviation of mood disturbances.

Hypothalamic hormones regulate diurnal cycles, and mood disturbances are clearly accompanied by changes in sleep-wakefulness and hormonal discharge cycles (Sachar et al., 1971a; Weitzman, 1974; Sachar, 1976; Carroll, 1978). The vegetative effects are well documented (Fulton et al., 1940; Haymaker et al., 1969; Lederis and Cooper, 1974; Salgado et al., 1976; Reichlin et al., 1978). The range of their clinical effects is impressive (Kastin et al., 1976b; Schally, 1976). Studies of ACTH, somatostatin, and the peptide fragments ACTH 4–10 and α-MSH find these hormones to have measurable effects on memory and recall functions (de Wied and Bohus, 1966; de Wied, 1969; Miller et al., 1977).

The clinical experience with two tripeptides is of special interest. TRH is a tripeptide (pyroglutamyl-histadyl-prolinamide) produced in the hypothalamus and carried to the anterior pituitary by the hypophyseal portal system where it stimulates the secretion of thyrotropin. In clinical trials, TRH induced a prompt but brief improvement in depressive symptoms, particularly in female patients (Kastin et al., 1972; Prange et al., 1972). On repeated administration, long-term clinical antidepressant activity was not demonstrated, although each observer noted the transient effects on mood with the administration of TRH (Takahashi et al., 1973; Ehrensing et al., 1974; Campbell, 1975; Gorden, 1975; Lipton and Goodwin, 1975; Hollister et al., 1977; Lipton et al., 1977; Prange et al., 1978a).

It is of some interest that TRH is distributed widely in the rat brain, being present in all areas except the cerebellum. About 30% of TRH was localized in the hypothalamus, using a sensitive and specific radioimmunoassay. The distribution suggests that TRH may have central actions in addition to its effects on the hypophysis (Winokur and Utiger, 1974).

More recently, a second tripeptide, prolyl-leucyl-glycinamide [MSH-release inhibiting factor (MIF-1) or hormone (MRIH-1)] was shown to have clinical antidepressant activity in two studies (Ehrensing and Kastin, 1974, 1978). In the first, these authors administered either 60 or 150 mg of the tripeptide as a single daily dose to 14 depressed women with endogenous unipolar depression. Four of the five patients who received 60 mg MIF-1 showed a clinical reduction in depression, while only two of four patients receiving placebo and two of five patients receiving 150 mg MIF-1 showed clinical improvement. In a second study, substantial improvement was seen in five of eight patients receiving 75 mg/day MIF-1, as compared to one of 10 receiving 750 mg/day MIF-1 or one of five taking placebo (Ehrensing and Kastin, 1978). Reviews of these findings and other effects of peptides on behavior have been published recently (Donovan, 1978; Prange et al., 1978b). While these studies of TRH and MIF-1 are not compelling evidence, they do indicate that peptides arising from central structures have direct effects on the CNS with behavioral consequences.

Additional evidence for the central effects of peptides is found in the studies of the endorphins, enkephalins, β-lipotropin, and similar substances for which specific brain receptors have been identified. These studies indicate that endogenous cerebral substances play active roles in the gross behavior of animals and man, and surely have the potential to influence mood and affect (Vale et al., 1978; Renaud, 1978; Moss, 1978). As these notes are written, new findings with synthetic and natural peptides are being reported with increasing frequency. The administration of β-endorphin elicited changes in behavior of schizophrenic and depressed patients (Kline et al., 1977). A synthetic analog of methionine enkephalin (FK 33–824, Sandoz) produced tolerance and cross-tolerance to morphine in monkeys and akinesia in rats and rabbits, effects that were abolished by naloxone (von Graffenried et al., 1978). In normal human volunteers, FK 33–824 elicited a diffuse syndrome consisting of feelings of heaviness in the limbs, oppression in the chest, tightness in the throat, and anxiety. Symptoms indicative of a histamine reaction were observed. Single doses of 0.1 to 1.2 mg slowed EEG alpha activity, increased beta activity, and increased total power, indicating a direct central effect for the compound.

de Wied et al. (1978) and Verhoeven et al. (1978) examined the effects of [des-Tyr¹]-γ-endorphin (DTγE) and found that this fragment of β-lipotropin exhibited neuroleptic activity in pharmacologic tests in rats and in the treatment of long-term psychotic patients. Hallucinatory activity and psychomotor hyperactivity disappeared on the fourth day after the daily administration of 0.5 to 1.0 mg DTγE i.m. in six patients. All patients improved, although the effects were short-lived in three.

There is some evidence that ECT affects CNS levels of endorphins. Emrich and Höllt (1978) reported that plasma levels of endorphin increased 10 min after the first to third ECT treatments in ten patients. This finding is consistent with the report by Green et al. *(in press)* that the met-enkephalin content of the caudate nucleus of the rat brain was increased after repeated ECS, while remaining unchanged in the samples from the cortex and the pons/medulla.

And, vasopressin has been implicated in a theory of manic–depressive illness (Gold et al., 1978). In discussing this hypothesis, de Wied (1978) presented some additional evidence for the central role in behavior not only of vasopressin but also a series of new analogs.

If convulsive therapy has a central brainstem locus of activity, with the ability to rapidly reverse the signs and symptoms of hypothalamic dysfunction, it is not too adventurous to seek hypothalamic-releasing substances as the core movers of mood and vegetative functions.

Anatomic Data

The role of the brainstem, particularly the hypothalamus and the visceral brain, in the elaboration of emotions has been extensively described (Papez, 1937; Scharrer and Scharrer, 1940; Hess, 1954; Harris, 1955; Magoun, 1958; Haymaker et al., 1969). The evidence of stimulation, ablation, and biochemical studies suggests that this anatomic region is actively involved in the autonomic regulatory functions of temperature, water metabolism, food intake, sexual activity, and cardiovascular and respiratory control. The hypothalamus is intimately involved in the expression of emotions, including rage, fear, and pleasure, and sites for self-stimulation for pleasurable and even painful stimuli have been identified.

The hypothalamus is a source of hormones, particularly those affecting the hypophysis. It is also a target organ for chemical mediators, derived from both the brain and the endocrine glands (Harris, 1955; Haymaker et al., 1969). Although most of our information is derived from studies in animals, supporting data are available from clinical studies, neurosurgical interventions, and pharmacologic and electrophysiologic studies.

The diencephalon is responsive to exteroceptive and interoceptive (hormonal) stimuli that activate pathways between the brain and the hypothalamus and the hypothalamus and the pituitary. Psychological stresses affect these interactions (Green, 1969). The diencephalon is the center not only for physiologic functions but of consciousness as well—the organism's awareness of the environment and its responses to changes in the internal and external milieu. Penfield (1975) summarized his neurosurgical experience by suggesting that:

> . . . there is much evidence of a level of integration within the central nervous system that is higher than the cerebral cortex. . . . I suggest that this region lies not in the new brain, but in the old—that it lies below the cerebral cortex and above the midbrain. . . . All regions of the brain may well be involved in normal conscious processes, but the indispensable substrate of consciousness lies outside the cerebral cortex, probably in the diencephalon.

An example of the interaction of external and internal stimuli by the hypothalamus is the integration of sexual behavior and the secretion of gonadotrophins (Sawyer, 1969):

> The regulatory mechanisms of secretion of gonadotrophic hormones are closely interwoven with mechanisms controlling reproductive behavior, a functional adaptation to insure survival of the species. This vital coordination is implemented by interposing the CNS in the feedback pathway by which the gonadal steroids influence pituitary secretion. The brain becomes at once a target organ for hormone action and an endocrine gland releasing internal secretions of which the adenohypophysis is the target via the hypophysial portal system. The reception and integration of hormonal feedback influences both on pituitary functions and on sexual behavior is the province of the hypothalamus.

Diverse stimuli may affect the hypothalamus:

> The pharmacologic stimulants, including catecholamines, histamine, metal ions and convulsant drugs, all activate central nervous rhinencephalic-hypothalamic function, and their action on the release of pituitary ovulating hormone is indirect and delayed. There is every reason to believe that the final pathway involves gonadotrophin releasing factor in all of the artificial ovulation-inducing procedures, excepting the administration of gonadotrophins themselves.

A review of clinical and psychopharmacologic data finds a close linked interdependence among estrogen and progesterone, psychopathology, and brain monoamine levels (Janowsky et al., 1971).

Similar analyses have been made for the control of other vegetative functions, such as lactation (Desclin, 1969), food and water intake (Stevenson, 1969), sleep and motor activity (Koella, 1969), and body temperature (Myers, 1969). Recent studies of hypothalamic regulatory peptides find these to have widespread endocrine, gastrointestinal, and behavioral effects, which probably can be implicated in the ECT process by further study (Vale et al., 1978; Renaud, 1978; Moss, 1978).

While the hypothalamus is sensitive to many stimuli, it is unclear whether an electrical or a biochemical stimulus (pentylenetetrazol and flurothyl) affects it directly or indirectly by releasing neurohumoral substances from other brain sites. Harris and George (1969) observed an increased release of TSH from direct stimulation of the anterior median eminence and the supraopticohypophyseal tract. Such stimulation resulted in enhanced thyroid activity. Electrical stimulation of the hypothalamus also released ACTH (Harris and George, 1969). The direct electrical or biochemical stimulation of the hypothalamus can elicit emotional responses of anger, fear, and pleasure (MacLean, 1969, 1974). In clinical studies, pathology involving the hypothalamus is accompanied by disturbances in affects, both anxiety and depression, indistinguishable from endogenous emotional disorders (Alpers, 1939). Electrical and emotional stimuli release catecholamines, acetylcholine, and possibly other neurohumoral mediators not only from the brainstem but also from a variety of cerebral structures, thereby stimulating the activity of the hypothalamus.

Monoaminergic transmission is integral to the secretion of the hypothalamic-releasing factors. There is a redundancy in the systems, with a number of aminergic systems operating in parallel. Catecholaminergic and cholinergic systems have both been identified (Kizer and Youngblood, 1978; Hökfeldt et al., 1978), although other neurohumors probably have direct effects on hypothalamic functions.

A recent study (Buckingham and Hodges, 1977) of the production of corticotrophin-releasing hormone by the isolated hypothalamus of the rat found that acetylcholine, 5-hydroxytryptamine, and angiotensin II were effective in releasing this hormone, while norepinephrine and glycine decreased its production. Other transmitters, such as dopamine, epinephrine, and histamine, failed to alter its production. This selective liberation, and the rich concentration of specific stimulating systems, provides the basis for the selective activity of different antidepressant treatments and their differential efficacy and time characteristics. The activity of these neurons probably provides the connection between the clinical antidepressant activity of ECT, tricyclic antidepressant drugs, and the MAO inhibitors. The difference in concentration in aminergic and cholinergic neurons may be responsible for the relative efficacy of these different treatments; the greater antidepressant efficacy of ECT reflecting its effects on numerous stimulating systems, whereas psychoactive drugs may affect only parts of the stimulating systems at any time.

Clinical Data

The best predictors of the treatment response to ECT are severity of the mood disorder and the symptoms related to hypothalamic functions (Chapter 6). ECT is specifically effective in endogenous depression, with a success rate greater than 90%, with a rapid relief of depressive mood, apathy, anorexia, insomnia, and glandular hypofunctions. Such specificity for ECT is in contrast with the lower efficacy of other therapies of depression and the distinctly lesser response of ECT in other psychiatric conditions.

Classifications of the depressions generally distinguish two types based on the presence or absence of physiologic dysfunction. It is this distinction that is most important in the decision of whether to use a biologic or a psychologic therapy (Pollitt, 1965a, b). In evaluating the clinical usefulness of ECT, the diagnosis of a psychological depression[3] is a poor prognostic sign. It may even be a principal contraindication to the use of ECT since the complication rate in such subjects may be substantial.

The response of endogenous depressed[4] patients to ECT is rapid and specific. We and others found the specificity to be so great that we suggested that changes in neurophysiologic or behavioral measures could be used to identify the members of a homogeneous population of patients with endogenous depression (Fink and Kahn, 1961). Roth (1951) and Roth et al. (1957) found that an increase in EEG slow wave activity to pentothal after the first seizure was prognostic of a good clinical outcome with few additional treatments. We interpreted their findings as evidence of the CNS sensitivity of this group of patients and confirmed their sensitivity to seizures (Fink and Kahn, 1957). In the intervening decades, no more valid classification of the endogenous depressed patient has been devised; we have restated this use of a therapeutic or a neurophysiologic response to ECT as a check on behavioral classification schemes (Fink, 1968, 1978a).

The specificity of the response to ECT in depressive psychosis may also be seen in the experience with tricyclic antidepressants in the treatment of depressed patients with delusions. In such cases, the tricyclic antidepressants are often ineffective, whereas ECT is rapidly effective.

Psychological Aspects

A theory of ECT should account for the differences in personality that characterize ECT responders from nonresponders. While the neurophysiologic and biochemical processes that characterize the brain changes of the therapeutic process provide the energy for changes in behavior, some other process must

---

[3] Psychological depression includes secondary, neurotic, personal, reactive, and justified depression in different classification schemes.

[4] Endogenous depression includes primary, psychotic, vital, somatic, and major depression in different classification schemes.

provide the direction in the behavioral adaptations that follow ECT. We are not yet able to translate cerebral biochemical and neurophysiologic events into psychologic constructs. It is tempting to assume that individual personality attributes, intelligence, mood, and affect are direct derivatives of differences in genetic strands, expressed through differing discharge rates and amounts of cerebral neurohumors, peptides, and hormones. But to relate micromolecular chemical changes to macrobehavioral events will require many more data and more viable constructs than now exist. Meanwhile, we are able to observe and measure the amnesia associated with ECT; we can describe and define personality attributes (as in the Rorschach, California F-scale, and perceptual tests) which bear some predictable relation to the behavioral and linguistic changes after ECT; and we can use the defense mechanisms of repression, regression, denial, and displacement that occur in patients during the ECT process for their therapeutic benefit. Until a better calculus of the biochemistry or physiology of behavior is defined, personality and psychological factors should remain significant aspects and important predictors of the therapeutic process.

MANIC PSYCHOSIS

ECT is an effective treatment for mania, particularly the manic phase of bipolar endogenous depression. In the early studies of ECT, its efficacy rate was similar to that found in the depressive psychoses. In later studies, manic patients required greater numbers of treatments than did depressed patients; often, the courses recommended for manic patients were comparable to those given schizophrenic patients. It is tempting to conclude that the early studies were successful with few treatments because the criteria for the selection of patients for ECT were more rigorous and the patients did, indeed, suffer from an endogenous mood disorder. In later studies, with the apparent safety of ECT defined, physicians were less discriminating and patients were selected for ECT who may have been suffering from manic-like disorders which were more related to schizophrenia than to a mood disorder. The classification of the mentally ill has changed in successive decades, often radically, and similarities in population samples remain a thorny problem in clinical research, awaiting a better image of the pathogenesis of the psychoses and genotypic classification criteria.

Present theories classify mania as a phase of the endogenous depressive syndrome. Some authors have examined the role of hormone dysfunctions in both the etiology and the manifestations of mania, and find that manic patients have hormonal patterns that are either similar to depressed patients or normal. For example, Gold (1977) reported that the GH response to l-dopa, the TSH response to TRH, and the urinary free cortisol production were increased in the depressed phase of bipolar depression but normal in the manic phase.

A parsimonious view of the mode of action of ECT in mania would assume that mania and depression are phases of the same illness. From the vantage of the hormonal theory of depression, the efficacy of ECT may also result from the stimulation of hypothalamic functions. It is equally plausible to suggest that mania results from an increased function of some hypothalamic nuclei; in such an instance, we need to seek elsewhere for an explanation of the efficacy of ECT in mania.

There are some interesting parallels in the treatment of mania by lithium and ECT. Electrophysiologic studies of patients receiving lithium therapy find synchronous slow wave activity, slowing of alpha rhythms, and increased EEG amplitudes associated with therapeutic levels of serum lithium. The changes become more prominent with toxic lithium levels (Small and Small, 1973). The EEG changes are consistent with either a diffuse toxic cerebral reaction or a localized dysfunction in brainstem structures similar to that seen with ECT. Further analyses and comparisons must await studies of ECT and lithium in patients with mania done under appropriate conditions and controls to assess their relative efficacy in different populations, with measurement of predictors of outcome, duration of treatment, and side-effects.

These views are speculative. There have been few recent trials of ECT in mania, and an assessment of the efficacy of ECT remains an academic exercise in the face of the general acceptance of the efficacy of lithium therapy, both for the relief of symptoms and as a prophylaxis. A theory of the efficacy of ECT in mania must await additional evidence as to its efficacy, studies of the hormonal patterns of mania and comparison with depression, and the direct measurement of neurohormonal changes after ECT in patients with mania.

CATATONIA

Although catatonia is described as a form of schizophrenia, its response to ECT is often so rapid and so dramatic that this classification should be reexamined. The symptoms of catatonia include negativism, withdrawal, hypotonia, stereotypy, stupor or excitement, and anorexia. Resolution with ECT is rapid, few inductions are needed, and the response is often long-lasting (Roth and Rosie, 1953; Sargant and Slater, 1963; Bernstein et al., 1977; Breakey and Kala, 1977; Regestein et al., 1977; Silverman, 1977).

Catatonia often arises from a matrix of a severe, generalized, inflammatory disease, such as typhoid fever or lupus erythematosus. While the cerebral manifestations are not well defined, there is evidence that cerebral dysfunction is a significant feature of the syndrome. EEG slowing and disorganization has been described during an acute attack; these resolve with clinical recovery (Walter, 1942; Rowntree and Kay, 1952; Breakey and Kala, 1977). Others find catatonia to arise in response to the central actions of some psychotropic drugs (Gelenberg and Mandel, 1977; Weinberger and Kelly, 1977; Weinberger and Wyatt, 1978).

Some authors find catatonic signs to be nonspecific, occurring in different psychiatric syndromes and generally having a good prognosis. In these analyses, the association with schizophrenia is only one of many associations. The association with mania is clearly defined; in such cases, catatonic signs are good prognostic indicators among patients treated by lithium, neuroleptics, or ECT. Catatonia, particularly the acute varieties, is prevalent among patients with bipolar affective disease (Abrams and Taylor, 1976a, 1977; Taylor and Abrams, 1977). Similar conclusions were proposed by others, including Kahlbaum (1874), Kirby (1913), Bonner and Kent (1936), Winokur et al. (1969), and Morrison (1973, 1974).

The acute onset and episodic nature of the illness, the absence of a long premorbid history of dysfunction, the lack of a progressive debilitating course, the high incidence among patients with affective illness, and the rapid and dramatic response to ECT distinguish this syndrome from that usually characterized as schizophrenia. It is likely that hypothalamic or centrencephalic dysfunction is a factor in the catatonic syndrome; and if so, the clinical efficacy of ECT may be related to the same mechanisms as in endogenous depression. The dysfunction of centrencephalic structures may arise from the exhaustion and stress of a severe life-threatening illness or the excitement and exhaustion of a manic state, rather than from the genetic or other unknown causes usually hypothesized for depressive states. In such conditions, ECT may directly stimulate the hypothalamus and act as if increasing the effective levels of cerebral monoaminergic activity. The continued classification of catatonia among the schizophrenias hampers the treatment of patients and limits our understanding of the syndrome. Further study should include assessments of hormone functions among catatonic patients and should seek parallels in dysfunctions of the affectively ill.

SCHIZOPHRENIA

Schizophrenia is a syndrome of protean manifestations and, probably, multiple etiologies. As a syndrome, it lacks the homogeneity in psychopathology, genetic and familial features, course, and responsivity to a defined therapy that characterize endogenous depression. The clinical efficacy of ECT is low, with a greater number of seizures given more frequently for a treatment response. Amnesia, confusion, and other aspects of an organic mental syndrome are usually important in the efficacy of ECT in such cases. Schizophrenic patients do not usually exhibit the vegetative symptoms or the altered hormonal functions described in depressive states; and improvement in the schizophrenic syndrome is not accompanied by systematic changes in these functions.

There is a great variation among the reports of the efficacy of ECT in schizophrenia. Since the diagnosis is so ill defined, it is probable that patients with other syndromes, which only superficially resemble schizophrenia, were included in samples treated with ECT. This is particularly true of patients with mania and catatonia. Manic patients with ideas of reference, motor excitement, hyperactivity, delusions, and affective disturbance are often erroneously classified as cases of schizophrenia. Catatonia is a syndrome that many authors define as a subtype of schizophrenia. However, both manic and catatonic patients respond to ECT rapidly with fewer treatments necessary for a course than for other types of schizophrenia. The underlying psychopathology of both mania and catatonia is more like that seen in the endogenous psychoses than in the schizophrenic syndrome. The reported efficacy of ECT in some schizophrenic populations probably is a result of the heterogeneity of the clinical samples selected for treatment rather than a reflection of a specific efficacy of ECT in schizophrenia (Fink, 1978c; in press).

It is also likely, considering the low efficacy of ECT, insulin coma, and leucotomy in schizophrenia, that the proclaimed success rate does not reflect a change in the pathophysiology of schizophrenia but results from a symptomatic alteration of the behavior of psychotic patients, so that they are more manageable and more tractable. In the initial surveys, the principal efficacy of ECT in schizophrenic patients was in the reduction in excitement, hypermotility, aggressivity, and delusional productions. The reduction in these symptoms is often accompanied by amnesia and a confusional syndrome, enhancing the patient's dependence and tractability (Weigert, 1940).

Drugs that are effective in the treatment of the depressive psychoses are either ineffective or even may exacerbate schizophrenia. Both the tricyclic antidepressant drugs and MAO inhibitors produce a worsening of the schizophrenic syndrome (Klein and Fink, 1962a; Kramer et al., 1961; Brune and Himwich, 1963; Pollack et al., 1965).

Biochemical theories of the pathogenesis of schizophrenia and of the mode of action of antipsychotic drugs focus on dopamine hyperfunction and its blockade rather than on the catecholamines and acetylcholine. Hypothalamic functions are altered by antipsychotic drugs, as evidenced by the heightened release of prolactin after the administration of effective antipsychotic drugs. A similar finding, an elevation of prolactin, has been reported in patients treated with ECT, suggesting that hormonal analyses may yet find other similarities between the antipsychotic drugs and ECT (Öhman et al., 1976; O'Dea et al., 1978).[5]

Studies of normal, psychoneurotic, and depressed psychotic patients often demonstrate a responsivity of hormonal measures to stress, but the same studies in schizophrenic subjects usually find a decrease in responsivity. For example, stress elevates the secretion of ACTH and the urinary levels of corticosteroids in nonschizophrenic populations (Spiegel and Spiegel-Adolf, 1953; Rubin and Mandell, 1966; Fawcett and Bunney, 1967). Schizophrenic patients fail to show a hypotensive response to subcutaneous methacholine and a hypertensive response to intravenous epinephrine, reflecting a decreased reactivity of the autonomic nervous system (Funkenstein et al., 1948; Gellhorn, 1956). Such lack of neurohumoral responsivity may be a factor in the decreased sensitivity to ECT and suggests that the action of ECT may not lie in the same neurohumoral mechanisms in these subjects as in depressive subjects.

In view of the different responsivity, need for a greater number of treatments, dependence on an organic mental syndrome, and absence of data reflecting hypothalamic or hormonal dysfunction in schizophrenia, it is difficult to encompass the clinical activity of ECT in schizophrenic patients in the same hypothesis

---

[5] For comment, see page 148.

that is useful in patients with endogenous depression. It is more likely that ECT is a nonspecific treatment in schizophrenic patients, not unlike the efficacy of insulin coma and leucotomy, depending more on confusion, amnesia, and generalized cerebral dysfunction to assure tractability, compliance, and reduced psychomotor activity than on specific neurohumoral mechanisms to alleviate a specific central dysfunction.

A number of authors cite the relationship of the efficacy of these treatments to the development of a severe organic mental syndrome. Thus Revitch (1954) and Fink (1957, 1962) emphasized the greater therapeutic success of insulin coma in patients who have suffered a prolonged coma. Success in leucotomy is related to the extent of the lesions, since many patients require multiple operations for efficacy (Freeman, 1967; Kalinowsky and Hippius, 1972). Regressive ECT is reported to be more effective than conventional courses of ECT in chronic schizophrenia.

If there is a central neurohumoral mechanism to ECT in schizophrenia, its elucidation will require more intensive study of the hormonal, biochemical, and physiologic features of both the schizophrenic process and the effects of seizures. Such a theory must await additional data, particularly regarding the efficacy of ECT in this syndrome.

CONCLUSION

ECT is a special intervention which increases the activity of central neurohumors and releases hypothalamic peptides for the relief of the primary depressive syndrome—a syndrome characterized by hypothalamic dysfunction. ECT may be viewed as a complex procedure of "diencephalic stimulation" to achieve a behavioral change.

The relevance of similar theories for the response of manic, catatonic, and schizophrenic patients is unclear. Considering their responsivity, the same mechanisms may operate for catatonic and manic patients. In schizophrenia, however, the significant physiologic and biochemical events for ECT probably differ from those in primary depression, since efficacy, specificity, frequency, and numbers of seizures differ, and dependence on defined vegetative symptoms is much less.

The rapid response of catatonic patients is noted, and a review of the classification and pathophysiology of these disorders is suggested.

TECHNICAL ISSUES

Convulsive therapy has undergone many modifications. Most have been of a technical nature in modifying the induction methods. Although many changes have been discarded and replaced by newer methods, much has been learned about the ECT process and about seizures during these trials (Chapter 15). The usage of ECT is also undergoing change, and it seems useful to relate experimental data to clinical practice to develop guidelines for treatment, as a reference for different tactics in patient care, and as a text for training (Chapter 16).

Chapter 15

Methods of Seizure Induction

PENTYLENETETRAZOL

Once Meduna (1938) conceptualized the value of inducing epilepsy in patients with schizophrenia, he experimented with various convulsants in animals and found intramuscular camphor to be safe. Patients were first treated in January, 1934, but missed seizures, panic, fear, and pain at the injection sites led to trials with other convulsants. Pentylenetetrazol [Metrazol, cardiazol, pentetrazol], a synthetic CNS stimulant, was safer and more reliable, and rapidly replaced camphor. From 5 to 7 cc of a 10% buffered solution was injected rapidly. If a seizure did not occur within 1 min, 8 to 10 cc was injected; and if that failed, dosages were increased by 1 to 3 cc.

To provide amnesia, treatments were often given with patients in a light coma induced by insulin or after barbiturate or nitrous oxide anesthesia. The convulsions were often severe and the risk of fracture high. Patients often experienced panic and fear between the injection and the onset of the seizure; and if a seizure did not occur, fear was intense. As described by Weigert (1940):

> The intravenous injection of metrazol was regularly followed by an aura that was marked by the facial expression of terror, and left in the patient a memory of helpless surrender to annihilation. After these moments—sometimes even minutes—of terror a seizure usually occurred, in occasional instances only a petit-mal, which was described by some patients as particularly dissatisfying, leaving them more restless and more excited. The usual seizure was similar to a typical epileptic grand-mal with unconsciousness and pathological reflexes; the tonic phase being sometimes introduced by irregular muscle-twitching, and followed by a clonic phase with impairment of breathing and typical circulatory changes. In the tonic phase the mouth was frequently widely opened even to the extent of jaw-dislocation; at the end of the tonic phase the mouth became tightly closed, persisting into the clonic and ensuing flaccidity-phase, so that it was often difficult to remove the mouth-gag inserted to prevent the typical tongue-bite. The other sphincter muscles frequently relaxed in this state of flaccidity, leading to urination, defecation and, in men, to emission without erection. Awakening out of unconsciousness most patients were confused, excited, restless, partly amnestic or aphasic. Becoming more or less aware of this impairment of ego-functions, the patients succeeded more or less quickly in regaining their orientation and self-mastery, sometimes after a short recuperative slumber. In this recovery-period we observed usually a heightened readiness of the patient to cling to personnel for help and support. Some patients complained of headache and nausea. The appetite was sometimes destroyed for the whole day; in other cases the patients experienced a heightened need for food. The repetition of the metrazol injection—three times weekly for several weeks—was experienced by almost all patients as a threat against life. One patient had an increase

in pulse rate up to 154 before injection. The repetition made the patients partly resistive, combative, partly subdued, intimidated in their further attitude towards the treatment [pp. 195–196].

Pentylenetetrazol treatments were found effective in patients with major psychoses (Bennett, 1938, 1939; Küppers, 1938; Müller, 1939; Delgado, 1939; Meduna and Friedman, 1939; Kwalwasser, 1940; Chase and Silverman, 1941). Treatments were given with varying frequency from daily to two or three times weekly. Complication rates were high, however, and there was much effort to find a more consistent convulsant, leading to the development of electric inductions.

Few studies compare pentylenetetrazol and electric inductions directly, and these find the treatments to have almost equivalent clinical efficacy (Küppers, 1938; Malzberg, 1943), although some find a greater efficacy for pentylenetetrazol (Bianchi and Chiarello, 1947). The ease and reliability of the induction of a seizure and the reduction in the incidence of incomplete petit mal seizures with ECT were so apparent that ECT rapidly replaced pentylenetetrazol. To reduce the dose of pentylenetetrazol, some authors used repetitive stimulation (such as intense flickering lights) to augment the cerebral stimulation of the drug. Some authors reported photopentylenetetrazol superior to ECT (Ulett et al., 1956), but most found no advantages over electric inductions.

Pentylenetetrazol is occasionally used today by some therapists for severe, chronic cases of schizophrenia and for patients with unusually high thresholds to an electric induction. In the latter instance, intravenous administration of 2 to 6 cc of 10% pentylenetetrazol is immediately followed by an electric induction in a fully anesthetized patient.

ELECTRIC INDUCTION

Before the development of the seizure therapies for the mentally ill, convulsions were induced electrically in experimental studies of epilepsy and to determine the efficacy of anticonvulsants (Bini, 1937; Spiegel, 1937; Merritt and Putnam, 1938). Similar studies by Cerletti and Bini in Italy provided the experience that led them to substitute an electric induction for pentylenetetrazol in psychotic patients. After experiments in animals which assured him of the safety of the method, Cerletti treated a catatonic schizophrenic patient, using frontoparietal electrodes and an alternating current of 80 V for 0.2 sec. The seizure was incomplete, and a second administration of 110 V for 0.2 sec was followed by a classic grand mal convulsion (Cerletti, 1956):

> We observed the same instantaneous, brief, generalized spasm, and soon after, the onset of the classic epileptic convulsion. We were all breathless during the tonic phase of the attack, and really overwhelmed during the apnea as we watched the cadaverous cyanosis of the patient's face; the apnea of the spontaneous epileptic convulsion is always impressive, but at that moment it seemed to all of us painfully endless. Finally, with the first stertorous breathing and the first clonic spasm, the blood flowed better

not only in the patient's vessels but also in our own. Thereupon we observed with the most intensely gratifying sensation the characteristic gradual awakening of the patient "by steps." He rose to a sitting position and looked at us, calm and smiling, as though to enquire what we wanted of him. We asked: "What happened to you?" He answered: "I don't know. Maybe I was asleep." Thus occurred the first electrically produced convulsion in man, which I at once named "electroshock" [p. 94].

The method of induction was the principal concern in the use of convulsive therapy. Many electric parameters were examined: (a) current type, wave form, and current characteristics (voltage, resistance or impedance, and milliamperage), (b) duration of the pulses and total duration of the application, (c) mode of onset, whether instantaneous or gradual *(glissando)*, (d) electrode size, and (e) location of the electrodes on the head.

Currents

Cerletti and Bini modified the 50-cycle alternating current obtained from a central electric utility by a timer (limiting the discharge of currents to 0.5 to 1.5 sec), a rheostat allowing the voltage to vary from 50 to 150 V, and a milliameter to measure the current flow. They defined the basic requirements for seizure induction as 80 to 115 V applied for 0.5 to 0.7 sec, which for a 50-Hz signal yielded 0.3 to 0.6 Amp (Cerletti and Bini, 1938). Others introduced a rectifier to allow unidirectional currents to reach the subjects. The design of most instruments used for ECT since 1940 has been based on these simple devices (Alexander, 1953; Davies et al., 1971). Electronic instruments have recently been devised which produce rectangular pulses of defined voltage, number, spacing, and duration, allowing a more accurate control of the electric parameters (Blachly, 1976; Weaver et al., 1977).

Although seizures were elicited safely and easily by unrectified alternating currents, the disturbing effects of amnesia, confusion, postseizure excitement, and agitation compelled researchers to alter the characteristics of the currents to forms deemed more "physiologic." The amperage was lowered and the currents rectified so that instead of 50 or 60 pulses alternating direction each second within the head, half the number of pulses would be discharged in one direction only (Delmas-Marsalet, 1942; Friedman, 1942; Friedman and Wilcox, 1942). This technique has come to be known as unidirectional sine wave currents. Others changed the shape of the waves to square waves of short duration with long interpulse intervals, the so-called brief-stimulus therapy (BST) (Liberson, 1945; Offner, 1946). Each instrument was progressively modified to decrease the amount of energy delivered, so that it is difficult to speak of a single set of characteristics for any wave form. Early unidirectional instruments were rated to deliver 40 mAmp of rectified current for 1.0 to 2.0 sec. As these required long durations to induce a seizure, irregularly spaced complex sharp wave spikes were superimposed on the rectified currents. These instruments were said to elicit seizures with only 6 mAmp of current for 2 to 3 sec (Alexander, 1953).

Brief Stimuli

Liberson (1953) decreased the duration of individual pulses in a brief stimulus instrument and added a resistance-estimating device that regulated the voltages delivered in accordance with changes in resistance. The energy delivered was further reduced by employing very brief square wave pulses of 0.2 to 0.5 msec, approximately 120/sec, which yielded about 350 mAmp of current when delivered for 0.5 to 1.0 sec (Alexander, 1953).

By the late 1940s, clinical trials found favorable reports for each of the three principal currents then in use—alternating currents (Cerletti-Bini, sine wave therapy), unidirectional rectified currents (Friedman-Wilcox), and BST (Liberson). Clinical equivalence was claimed for unidirectional and alternating current seizures, with fewer complaints or evidence of amnesia and confusion, especially in elderly patients, and a more rapid awakening for the unidirectional currents (Goldman, 1949; Epstein and Wender, 1956). BST engendered greater amounts of fear, which could be controlled by an anesthetic before treatment. Unidirectional current treatment was reported to be clinically effective: 86% recovered and improved among depressive, 66% among schizophrenic, and 22% among neurotic patients (Impastato et al., 1951, 1952). The mean number of treatments was 8.9, which was comparable to an average of 10 treatments for the alternating current instruments. Fractures, flexor spasm, postconvulsive apnea, and memory impairment were less than in an earlier period when an alternating current instrument had been used. Many patients, however, required multiple applications; i.e., missed seizures were common with unidirectional currents, even when repeated or maintained in an extended application.

BST was associated with a lesser organic mental syndrome, more favorable patient acceptance, and a greater opportunity for psychotherapy than alternating current treatments (Medlicott, 1948; Liberson et al., 1956). Unidirectional and brief stimulus currents were estimated as clinically equal to the alternating currents, with lesser evidence of an organic mental syndrome. The modified currents made maintenance treatments possible, but also:

> [a] much more vivid antipathy toward and apprehension of treatment is noted with brief stimuli treatment, a problem which is sometimes overcome by giving treatment after the intravenous injection of pentothal sodium [Alexander, 1953, p. 64].

Other Wave Forms

Bayles et al. (1950) compared sine wave stimuli (110 to 135 V for 0.2 to 0.4 sec) and brief pulse stimuli (0.5 to 0.7 msec, 8 msec interpulse interval, peak of 250 to 500 mAmp, and average of 20 to 60 mAmp for 1.3 to 2.0 sec), finding that the clinical evaluations were equivalent in patients with depression. Memory loss and confusion, however, were less in those patients who were treated with brief stimuli (66 versus 90%). The severity of the seizures was the same, but the EEG records after alternating current treatments showed more severe abnormality than after BST, a finding consistent with the clinical measures of confusion.

The effects of unidirectional sawtooth-shaped waves (5 msec duration, 15 msec interval) were compared to ultrashort square waves (0.1 msec duration and 67 msec interval) by Cronholm and Ottosson (1963a, b). A third sample of the patients received the unidirectional current induction with lidocaine premedication. Seizures of equal length were induced by both modified currents, although the amount of energy was less with the ultrashort (BST, Elther instrument) currents. There was a lesser interference with memory tests and lesser clinical efficacy for the BST treatments compared to the currents derived from the unidirectional sawtooth waves from the Siemens Konvulsator III instrument. They also noted that seizures were subtotal in four subjects receiving BST treatment, and there seemed to be a more rapid postseizure recovery.

The clinical and electrographic effects of seizures induced by alternating currents at both suprathreshold and threshold voltages were compared with those of unidirectional currents (Fink et al., 1958b). Assessments were made after four to six, seven to nine, and 10 to 12 treatments. While each treatment induced EEG slow wave activity, suprathreshold alternating currents elicited greater degrees of slowing earlier than treatment with either modified current, the latter showing no distinctions. Clinical assessments of improvement followed the same patterns, with greater improvement found after the alternating current suprathreshold treatments.

Various other authors have compared alternating, unidirectional, and brief stimuli currents, generally finding equivalent clinical efficacy and some small differences in effects on memory or physiologic indices (Proctor and Goodwin, 1945; Moriarty and Siemens, 1947; Wilcox, 1947; Gayle and Josephs, 1948; Lindner and Brouschek, 1953; Epstein and Wender, 1956; Kendall et al., 1956). Where differences are observed, the findings show that alternating currents produce better clinical results in shorter time and with greater disturbances in memory tests and EEG than the unidirectional and BST methods.

In other physiologic studies, the unidirectional and brief stimulus currents elicited lesser EEG changes than after alternating currents (Proctor and Goodwin, 1943; Liberson, 1953), lesser neurovegetative side-effects associated with the convulsion (Alexander, 1953), and memory scores were less affected (Liberson, 1953).

Despite the favorable encomia for the modified currents, however, alternating current instruments continued to enjoy clinical favor as providing more predictable seizures and more reliable clinical results.

Subconvulsive Currents

The clinical efficacy of subconvulsive currents has been examined. At first, such low voltage currents were found to be as effective as seizure-inducing currents in uncontrolled studies (Androp, 1941; Berkwitz, 1942; Delmas-Marsalet, 1946; Alexander, 1953). In studies comparing subconvulsive with convulsive currents, the efficacy of the convulsive treatments was superior (Miller et al., 1953; Ulett, 1953; Ulett et al., 1956; Fink et al., 1958b; Sainz, 1959). At one time, it was thought that subconvulsive or petit mal responses would be useful in the elderly, weak, or physically incapacitated patients in whom a softer treatment would be safer. However, petit mal responses are not clinically effective (Kalinowsky et al., 1942; Ziskind et al., 1945) and have been associated with death (Cropper and Hughes, 1964).

Others sought to give extended electric stimulation at subconvulsive levels, either following or in the absence of a seizure. This extended stimulation was termed electronarcosis and was initially thought to be effective in cases of schizophrenia. In these treatments, stimulation was continued for 5 to 7 min or longer at settings of unidirectional instruments to deliver 45 to 150 mAmp currents, often to maintain conditions of stridor for the stimulation period. The treatments were described by Frostig et al. (1944), Tietz (1947), Alexander (1953), and Paterson (1963). Many authors saw electronarcosis as an analog to insulin coma and suggested it be used in refractory cases, either alone or with insulin. With the appearance of psychotropic drugs, these special nonconvulsive treatments were rapidly replaced.

The persistence of complaints of amnesia has led to a number of recent studies of modified currents. Valentine et al. (1968) compared the clinical results and side-effects of two currents to induce convulsions—a pulse current of low power (0.2 msec width, 45 msec interpulse width, 300 mAmp, 5 sec, 10 joules; Ectonus Mark III) with a sinusoidal current (260 V peak to peak for 1 sec = 30 joules; Ectron A. C. Mains). They also compared bilateral bitemporal and unilateral nondominant placement of electrodes in the same experiment. They studied 24 depressed patients and found the same reduction in depressive ratings regardless of current type or electrode placement. The number of treatments given for the bilateral placement was 8.8 and for unilateral placement 7.2, which they considered equivalent.

Carney and Sheffield (1974) studied the effects of six or more treatments with brief pulse currents [similar to that of Valentine et al. (1968)] with bilateral electrode placement in both neurotic $(N = 22)$ and psychotic $(N = 53)$ depressed patients. They found a greater efficacy in endogenous depressed patients (72% recovered) than in neurotic depressed (32%) and concluded that pulse ECT was beneficial in endogenous depression.

Following the observations of Ottosson (1960) that the antidepressant and amnesic effects of ECT could be separated by the use of currents with minimal energy, Maxwell (1968) described the current characteristics of a number of instruments. Using a solid state thyristor modified current, he reported that seizures could be induced in 59% of inductions with current density of 28 joules, and that by increasing the voltage to 240 V, seizures could be induced in 99% of inductions at 96 joules using currents with a narrow pulse width (2 msec), fast rise and sharp turn-off, high repetition rate (> 100 Hz), and peak voltage of 200 to 600 V. Maxwell (1968) notes that a similar instrument had been designed by Strauss and MacPhail (1946) using a mechanical vibrator to achieve the short pulses needed for minimal current therapy.

Low Energy—Brief Pulse Current

Weaver and his co-workers designed an electronic instrument to control the current parameters for a low energy-brief pulse (LEBS) treatment. Weaver et al. (1974) found that seizures could be induced in rats by combinations of number of pulses, pulse duration, current, and interpulse interval that exceeded a defined threshold for total energy delivered. Contrary to Liberson (1948, 1953), Weaver et al. found that a single pulse of high amperage could produce a seizure, provided the energy was at least 0.5 to 1.0 joule. For 10 or more pulses, the total energy needed was 0.15 to 0.20 joules. Trains of discrete pulses produced satisfactory seizures, and pulse widths greater than 1 msec did not enhance seizure induction. Interpulse intervals had no effect up to 20 msec. From these studies, they confirmed that pulsed unidirectional stimuli produce adequate seizures at energy levels that are significantly less than conventional alternating currents.

In a clinical study, Weaver et al. (1977) compared seizures produced by two types of currents in 20 depressed, hospitalized patients; 17 met and two almost met the diagnostic criteria for primary depression, and one for secondary depression. Standard treatment used a Medcraft B-24 (AC) instrument which delivered 150 V RMS for 0.5 sec and, by their calculation, delivered 29 joules. An experimental instrument (LEBS) delivered 150 square wave pulses of alternating polarity, each pulse width 1 msec, interpulse interval, 10 msec, and, by calculation, it delivered 16 joules. They reported an equivalent clinical reduction in depression, anxiety, and other clinical scores and equivalent changes in psychological performance tests for the two inductions. Both methods induced seizures reliably, with 53% total energy and 18% peak current for the brief stimulus instrument compared to the alternating current instrument. They concluded that (a) neither alternating currents nor glissando were necessary for ECT; (b) measured currents of defined dosage (joules) could be used successfully; and (c) modified currents reduced the risks of the direct effects of larger currents. In another report, Weaver et al. (1978) examined the minimum number of LEBS pulses required to induce a seizure in bilateral and unilateral ECT. Fewer pulses were required with unilateral electrode placement than with bilateral.

Blachly, as an outgrowth of his interest in EEG monitoring of seizures, developed an electronic device for EST in which pulse width (0.15 to 1.5 msec), interpulse interval (7 to 25 msec), and duration (0.5 to 20 sec) could be varied. The instrument (MECTA) is designed to deliver a constant current (800 mAmp), varying the voltages to deliver energy levels of 0.6 to 80 joules. The MECTA has built-in, fail-safe features, including a device to measure the impedance between electrodes and to prevent a discharge of the instrument if the resistance is outside a preset range. The instrument also has two built-in oscillographs and amplifiers to record EKG and EEG during each treatment, providing an accurate record of changes in these measures, particularly of seizure duration. The clinical efficacy and relative usefulness of the instrument, like that of Weaver (LEBS), is yet to be demonstrated.

These studies find the therapeutic results and the physiologic effects of seizures induced by modified currents to be virtually equivalent to alternating currents. When differences are determined, the modified currents are associated with lesser physiologic and behavioral effects. These observations are inconsistent with beliefs that seizures are all-or-none phenomena, as seizures with modified currents consistently show earlier awakening, variations in seizure pattern, decreased EEG abnormality, and decreased amnesia. The lesser efficacy may be related to a modified seizure activity, which unfortunately has not been carefully studied by EEG methods. The studies leave unresolved whether direct effects of the currents and total energy contribute to the therapeutic (antidepressant) and amnesic processes of ECT, or whether the differences are wholly explained by differences in the seizure pattern (Cronholm and Ottosson, 1963a; Ottosson, 1960). The studies emphasize the merit in the use of minimal doses to elicit seizures, but it is clear that the available instruments have built-in limitations—modified currents bring with them a reduction in therapeutic efficacy. New instruments need to be developed that deliver brief pulse stimuli, as described by Maxwell (1968), with the instruments calibrated in joules rather than the intermediate measures of voltage, duration, or milliamperage. In the interim, the available instruments used for ECT should be examined to be sure that they function according to specifications while new instruments meeting better physiologic criteria are designed and tested (Davies et al., 1971).

Electrodes

Therapists exhibited as much ingenuity in locating the stimulating electrodes as they did in devising different wave forms to elicit seizures. Cerletti and Bini (1938) used large, flat disc electrodes applied to the frontoparietal regions in their first treatments. In a discussion of the effects of modified currents, Friedman (1942) noted that bitemporal and unilateral temporal-vertex electrodes were in general use:

> Admittedly a number of other leads were just as effective though not nearly as practical. For example, the pharyngeal-vertex, the bi-occipital, the shoulder-vertex (using a large negative pole on the shoulder or back) electrode placements have been tried in a number of cases and found to be quite effective and the corresponding convulsive doses just as low. But each of the placements seemed to have special disadvantages. Cooperation of the patient was usually difficult to obtain to place an electrode in the oropharyngeal mucosa. Unusually severe inspiratory gasps resulted from low bi-occipital placements, suggesting medullary stimulation. Shoulder-vertex directions were deemed inadvisable when simultaneous EKG tracings indicated passage of current through the cardiac axes [p. 218].

For the most part, the treatments were given through temporal-vertex, bilateral temporal, or bilateral frontoparietal electrodes, as these were easy to apply. The skin was readily accessible for cleansing and for the application of electrode contact materials, and the side-effects (other than burns under poorly applied electrodes) were minimal. When electrodes were placed posteriorly, patients often complained of diplopia, ataxia, nausea, and vomiting, and such locations were generally avoided (Cannicott, 1962). The persistence of amnesia, confusion, postseizure anxiety, and fear in ECT, however, led to trials with focal stimulation technics (Impastato and Pacella, 1952; Impastato et al., 1953; Pacella and Impastato, 1954), monopolar stimulation (Epstein, 1955), and various unilateral electrode placements (Blaurock et al., 1950; Thenon, 1956; Lancaster et al., 1958; Cannicott, 1962; Dolenz, 1964; Gottlieb and Wilson, 1965; Martin et al., 1965) to reduce these complications.

Focal Seizures

Paterson (1952) experimented with techniques to limit the spread of the currents to an area between electrodes. A description of his experience led Impastato and Pacella (1952) to induce a unilateral fit, placing electrodes about 2 inches apart on one side of the head, with continuous, low voltage unidirectional currents. In anesthetized patients, a unilateral (focal, Jacksonian) fit was limited to one side, without spread to the other side or the development of a grand mal convulsion. The focal seizures were less effective than grand mal treatments (Impastato et al., 1953; Pacella and Impastato, 1954). In EEG recordings, persistent focal changes did not occur, and the number of abnormal records (those with slow wave activity) was significantly less than in patients after a grand mal seizure, whether through unilateral or bilateral electrodes (Bergman et al., 1953).

Electrostimulation of discrete cortical sites through very fine electrodes was described by Heath and Norman (1946), who noted that it was possible to elicit specific focal neurologic effects from scalp electrodes by carefully controlling the intensity of the currents and the location of the electrodes. Negrin (1957) also describes stimulation through intracerebral electrodes, but he presents no compelling data to encourage this approach.

In another modification, both convulsive and subconvulsive stimulation treatments were given through a hand-held, insulated, active disc electrode held over different parts of the head and a large, indifferent electrode over the right forearm (Epstein, 1955). With unidirectional currents of low amperage, Epstein maintained subconvulsive stimulation or elicited focal or grand mal convulsions; as the modification lacked advantages over conventional electrodes, however, it was rarely used.

To stimulate the diencephalon directly, Breitner (1957) induced seizures through a fine intranasal needle electrode placed in the retropharyngeal wall using continuous subconvulsive stimulation. He placed a second large electrode on the scalp at the vertez. Although he described some favorable results, difficulties with the procedure precluded controlled testing.

In administering focal or monopolar treatments, the spread of currents was not always confined, and typical bilateral grand mal convulsions often developed, with an improvement in clinical status and the development of amnesia and EEG abnormality. Others sought to elicit grand mal convulsions with unilaterally placed electrodes, believing that the severity of the amnesia was related, in part, to the passage of the current. It was soon apparent that convulsions induced through unilateral electrode placements were clinically effective and, indeed, produced less amnesia.

Unilateral Electrodes

The efficacy of seizures induced through unilateral electrodes over the dominant or nondominant hemispheres were compared to seizures induced through conventional bilateral (bitemporal) electrodes. The effects on memory function, performance tests, and EEG in different clinical conditions have been studied extensively. The reviews by d'Elia (1970a, b, 1974), d'Elia and Raotma (1975), Sand-Strömgren (1973), and Squire (1977) summarize the experience well.

The clinical results in 19 studies of unilateral and bilateral ECT were compared; although the studies were hardly comparable in patient selection, number and frequency of treatments, electrode position, or criteria of outcome, they did reflect the marketplace of experience (d'Elia, 1974). The mean number of treatments for bilateral ECT was 7.14 and for nondominant unilateral ECT, 6.95. In overall antidepressant efficacy, a judgment made on reviewing the clinical data in each study, d'Elia found one study in which unilateral treatments were less effective, six in which the results were not completely equal with some advantage for bilateral ECT, and 11 in which the treatments were clinically equal.

Sand-Strömgren (1973) reported no statistical difference in therapeutic effect between bilateral and unilateral nondominant ECT, but she qualified her findings: (a) the therapeutic results were better among the older patients suffering from endogenous depression; (b) efficacy of the first six treatments was slightly better for bilateral than for unilateral treatment; and (c) unilateral-treated patients required an average of 0.5 more treatments before termination.

In a second assessment of the relative clinical efficacy of the two electrode placements, d'Elia and Raotma (1975) summarized the findings of 29 studies, 10 more than in the earlier summary (d'Elia, 1974). They divided the studies into five groups, according to the use of controls: no control group ($N = 5$); nonsimultaneous control ($N = 3$); simultaneous controls, with random assignment, double-blind assessments, but heterogeneous groups ($N = 8$); with homogeneous groups and a fixed number of treatments ($N = 5$); and with a free number of treatments ($N = 8$). Fourteen studies reported equal antidepressant efficacy;

13 found nondominant unilateral treatment somewhat less effective (in one study, unilateral ECT was rated as decidedly less effective); and two studies found unilateral treatment somewhat more effective than bilateral treatment (Table 15.1).

Follow-up data in five studies showed the efficacy of the treatments equal in three studies and slightly more effective for unilateral nondominant treatment in two studies. Follow-up periods were 1 to 3 months in four studies and 3 to 12 months in one study. d'Elia and Raotma concluded that nondominant unilateral ECT has the same antidepressive effect as bilateral ECT.

Among the more recent reports, Reichert et al. (1976a, b) found the clinical efficacy of bilateral and unilateral nondominant ECT in patients with psychotic depression equal on physicians' rating, but the patients' self-rating found bilateral ECT superior in symptom relief. More patients in the unilateral ECT group (26%) required additional ECT within 1 month of the assessment than did those in the bilateral ECT group (3%).

Technically, nondominant ECT may be less simple to administer than bilateral ECT, and they considered that much of the clinical dissatisfaction with the efficacy of unidirectional ECT was related to the provocation of submaximal seizures. The average number of seizures differed in the two treatments, with 6.4 for bilateral and 7.3 for nondominant unilateral treatments among patients rated as severely depressed, and 6.0 for bilateral and 6.7 for nondominant unilateral among patients rated as mildly depressed. In assessing other criteria of seizure activity, such as duration of the seizure and the EEG seizure and postseizure patterns, d'Elia and Raotma also found differences among the electrode placements.

My own review of the many studies of unilateral and bilateral ECT agree with the assessment by d'Elia and Raotma (1975). The clinical data clearly define the efficacy of ECT to be related to the induction of the seizure. It is more difficult to achieve a successful seizure of equivalent length through unilateral electrodes; yet it is probable that, were seizure duration monitored, the efficacy of the two electrode placements would be equivalent. The one study in which the efficacy of unilateral nondominant electrode placement was rated as decidedly less effective than bilateral ECT was that reported by Abrams et al. (1972). The study was done in my laboratory, in patients in a private mental hospital in New York. Assignment of patients to treatment was not random; the diagnoses were complex and quite heterogeneous; and the treatments were not administered uniformly. Evidence for the latter is clearly evident in the lesser EEG abnormality and the shorter duration of EEG seizure activity (61.9 versus 51.5 sec) for patients treated through unilateral electrode placements (Abrams et al., 1973b).

Comparisons of the efficacy of the two electrode placements for patients with schizophrenia find the efficacy equivalent (Abrams, 1967; El-Islam et al., 1970; Doongaji et al., 1973). In a study of the EEG findings of unilateral and bilateral

TABLE 15.1. *Immediate antidepressant efficacy*

Authors	No. of patients BI-ECT	ND-ECT	No. of ECTs BI-ECT	ND-ECT	−2	−1	0	+1	+2
Group I									
1. Bilikiewicz and Krzyzowski, 1964	—	13	—	4.8		X			
2. Impastato and Karliner, 1966	—	42	—	11	X				
3. Jensen, 1968	—	46	—	—	X				
4. Rinaldi, Manacorda, and Mazzarella, 1967	—	—	—	—		X			
5. Pancheri, 1969	—	20	—	11		X			
Group II									
6. Cannicott, 1962	51	40	7.2	6.3		X			
7. Abrams, Fink et al., 1972	43	33	—	—	X				
8. Hinterhuber and Nowak, 1973	61	85	6.8	8.6		X			
Group III									
9. Di Perri, Meduri, and Messina, 1969	18	18	6	6	X				
10. Giberti, 1969	16	16	8	8	X				
11. Halliday, Davison et al., 1968	18	18	4	4	X				
12. Lancaster, Steinert, and Frost, 1958	15	21	4	4	X				
13. Pavan, Semerano, and Agius, 1969	30	30	6	6		X			
14. McAndrew, Berkey, and Matthew, 1967	12	12	8.0	7.8		X			
15. Small, Small, et al., 1970	65	12	22	22	X				
16. Sutherland, Oliver, and Knight 1969	14	13	5.6	5.5		X			
Group IV									
17. Abrams and de Vito, 1969	10	11	6	6		X			
18. Cronin, Bodley, et al., 1970	15	16	8	8	X				
19. Fleminger et al., 1970	12	11	6	6	X				
20. Levy, 1968	39	40	6	6	X				
21. Martin, Ford, et al., 1965	20	20	10	10					X
Group V									
22. Bidder, Strain, and Brunschwig 1970	7	7	10.4	8.2		X			
23. Cannicott, 1962	20	30	6.7	7.0	X				
24. Costello, Belton, et al., 1970	10	10	—	—		X			
25. d'Elia, 1970	29	30	6.2	7.0		X			
26. Sand-Stromgren, 1973	48	52	8.7	8.9		X			
27. Strain, Brunschwig, et al., 1968	46	50	7.5	8.4	X				
28. Valentine, Keddie, and Dunne, 1968	—	—	8.8	7.2		X			
29. Zinkin and Birtchnell, 1968	20	24	8.0	8.3				X	

From d'Elia and Raotma, 1975 (page 84).
−2 = ND-ECT decidedly less effective
−1 = ND-ECT somewhat less effective according to clinical impression
 0 = equal efficacy
+1 = ND-ECT somewhat more effective according to clinical impression
+2 = ND-ECT decidedly more effective

ECT among depressive and schizophrenic patients, Marjerrison et al. (1975) found significantly less EEG change (variance of amplitude integration) after nondominant unilateral ECT than after bilateral ECT in schizophrenic patients. The clinical response, however, was not distinguishable, leading the authors to question whether their sample of schizophrenic patients may not have had some unique sample characteristics (Reichert et al., 1976 a, b).

There are differences in the seizure and the interseizure EEG and in effects on memory and performance tests between seizures induced through unilateral and bilateral electrode placements. These are discussed among the experimental studies (see Chapter 8 for EEG and Chapter 9 for memory and performance tasks).

Various other locations for electrodes have been examined in efforts to improve efficacy or minimize amnesia. Anterior bifrontal placements, in which currents were thought to bypass the temporoparietal speech centers, were tried (Inglis, 1969; Abrams and Taylor, 1973). Four and eight seizures successfully reduced depression rating scale scores, and the effects were concluded to be intermediate between unilateral and bilateral ECT. Neither changes in Wechsler memory tests nor confusion or clouding of consciousness were observed, similar to their experience with unilateral nondominant ECT. Abrams and Taylor (1974) also compared the effects of two nondominant unilateral seizures, a unilateral nondominant and a unilateral dominant, and a conventional bilateral treatment; they found no difference in depression rating scale scores after four treatments or in the global estimate of treatment response after the treatment course.

As a further test of the path of current on antidepressant efficacy and amnesia, Abrams and Taylor (1976b) compared conventional bilateral ECT with treatment through simultaneous unilateral electrode placements to both sides of the head in 20 patients with endogenous depression. They found that six bilateral ECT were more effective than dominant/nondominant unilateral ECT in reducing depression rating scale scores. Furthermore, 10 of the 11 patients in the simultaneous unilateral ECT group required additional treatment (average 4.2 treatments), whereas only three of nine in the bilateral ECT group required more treatment (average 1.8 treatments).

A comparison of frontoparietal and temporoparietal placements for unilateral ECT found little difference in intensity of currents necessary to induce the seizure, although the duration of seizure activity was notably shorter for the frontoparietal placement (50.5 ± 23.7 versus 56.7 ± 20.6 sec, $p \leq 0.01$) (d'Elia and Widepalm, 1974). The effects on memory were indistinguishable. It was also more difficult to elicit a grand mal seizure through frontal electrodes.

Path of Currents

An important question regards the influence of the path of the current on the antidepressant and amnesic effects of the seizure. Brain structures, such as parenchyma, neuronal tracts, ventricular spaces, vascular tree, meninges, galea, and skull, provide media with different current-transmitting qualities. Do currents pass preferentially through brain parenchyma in essentially straight lines, along neuronal tracts (particularly the intracerebral connecting pathways), or along cerebrovascular pathways?

The high resistance of the skull and a shunting of the major portions of the current through extracranial tissues and meninges left little that actually passed through brain tissues (Alexander and Löwenbach, 1944; Smitt and Wegener, 1944; Hayes, 1950). The remaining current was believed to follow a direct path between the electrodes, with the magnitude varying with the conductivity of the tissues (Smitt and Wegener, 1944; Delgado et al., 1952). Some authors emphasize the lower conductivity of the great neuronal tracts (Lorimer et al., 1949) and some the vascular tree (Aird et al., 1956a, b) as providing the pathway for the flow of residual currents to the brain. Following a series of studies in cadavers and living dogs, Roubicek (1949) concluded that current characteristics were highest in the basal ganglia and mesodiencephalic regions.

None of the studies examined the pathway of the current after unilateral electrode placement, but a number of inferences can be made from the clinical data. Much of the energy is probably dissipated through skull and extracerebral tissues, with only small amounts reaching the brain substance. A greater current density is needed to elicit a seizure from unilateral electrodes placed together, with the density of the current falling as electrodes are further separated. The type of psychological test deficit varies with the location of the electrodes, suggesting that the deficit is related to direct effects of currents passing between the electrodes. Only a small portion of the energy reaches centrencephalic nuclei essential first for the bilateral seizure and second for the change in mood and illness.

Chemical Induction

The first inductions of seizures were chemical: camphor, pentylenetetrazol, cyclohexylethyltriazol, and picrotoxin (Meduna, 1937; Mayer-Gross and Walk, 1938; von Braunmühl, 1942). To enhance the seizure induction properties of the chemicals, concurrent repetitive stimulation with high intensity light was added (Gastaut and Cossa, 1949; O'Flanagan et al., 1951; Ulett, 1957; Driver and Edenberg, 1960). These inductions were not easier than ECT, however, and the complications were not less. In addition to the effects on memory, patients exhibited status epilepticus and recurrent spontaneous seizures. Other compounds were examined for the effects on EEG and behavior, including Lilly 22451 and 31777 (Friedman, 1960), PM 1090 (Edwalds, 1956), and bemegride (Green and Fink, 1958; Lüttke and Koch, 1962). Their usefulness appeared to be no better than ECT, and none became established.

Flurothyl (hexafluorodiethyl ether, Indoklon) is a halogenated derivative of the anesthetic diethyl ether; it exhibits both anesthetic and seizure-inducing properties on inhalation and after intravenous administration (Krantz et al.,

1953, 1959; Adler, 1975). In the first psychiatric clinical trials, flurothyl was described as an easy way to develop seizures with good patient acceptance and was recommended as a substitute for ECT (Esquibel et al., 1958). During the next decade, many studies assessing the clinical, memory test performance, and EEG effects of flurothyl were published; the findings were consistent among the different investigators, and recent reviews summarize the findings (Laurell, 1970; Small and Small, 1972; I. Small, 1974).

Numerous open clinical trials found flurothyl, both by inhalation and by intravenous administrations, an effective convulsant, with effects in patients with depression and schizophrenia that were similar to ECT (Krantz et al., 1957; 1958; Karliner and Padula, 1959a, b, 1960, 1962; Kurland, Krantz and Truitt, 1960; Freund and Warren, 1965; Regestein and Roper, 1966). These observations led to direct comparisons of ECT and flurothyl. In the short-term evaluations of improvement and number of seizures, the studies found the two treatments equal (Kurland et al., 1959; Fink, et al., 1961; Spreche, 1964; Rose and Watson, 1967; Gander et al., 1967; Kafi et al., 1969).

In our study, 27 patients were randomly assigned to flurothyl ($N = 15$) or to bilateral ECT ($N = 12$) using suprathreshold alternating currents (Fink et al., 1961). Premedication was limited to sublingual atropine. The flurothyl was administered using the methods described by Esquibel et al. (1958). Seizures were regularly induced by both methods, and except for some differences in the induction, the seizures were seen as very similar. The behavioral changes were also similar with equivalent ratings of short-term improvement (Table 15.2). Complication rates, including the incidence of fractures seen on repeat X-ray films (20% and 25%) were equivalent. Physiologic measures, including EEG (Table 8.6) and memory and performance tests (Tables 9.6 to 9.9) showed equivalent changes in degree and in time. The lack of any clinical advantage or differences in physiologic measures led us to discard flurothyl since the induction was less secure and considerably more cumbersome than ECT.

These results were confirmed by subsequent studies. In a double-blind compari-

TABLE 15.2

	Flurothyl ($N = 15$)	ECT ($N = 12$)
Clinical assessment		
Recovered, much improved	7	6
Improved	5	5
Unimproved	3	1
Behavioral patterns		
Euphoria, denial	6	7
Somatization, withdrawal	6	2
Confusion, memory loss	3	3
Fracture (spine)	3	3

From Fink et al., 1961.

son, Small et al. (1968) randomly assigned 100 schizophrenic patients to either ECT or flurothyl. Atropine premedication and methohexital and succinylcholine anesthesia were used. Assessments were made by an independent team of clinicians. The average number of treatments were 26 for ECT and 23 for flurothyl, with similar outcome assessments at 2 and 3 months after treatment. In a similar detailed study in 59 depressed patients, Laurell (1970) found the two treatments equivalent in antidepressive effects, as measured by the Cronholm and Ottosson depression rating scale and global ratings 1 month after treatment ended. Total seizure time was longer for flurothyl than ECT (using maximal AC currents), averaging 280 sec (range = 189 to 849; s = 160) for flurothyl. Other investigations also reported longer seizure time for flurothyl (Karliner and Padula, 1962; Gander et al., 1967; Small and Small, 1968).

Flurothyl seizures elicited the same incidence of fractures and changes in physiologic indices as ECT. Some authors found patient acceptance of flurothyl high, with a psychological advantage to being able to describe the treatments as an "inhalation" or a "drug" treatment, rather than "electroshock" (Sandifer et al., 1962; Karliner, 1964; Kafi and Dennis, 1966). Sebag-Montefiore (1974) found equivalent clinical efficacy for patients treated with flurothyl or ECT, each either alone or combined with antidepressants. In statistical analyses of the data, however, after the first four treatments both the raw Hamilton scores and the change in the scores were significantly better for the patients treated with flurothyl than for those treated with ECT, but the advantage was lost at the end of the trial. But others found flurothyl treatment more cumbersome, the anxiety and reluctance of the staff a handicap, and the neurologic sequellae greater (Fink et al., 1961; Spreche, 1964; Gander et al., 1967). For example, if patients were anesthetized with adequate doses of succinylcholine and methohexital, then the delivery of flurothyl was under forced ventilation and the minimum dosage was difficult to define. The seizures were apt to be supramaximal and prolonged. If the patient was allowed to breathe for himself, the dosage of flurothyl was less, but seizure intensity, particularly the tonic phase, was greater and the likelihood of fracture increased. To circumvent these difficulties, intravenous flurothyl was used, with its own complications of dosage, unpredictability of seizure intensity and duration, and venous thrombosis (Karliner and Padula, 1959a, b; Nussbaum and Kurland, 1962, 1963; Karliner, 1963, 1964; Dolenz, 1965; Tetlow et al., 1968; I. Small, 1964; Small and Small, 1975).

Spontaneous seizures and prolonged status epilepticus have been described after flurothyl. While it is difficult to assess the incidence of these complications in small studies, the incidence seems higher with flurothyl, reflecting perhaps the possibility of storage and later release of flurothyl if dosages are excessive (Karliner and Padula, 1959; Nussbaum and Kurland, 1963; Spreche, 1964). Headache is more common after flurothyl (Gander et al., 1967; Rose and Watson, 1967; Small et al., 1968).

In direct comparisons, flurothyl seizures elicited greater increases in cerebrospinal fluid pressure (Gunn et al., 1966). Cardiovascular effects were similar

(Gravenstein et al., 1965; Tetlow et al., 1968), as were the effects on pulmonary diffusion (Rozman and Kurland, 1970). In animal studies, the effects on brain tissues and cardiovascular functions were similar for seizures induced by flurothyl and electrically (Adler et al., 1965; Adler, 1975).

In comparative studies, flurothyl and ECT exhibited similar effects in the EEG (Chapter 8) and memory and performance tests (Chapter 9). The similarities in clinical and physiologic effects led therapists and patients to prefer ECT because of its ease of administration, and lesser incidence of missed seizures.

Frequency, Number, and Duration of Seizures

Repeated treatment was a feature of the early reports of the development of convulsive therapy. But the criteria for determining the frequency and total number of seizures needed for a course of therapy in an individual patient remained experimental.

Frequency

Seizures induced two or three times a week were clinically effective in the first studies, and this frequency remains a standard. More frequent seizures are given when patients are more acutely and severely ill, so that in severe depressions with suicidal risk, pernicious catatonia, and hyperexcitable mania, the initial treatments are often given daily for three to five treatments, or in some instances twice or three times a day for two to three days. There is a direct relationship between frequency of treatment and severity of the organic mental syndrome, however, and a balance must be struck between the need for a rapid clinical response and the risk of confusion, disorientation, and amnesia. In typical cases of endogenous depression, without severe threat to life, three treatments the first week, two the second, and one for one or two subsequent weeks is a rate which is clinically effective with minimal mental changes (Sargant and Slater, 1964; Kalinowsky and Hippius, 1972; Ilaria and Prange, 1975; Frankel, 1978).

The rate of seizure induction is also influenced by factors other than diagnosis and clinical severity: currents, electrode placement, and seizure duration. When the induced seizures are complete and of long duration, the frequency may be decreased; when seizures are incomplete and short, their frequency need be increased. Seizures elicited by suprathreshold currents through bitemporal electrodes, under hyperoxygenation and light anesthesia are usually complete and of long duration; while seizures produced with unidirectional and brief stimuli or threshold currents, through unilateral electrodes, under deep anesthesia are likely to be incomplete and of short duration (Liberson, 1953; Holmberg, 1955; Fink et al., 1958; Ottosson, 1960; d'Elia and Raotma, 1975).

Regressive ECT (REST). Some authors, dissatisfied with the clinical results in some patients using these frequency rates, increased the rate to a few times daily for 7 to 15 days, so that patients received courses of 20 to 45 treatments within 2 weeks. These treatments elicited a severe organic mental syndrome in which the patients were disoriented, confused, incontinent, and unable to feed or care for themselves. With the termination of the course, patients usually became even more regressed for a number of days and then, gradually, in a period of 2 to 6 weeks, recovered to a more normal, oriented mental state with few residual neurologic signs. Memory tests and EEG records usually exhibited pretreatment patterns within 1 to 3 months.

The treatment was recommended in chronic psychotic patients, unresponsive to regular courses of ECT or insulin coma, and was termed "regressive therapy" (REST), "annihilation therapy," or "depatterning" by different authors (Milligan, 1946; Bini and Bazzi, 1947; Tyler and Lowenbach, 1947; Kennedy and Anchel, 1948; Cameron et al., 1962). The treatments were at first thought to be effective, but follow-up studies failed to show an advantage of these regimens over conventional treatment. The use of antipsychotic drugs replaced REST as the drugs were found to be effective and without its unpleasant features and risks.

Multiple ECT (MECT). Some authors, concerned with the risks of anesthetic induction, recommended the administration of multiple seizures, up to six, one after the other with intervals of a few minutes, with only one anesthetic induction (Blachly and Gowing, 1966). To improve the safety of the procedure, they recommended continuous monitoring of the EKG and the EEG, thus providing evidence of the intensity and duration of the cerebral seizure. Following the reports of Holmberg (1953, 1955), they determined to further reduce the risk of anesthesia by forced ventilation of the patient with oxygen. The treatment was termed "multiple monitored ECT" (MMECT) and was found safe. We found that monitoring was not essential, so we adopted the term "multiple ECT" (MECT) followed by a digit for the number of seizures in a treatment (Abrams and Fink, 1972).

In their initial report, Blachly and Gowing (1966) treated 46 patients with MECT-3 to MECT-8, and they estimated amnesia to be similar to that seen after one to two conventional ECT. White et al. (1968) gave MECT-5 to 29 patients with a variety of diagnoses and reported a satisfactory therapeutic effect with less amnesia than after six to eight conventional ECT. Bidder and Strain (1970) gave two sessions of MECT-4, 48 hr apart with an excellent clinical result in one patient, a good response in nine, and fair to poor in four patients, but the clinical responses seemed delayed as with conventional ECT. They reported two complications: one patient exhibited a severe organic mental syndrome after each session of MECT-4, and one patient developed prolonged status epilepticus after the first session of MECT-4 (Strain and Bidder, 1971).

In an assessment of MECT in schizophrenic patients, Bridenbaugh et al. (1972) treated 17 patients with MECT-5 twice weekly. After an average of 4.5 sessions, 14 patients were improved and three were not. They related the clinical outcome to the total seizure duration, although their findings were clouded by many seizures recorded for more than 15 min, and one longer than an hour. One patient developed pulmonary aspiration and pneumonitis after the first MECT-5 session.

In our own studies, we treated 38 patients who received either unilateral or bilateral MECT-4 or MECT-6 (Abrams and Fink, 1972). Improvement after one session occurred in only one patient, and in several patients we believed that the clinical effects were accelerated. In two patients with endogenous depression, bilateral MECT-6 failed to elicit improvement, but they did recover with additional seizures on alternate days. Patients exhibited post-seizure confusion and agitation more frequently than we anticipated, and two patients developed confusional states with disorientation and increased, persistent EEG slowing. For most patients, however, the memory effects on the day after MECT were no more than after a single seizure. We also failed to find changes in EEG after MECT that differed from those usually recorded after a single seizure (Abrams et al., 1973). We concluded that MECT, as now applied, carried more risks and fewer benefits than conventional ECT for our patients.

Maintenance ECT. At the other end of the frequency spectrum is the use of ECT at weekly, bi-weekly, and monthly intervals for patients who have recurrent illnesses. Such "maintenance" or "prophylactic" therapy was recommended by some authors (Moore, 1943; Geoghegan and Stevenson, 1949; Stevenson and Geoghegan, 1951; Bourne, 1956; Hastings, 1961; Karliner and Wehrheim, 1965; Holt, 1965). Bourne (1954, 1956) described patients who required regular convulsions, as often as every few days or every few weeks, to maintain their "normal mental health." With the availability of psychoactive drugs, interest in this use of ECT waned, particularly after the demonstrations that maintenance drug therapy was useful in reducing relapse (Seager and Bird, 1962; Imlah et al., 1965; Kay et al., 1970). There is little evidence, however, that treatments spaced so widely apart bear special risk, nor is there evidence of their usefulness.

Number

A principal concern in every treatment course is the question of the adequate number of treatments for a maximum therapeutic effect. The determination of the endpoint is a most difficult decision in clinical practice, and no objective guides exist. The number of treatments is related to diagnosis, severity of illness, and the mode of induction. A principal reason for treatment failure or early relapse is an insufficient course of treatment (Kalinowsky, 1948, 1954).

Patients with endogenous depression are usually treated successfully with four to eight treatments, although some authors find that six to twelve may be required. Cases of mania were responsive to similar numbers of treatments, but in more recent assessments, a course of 12 to 20 treatments seems necessary. Catatonic patients require fewer treatments when the catatonia is severe. It is in the treatment of schizophrenic and neurotic patients that the longest series of treatments are reported. Fewer than 12 to 20 treatments are rarely successful in schizophrenia, and series up to 35 treatments are common (Sargant and Slater, 1964; Kalinowsky and Hippius, 1972; Ilaria and Prange, 1975; Frankel, 1978).

Some authors cite courses of ECT into the hundreds of treatments, but one wonders now whether the patients obtained a benefit from such a heroic treatment that could not be achieved by other, less dramatic, means. Wilcox (1947), in an analysis of the course of treatment of more than 500 chronic mentally ill who received more than 23,000 treatments, found that the cumulative percentage of patients who improved with ECT did so rapidly as more treatments were given, up to an asymptote of 20 to 30 treatments. Beyond that number in a course, there was no increase in the number who improved or were rehabilitated regardless of the number of further treatments given.

The clinical endpoint that is most often used is the relief of the vegetative symptoms of the depression. When patients cease to ruminate about suicide, take food voluntarily, and sleep continuously during the night, the treatment may be terminated. At such times additional treatments do not provide additional benefit (Barton et al., 1973). In part, this may be related to the usual delay in the development of the biochemical events that are central to the therapeutic process, so that at the time that the clinical manifestations of mood elevation and change in the endogenous features of the illness are clearly defined, additional treatments have already been given.

Some therapists wait until a patient refuses further treatment, insisting that he is well, before terminating treatment. Others wait on the development of early signs of an organic mental syndrome, equating the development of brain change with evidence that an adequate course has been given. But these indices are poorly related to outcome, and since these usually occur after more treatments than are ordinarily necessary, their use is not reasonable. A few authors have used EEG criteria, the changes in language, and the EEG or language response to barbiturate as a guide to the number of treatments, but these studies are insecure (Chapters 8 and 10).

The number of treatments varies with the mode of induction. In general, induction with unidirectional and brief stimuli instruments are reported to require more treatments than induction with alternating current instruments; and unilateral electrode placements may require more treatments than bilateral electrode placement (Proctor and Goodwin, 1943; Liberson, 1953; Green, 1960). Such observations may best be understood by reflecting that most studies fail to monitor the presence or duration of a seizure, and under threshold currents and unilateral electrode placement, the likelihood of incomplete and missed seizures is high. The inefficacy of incomplete seizures is well documented. In the comparisons of unilateral and bilateral ECT from research settings, the number of seizures for a course is usually the same, particularly if the duration of each seizure is used as evidence of the development of a typical grand mal seizure (d'Elia, 1970a, b; Small and Small, 1971; Volavka et al., 1972; Sand-Strömgren, 1973; Abrams et al., 1973).

Duration

The duration of the seizure is a measurable feature of ECT which has been examined for its significance to outcome. Seizure duration has usually been measured by timing each phase of the convulsion observed visually, or by EEG or EMG measures. Estimates of the duration of the seizure may differ by these different methods, particularly if the convulsion is modified by succinylcholine and anesthesia.

The duration of the first seizure is longer than subsequent seizures, regardless of the mode of induction, diagnosis, or method of observation (Finner, 1954; Holmberg, 1954a, b, 1955; Green, 1960; Abrams et al., 1973). This is also a feature of ECS (Pollack et al., 1963). Seizure duration is influenced by the induction method, with suprathreshold currents eliciting longer seizures than threshold currents (Green, 1960); and flurothyl seizures longer than those induced in ECT (Fink et al., 1961; Laurell, 1970). The data for unilateral ECT is less clear. d'Elia (1970a, b) and Small et al. (1970) found seizures in unilateral ECT to be shorter, but the differences from bilateral ECT were not significant. We found seizure duration after bilateral ECT to be longer (61.9 sec) than after unilateral ECT (51.5 sec) (Abrams et al., 1973). d'Elia and Widepalm (1974) examined seizure duration and found it to be shorter when unilateral electrodes were placed in frontoparietal locations (50.5 $\pm$ 20.6 sec) than in temporoparietal locations (56.7 $\pm$ 23.7; $F = 6.53$, $p \leq .01$), suggesting that location of electrodes may also influence the duration of the seizure.

With increased number of seizures, the threshold rises in patients (Finner, 1954; Green, 1960) and in animals receiving ECS (Pollack et al., 1963). The rise in threshold was not related to clinical outcome or EEG change (Green, 1960). The amount of EEG slowing was related to seizure duration, with longer seizures eliciting greater degrees of EEG change (Green, 1960; Ottosson, 1960; Laurell, 1970).

Diagnosis may affect seizure duration, with seizures in schizophrenic patients being shorter than in depressed patients (Finner, 1954). Sex and age have no effect on seizure duration (Finner, 1954; Holmberg, 1954b, 1955).

Seizure duration is increased by oxygenation, and prolonged durations may occur if patients are maintained under forced ventilation with oxygen during the seizure (Holmberg, 1953a, 1955; Haard et al., 1956; Bridenbaugh et al., 1972). The lengthened duration of the seizure was thought to reduce the number of seizures needed for a treatment course (Holmberg, 1955). Duration of the seizure was reduced by lidocaine, and such modified seizures were clinically less effective than unmodified seizures (Ottosson, 1960).

The relation to clinical outcome is not clear. Ottosson (1960) found that seizures shortened by lidocaine were less effective. Finner (1954) and Green (1960) found no relation to outcome. But Maletzky (1978), examining the findings of MMECT, noted that while no linear relationship between duration and outcome existed, patients with less than 210 sec or more than 1,000 sec of seizure time did less well in clinical assessments than patients whose duration of seizure time, as measured by EEG monitoring, was between these figures. The suggestion of a therapeutic window is an interesting one, and is consistent with other aspects of ECT: the relation between outcome and amnesia, and outcome and degree of EEG slowing. In these relationships, the seizure parameters are not directly related to outcome in themselves, but their change indicates that the biochemical events necessary for improvement have been stimulated.

Adjunctive Measures

The incidence of fear, panic, fracture, spontaneous seizures, and death in ECT has been sharply reduced by modifications of the treatment process— particularly the use of anesthesia, muscle relaxants, anticholinergic drugs and oxygenation. The early methods for anesthesia and muscle relaxation brought with their use some unpleasant side-effects of their own—prolonged apnea, sensations of choking in inadequately anesthetized subjects, laryngospasm, hypersalivation, post-anesthesia excitement, and cardiac arrhythmia. Anoxia was a common accompaniment of prolonged anesthesia and unmodified treatments. Some authors, notably Kalinowsky and Hoch (1961) and more recently, Kalinowsky and Hippius (1972) find the risks of the use of anesthesia considerable. But with improvements in the drugs available, and experience in the technique of administration, the use of adjuvants has become an integral part of the ECT process.

Anesthesia

While many treatments with pentylenetetrazol and ECT were given without anesthesia, most early descriptions indicate that sedatives and a short-acting anesthetic were useful, particularly in anxious and fearful patients. Barbiturates, particularly amobarbital, thiopental and hexobarbital, subcoma doses of insulin, and mixtures containing scopolamine and an opioid were frequently used. Barbiturates were also used to reduce post-convulsive excitement and delirium. However, complications of anesthesia, particularly laryngospasm, loss of the gag reflex and vomiting, cardiovascular effects, and death, as well as the time needed for the proper administration of an anesthetic, led to the infrequent use of anesthesia.

With the introduction of short-acting and safe muscle paralytic agents such as succinylcholine in 1952, the conditions of treatment changed. Succinylcholine is rapidly effective, and a dose sufficient for paralysis of spinal muscles also paralyzes respiration, leading in the awake patient, to feelings of choking, helplessness, dyspnea, and acute panic. By the early 1950s, the question was no longer whether to use an anesthetic, but which anesthetic was short acting, safe and easy to administer in conjunction with succinylcholine.

Havens (1958) and Huggins et al., (1964) compared treatments given with and without anesthesia and succinylcholine, and found no differences in number of treatments, duration of hospitalization, or measures of outcome. They also found little difference in the patients' attitude to the two treatments. Fractures (28% to none), organic psychotic reactions, and restlessness were more frequent in the unmodified treatment group. They also noted that the patients receiving anesthesia had more venous thrombosis, aspiration pneumonia, and transient hypotension than the patients in the unmodified treatment group. Based on a historical comparison of the clinical results in patients who were treated with unmodifed or modified ECT, Seager (1958) concluded that the patients treated with unmodified ECT were in the hospital for a shorter period, received less treatments and were more likely to remain well than those treated with ECT modified with anesthesia and succinylcholine. Seager (1959) then carried out a controlled comparison in 118 depressed patients given unmodified ECT, ECT modified by thiopental alone, or modified by thiopental and succinylcholine. There were no differences in length of stay, number of treatments, and clinical outcome at discharge or after 6 months. Similar findings were also reported by Little and Reid (1957).

Pitts and his co-workers undertook systematic studies of anesthesia for ECT (Pitts et al., 1965; Pitts et al., 1968; Woodruff et al., 1968; Woodruff et al., 1969; Pitts, 1972). They divided their patient sample into those with and those without cardiac disease, based on the experience that cardiac arrhythmias after anesthesia were more common in patients with cardiac disease. They compared anesthesia inductions with thiopental and methohexital and found that the methohexital induction had a lower incidence of arrhythmias and EKG abnormalities, particularly in the patients with prior cardiac disease. Pre-oxygenation had no effect on the incidence of cardiac dysfunction with either anesthetic. They also varied the dosage of methohexital and recommended a dose of 0.75 mg/kg body weight as effective and safe.

One limitation of the use of barbiturate anesthesia has been the associated elevation in the seizure threshold. Current intensity must be increased to obtain a seizure. In conventional bilateral ECT, the elevation in seizure threshold may not be a significant limitation in achieving a seizure, but in unilateral ECT, the elevation in threshold may preclude a successful seizure. This has led some authors to recommend lower doses of anesthetics for unilateral ECT (d'Elia and Raotma, 1975).

Muscle Relaxation and Paralysis

Fracture was the principal complication of the early inductions of seizures, and was so frequent that some authors recommended treatment be given under spinal anesthesia. Bennett (1940) demonstrated that the body musculature could be sufficiently relaxed by natural extracts of curare that the incidence of fractures could be reduced. But the use of both the natural and synthetic curare (Intocostrin, tubocurarine) was associated with many problems that precluded their routine use. Prolonged muscle paralysis, delayed induction, and symptoms of bronchospasm, urticaria, and hypotension due to the release of histamine were frequent. When prostigmine was used as an antidote, hypersalivation ensued (Holmberg and Thesleff, 1952). Fatalities occurred (Ebaugh et al., 1943; Cash and Hoekstra, 1943). Other drugs were studied, including diphenylhydantoin, mephenesin, gallamine triethiodide (Flaxedil), decamethonium bromide (Syncurine) and succinylcholine (Anectine, Scoline).

While most authors sought to reduce the risk of fracture in ECT by muscle paralysis, others sought to raise the cerebral threshold to facilitate partial seizures by administering anticonvulsant drugs (Hemphill and Walter, 1941; Holt and Borkowski, 1951). Diphenylhydantoin was given for 6 days, raising the seizure threshold so that grand mal convulsions could not be obtained. The clinical efficacy of the modified seizures was less than the unmodified (Hemphill and Walter, 1941). Holt and Borkowski (1951) gave their patients 100 to 600 mg diphenylhydantoin a day until toxicity occurred. ECT was given and of 300 seizures, 197 were partial and 103 were complete in 26 patients. The treatment course was generally incomplete because of toxicity to diphenylhydantoin, and in only 3 of 23 cases were the modified treatments deemed effective. With this failure, they treated another group of patients with diphenylhydantoin and mephenesin combined, the latter being given as an intravenous bolus 15 min before ECT. The clinical results of the combination were better than diphenylhydantoin alone, but not sufficiently superior to unmodified ECT to be recommended.

The early trials with succinylcholine found it safe, reliable, short-acting and rapid in onset (Arnold and Böck-Greissau, 1952; Holmberg and Thesleff, 1952; Fisher and Bannister, 1953; Murray, 1953; Wilson et al., 1954). In their initial report, Holmberg and Thesleff (1952) described 512 successful inductions in 136 patients. The principal complaints were of choking sensations, muscular aches, and tenderness of the jaw but the patients suffered no fractures. They found that succinylcholine could be safely combined with a short acting barbiturate anesthetic.

Comparisons with gallamine triethiodide found succinylcholine superior in the relaxation induced and the duration of its effect (Holt et al., 1953). In the comparative studies of modified and unmodified ECT by Havens (1958) and Huggins et al., (1964), succinylcholine was a feature of modified ECT, and contributed to their conclusion that modified ECT was preferred.

Succinylcholine is a specific depolarizer of the myoneural membrane, and it is rapidly degraded by pseudocholinesterase normally present in human muscle tissues. Except for individuals with a hereditary enzyme deficiency or those with one derived from hepatic disease, the duration of action is short with a rapid onset when given intravenously. But prolonged muscle paralysis may occur, and various techniques have been suggested to avoid this risk (Chapter 16).[1] Paralysis may affect the gag reflex and patients may regurgitate gastric contents and drown in these fluids or develop pneumonia. Death has been associated with its use (Robinson and de Mott, 1954).

Succinylcholine may also reduce the cardiovascular effects of the seizure. A rise in blood pressure, a marked Valsalva effect, and tachycardia occur during the seizure and for some minutes thereafter (Gordh and Silfverskiöld, 1943; Altschule et al., 1947a; Brown et al., 1952; Brown et al., 1953a, b). Arrhythmias are common, particularly in patients with preexisting cardiovascular disease (Bellet et al., 1941; Altschule et al., 1947b; Craddock and Gilbert, 1948). Holmberg et al. (1954) examined the cardiovascular effects of ECT modifed by anesthesia, succinylcholine and oxygen and found the rise in blood pressure during the seizure to be slower and more even, the pulse pressure remained within normal limits, the usual rise in venous pressure was sharply reduced, and the cardiac rate remained slow and regular.

Oxygenation

Amnesia was a feature of many early theories of the mode of action of ECT. Since hypoxia contributed to amnesia, little effort was made to reduce it. Holmberg (1953a, b) reported that hypoxia could be eliminated by the inhalation of pure oxygen for 1 min before the treatment. Such inhalation of oxygen resulted in a prolongation of the duration and an increase in the intensity of the seizure by 20 to 30%. It also increased the frequency of tonic jerks. But, the greater intensity of the seizure probably increased the risk of fracture. In a test of the effects of succinylcholine, Holmberg et al. (1954) reported that muscle paralysis could prevent fracture even as oxygenation had precluded hypoxia. Indeed, the duration of the seizure was further increased by oxygenation and could be prolonged for minutes (Haard et al. 1956; Holmberg et al., 1956). Others confirmed the clinical value of succinylcholine and oxygenation (Wilson et al., 1954).

These observations led to the routine use of oxygen inhalation prior to ECT, especially in patients receiving modified treatment. In their experiments to induce many seizures in one session, Blachly and Gowing (1966) reduced the amnesia, confusion, and disorientation of multiple seizures by increased oxygenation. They provided forced ventilation with oxygen before, during, and after each seizure. Their subjects receiving two to six seizures exhibited no more effects on memory in self reports, clinical assessments, and psychological performance tests than patients receiving a single ECT—a finding confirmed by others (Bidder and Strain, 1970; Abrams and Fink, 1972). In his analysis of MMECT, Abrams (1974) suggests that the limited effects on memory functions may not be the

---

[1] Prolonged apnea may occur in patients receiving organophosphate cholinesterase inhibitors for the treatment of glaucoma (Chessen et al., 1974; Packman et al., 1978).

result of oxygenation as much as the reduced number of anesthetic inductions, or that amnesia, like the antidepressant activity of ECT, requires time for the biochemical events that are the basis for amnesia to occur.

Anticholinergic Drugs

Anesthetic agents induce increased salivation, and atropine was recommended to reduce nasopharyngeal secretions. It was also thought that vagal stimulation during ECT may be a cause for cardiac arrest, and atropine was recommended as a prophylactic. Some authors, notably Kalinowsky and Hoch (1961) found little merit in these indications, and did not use atropine for ECT inductions. But others regularly use atropine as premedication, either parenterally 1/2 to 1 hr before treatment or intravenously as the first agent in modified ECT. In a systematic study of atropine dosage, Rich et al. (1969) found that 1.0, 1.5, 2.0, and 2.5 mg atropine given 45 to 60 min before ECT produced no differences in the cardiac variables measured, and they concluded that the minimal dosage of 1.0 mg was adequate. But we lack substantive studies defining the merit of its use.

Some adverse reactions have been reported. Tachycardia often occurs and in patients with cardiac disease their decompensation may be exaggerated. And overdose or sensitivity may induce a toxic delirium, particularly in patients who are concurrently receiving antiparkinson and antipsychotic drugs (Frankel, 1978).

Chapter 16

A Manual for Convulsive Therapy

> . . . convulsive therapy is a surgical treatment in psychiatry, and the general rules governing the admissability of surgical intervention apply . . .
> . . . it should never be employed as a mere placebo.
> . . . When the treatment is eventually carried out, every method should be used to minimize the risks which can never be entirely excluded.
>
> Sargant and Slater, 1964.

ECT has undergone many modifications, and the therapist is faced with decisions regarding the instrument and current parameters (dosage), electrode placement (unilateral or bilateral), anesthetic and its administration (bolus or drip), EKG and EEG monitoring, oxygenation, single or multiple seizures in a session, and frequency and number of treatments. To these must be added the concurrent and sequential use of drugs, maintenance treatments, and the advice to be given the patient and the family to minimize the risks of treatment.

There is no single, accepted procedure for ECT, and each patient represents a unique therapeutic problem. Procedures vary with the age and medical status of the patient, severity and duration of the illness, and availability of trained personnel and specialized treatment facilities in the community. The following procedures are derived from many experiences and provide a safe and effective treatment. Few manuals for ECT have been published, although some training institutions have distributed guidelines locally (Seidman et al., 1956; Kindwall, 1966; Abrams and Fink, 1969; Blackman, 1974). Some authors have written uncritical testimonials to ECT that attempt to allay the anxiety of patients and their families (Cammer, 1969; Peck, 1974). The procedures are also described in texts (Paterson, 1963; Sargant and Slater, 1963; Kalinowsky and Hippius, 1972). The indications for ECT are discussed by many authors, most notably Kalinowsky (1962). The aspects of anesthesia that are important for ECT are detailed in a report by Pitts (1972). Salzman (1975) and Frankel (1978) present specific descriptions of treatment procedures that are generally consistent with those presented here. Shaw (1977) discusses the management of affective disorders by the various antidepressant treatments, including ECT, clearly and with specific recommendations.

INDICATIONS FOR THE USE OF ECT

Selection Criteria

ECT is a treatment for patients who are severely ill. It is a major treatment in psychiatry and should usually be reserved, in the first instance, for patients ill enough to be hospitalized. In patients who have successive episodes of illness, particularly those who have responded to ECT, treatments may be considered on an outpatient basis. The primary indications for ECT are severe depression, particularly when suicide is a risk, refusal of food, hyperactivity leading to exhaustion, and stupor. In these conditions, ECT is a primary treatment, and its early use may be lifesaving.

ECT is effective over a wide range of affective disorders, including the psychotic depressions, mania, and catatonia (Table 16.1). There is no decrement in efficacy with age (indeed, the efficacy seems to improve in the elderly). Results are likely to be better in patients with an acute onset of illness, short duration of decompensation, and greatest severity of disturbance.

ECT is also indicated, largely as a secondary treatment, in affectively disturbed patients who have not responded to other treatments, in manic patients who are not responsive to psychoactive drug treatments, and in patients in whom catatonic symptoms secondary to medical disorders have developed. Some therapists use ECT in cases of schizophrenia, either in acutely disturbed patients whose behavior has become unmanageable or in those in whom other treatments have failed.

TABLE 16.1. *Diagnostic indications for ECT*

Primary
Primary (major) affective disorder
Psychotic depression (endogenous, primary, S-type, vital)
Unipolar, bipolar depression
Involutional depression
Depression in the elderly
Postpartum depression

Secondary
Mania
Catatonia
Schizophrenia, unresponsive to other therapies

There are many symptomatic indications for ECT. Vegetative symptoms accompanying severe mood disorders are particularly important (Table 16.2). The results with ECT seem to parallel the extent and severity of vegetative symptoms; for example, the more prominent the weight loss and insomnia, the better the outcome with ECT. In behavioral symptoms, there is evidence that patients with psychotic depression who also exhibit somatic and guilt delusions do badly with tricyclic antidepressant drugs and respond rapidly to ECT; in such instances, ECT may be considered a primary treatment.

In patients who are depressed and have a severe medical illness, ECT may be preferred to drug treatment for their mental state. This is particularly true

TABLE 16.2. *Symptomatic indications for ECT*

Vegetative
Insomnia
Early morning awakening; diurnal mood swing (worse in morning)
Anorexia
Weight loss
Constipation
Low salivation rate
Amenorrhea
Loss of libido
Retardation
Inability to cry
Inability to concentrate

Behavioral
Stupor
Catatonia
Suicidal thoughts, activity
Refusal of food
Delusions: worthlessness, guilt, somatic
Uncontrollable excitement, exhaustion

of patients with recent myocardial infarction, cardiovascular disease, renal disease, and recent surgery or fracture.

The safety of ECT in pregnancy has been reported in a number of studies (Chapter 4). Use is to be considered in those women who are severely depressed and psychotic and for whom high doses of antidepressant medications may be contraindicated, particularly because of the risk to the fetus early in pregnancy. Some special considerations in administering ECT in pregnancy have recently been suggested, including external fetal monitoring (Remick and Maurice, 1978).

ECT may also be useful in those clinical conditions in which other therapies are unavailable and where ECT has, on occasion, been gratifying, such as in depressed patients with parkinsonism, syndromes of thalamic pain or trigeminal neuralgia, and the psychoses associated with lupus erythematosus.

Although many authors cite favorable predictive experiences with psychological and physiologic predictors, these have generally not been validated. The tests were developed at times when the efficacy of ECT was thought to be related to its effects on autonomic measures (e.g., sedation threshold, methacholine test, GSR responsivity) or on psychological mechanisms (e.g., denial scale, California F-scale, MMPI, Rorschach). Dynamic tests of neuroendocrine integrity may also be predictors for ECT (e.g., tests of suppression, stimulation, and periodicity of hormone release) (Chapters 11 and 14). Although these tests are not usually used in uncomplicated cases, they provide useful information for the experienced clinician.

Exclusion Criteria

Psychiatric

There is much evidence that ECT is a specific treatment for mental syndromes characterized by severe mood disorder and vegetative dysfunction. Patients who fail to meet the clinical criteria are clearly not suitable candidates. The principal diagnostic problems are in differentiating neurotic from psychotic depression, the former doing poorly with ECT. Poor responders are usually classified as suffering from neurotic (secondary, reactive, J-type, personal) depression and other states in which anxiety is prominent (Table 16.3). In general, patients with schizophrenia also do poorly, except for the few patients with catatonia or prominent disturbances in mood (schizoaffective syndromes). Age is an important criterion, with patients under 35 years of age not responding as well as older patients.

In addition to these diagnostic criteria are symptoms associated with a poor response to ECT or a particularly distressing response with prolonged complaints of amnesia or agitation (Table 16.3).

TABLE 16.3. Exclusion criteria

Diagnostic
Depression, reactive (neurotic, personal)
Schizophrenia
Paranoid
Simple
Hebephrenic
Psychoneurosis
Hysteria
Anxiety state
Hypochondriasis
Personality disorders
Drug dependence, all types

Symptomatic
Age under 35 years
Anxiety
Initial insomnia
Worsening in p.m.
Fluctuating course
Tearfulness
Self-pity
Hypochondriasis
Hysteria
Paranoia
Mildness of symptoms

Physical

There are no absolute medical contraindications to the use of ECT. In patients with serious medical liabilities, it is necessary to modify the ECT procedures, but treatment may be given. In some texts, brain tumor is considered an absolute contraindication; excluding the rare need for ECT in such a patient, there are records of successful ECT treatment even in this condition of very high risk. In addition, there are many other medical conditions in which ECT should only be considered and given with consideration for the special precautions that would improve the safety of the treatment (Table 16.4). Patients with cardiac pacemakers may be treated safely (Abiuso et al., 1978).

TABLE 16.4. Conditions of special consideration

Symptom	Complication
Increased intracranial pressure	Cerebral and vascular hypertension
Recent myocardial infarction	Vascular hypotension; cardiac failure
Cardiac arrhythmia	Exaggerated arrhythmia
Porphyria	Barbiturate toxicity
Low cholinesterase activity	Succinylcholine toxicity
Recent fracture	Fracture
Liver disease, malnutrition	Low cholinesterase activity
Organic mental syndrome	Organic psychosis, confusion
Glaucoma	Ocular hypertension with atropine; prolonged apnea

CONSENT AND ADVICE TO PATIENTS

ECT is a major treatment in medicine, with defined risks. While the risks may have been exaggerated and unmodified ECT embellished for dramatic effect in the communication media, the risks inherent in the treatment are sufficient to encourage therapists to fully inform each patient of the nature of the treatment and for the patient to assent to or refuse treatment. There was a time when the diagnosis of a psychosis was considered sufficient for the judgment that the patient was incapable to give consent, that as a ward of the state, the patient's agents (physicians) could apply remedies, even dangerous ones, without the patient's consent. Recent judicial decisions find that the patient has a right to as much information as is available to allow consent or refusal of treatment, and that physicians have no special duties or privileges to impose their judgment, even for the patient's welfare (Frankel, 1978).

Trust between patient and physician is integral to the optimal application of consent procedures. A favorable doctor-patient relationship provides the basis for the physician to select the best treatment for the patient and for the patient to allow that which is necessary with a minimum of anxiety and fear. Consent procedures cannot be defined in absolute terms. The physician must exercise his or her best judgment as to the way that the risks of therapy are explained; the aim is to inform adequately and yet to avoid an undue concern which could preclude assent from a patient for whom treatment may be lifesaving.

A consent form is proposed, which presumes the competence of the patient to understand the information and the ability to voluntarily make a decision (Fig. 16.1). Where a competent patient agrees to treatment after a reasonable explanation of benefits and risks, there is no conflict in undertaking treatment.

In the instance in which a voluntary, competent patient does not consent to treatment, it is not reasonable for the physician, the family, or institutional officials to insist. An alternate treatment, and presumably an alternate therapist, should be provided.

It is difficult to invoke these consent procedures in patients of dubious competence to understand the intent, benefits, and risks of treatment. When hospitalized involuntary or incompetent patients consent to treatment, and particularly when relatives and the psychiatrist agree that ECT would benefit the patient, good faith, and the history of doctor-patient relationships should insure that the treatment be administered. A prudent therapist, however, should support his or her judgment by an independent consultation with a psychiatrist who can give the family an arm's length consultation.

The most complex situation for consent is with the involuntary incompetent patient who refuses consent and resists treatment. In such situations, treatment can only be given by following the special procedures that may govern in each community. The issues are complex and are undergoing continuing study. The present interpretations of voluntary informed consent preclude a medical resolution of the dilemma; nor is it acceptable to substitute an agreement by family, institutional authorities, psychiatrist, or consultants. The problems are considered more fully in the report of the American Psychiatric Association Task Force on Convulsive Therapy (Frankel, 1978), the Royal College of Psychiatrists' (1977) memorandum on the use of electroconvulsive therapy, and a survey by Roth (1977). A recent example of the value of ECT in a disturbed, nonconsenting patient and the legal issues is discussed by Weitzel (1977).

The treatment should be described in detail to patients and relatives, who should be advised of the common occurrence of amnesia and headache and the rarity of death, fracture, and spontaneous seizure. Psychiatrists should consider a tape or video recording of the consent discussion, although personally disagreeable, for record purposes.

Treatments must be described and given with compassion. After all, patients are likely not to be stupid, insensitive, deaf, or blind. They fear the currents that will pass through their body; they fear pain and brain damage; they anticipate and dread the loss of memory. After the first treatment, they are concerned about their feelings of unreality, confusion, unsteadiness, headache, and nausea. A special concern may be for the feeling of being conscious and unable to breathe, of suffocation, particularly when the anesthesia has been ineptly administered (Gomez, 1975; Clare, 1976; Spencer, 1977). It is of little help to a waiting

FIG. 16.1.

CONSENT for ELECTROTHERAPY

I, _____, M.D. (and _____ _____, M.D.) recommend electrotherapy (brain stimulation, electroconvulsive therapy) for your present mental symptoms. These treatments have been given to thousands of mentally ill patients since 1938, with many improvements in the treatments and greater success in helping patients since then.

Treatments are given in the mornings before breakfast, in a specially equipped treatment room. You will be attended by an anesthetist, a nurse, and a physician.

A needle will be placed in your vein (like you may have had when samples were taken for blood tests) and an anesthetic will be injected. You will be asked to count backwards and you will become drowsy and fall asleep. Other medicines will be given to relax your muscles and reduce the irritability of your heart. The anesthetist will help you breathe with pure oxygen through a mask.

The treatment is given while you are asleep. Momentary electric currents are passed through electrodes on the scalp to stimulate the brain. When the brain is stimulated, there are muscular contractions for up to a minute; but with proper relaxation, the contractions are barely measurable.

The treatments take only a few minutes. You are then moved to the recovery room where you will gradually wake up as after a deep sleep. You may feel groggy, probably have some muscular aches like after a lot of exercise, and some headache. You will return to your room, usually within an hour of the treatment. You may be hungry and will be given your breakfast and you will spend the rest of the morning on the ward with your nurse or attendant.

Treatments are given every other day for up to 12 treatments. Many patients improve rapidly and require fewer treatments; some require more than 12, but these will not be given without another discussion with you and your family.

There are some risks in the treatment. Much is related to the anesthesia, and treatments are given in a room where special equipment and supplies for emergencies are available. Patients often become confused, and may not know where they are when they awaken. This may be frightening, but the confusion usually disappears within a few hours. Memory for recent events may be disturbed, and dates, names of friends, public events, telephone numbers and addresses may be difficult to recall. In most patients, the memory difficulty (amnesia) is gone within four weeks after the last treatment, but in about 1 in 200 patients, the problems remain for months and even years. Death is a rare complication, occurring once in 40,000 treatments. Equally uncommon with modern anesthesia are bone fractures and spontaneous seizures after the treatment is over, but these may occur.

You may discontinue the treatments at any time, although you will be encouraged to continue until an adequate course is completed.

I, _____, have read this description of the treatments, and these have been explained to me by _____.

I agree to have the treatments and understand that Dr. _____ will be the physician in charge of my treatment.

_____

Dated, _____
Witness: _____
Agreed _____
Relationship to Patient _____

and anxious patient to hear the bustle and comments associated with the treatment of another patient or to see a patient in post-ECT confusion or delirium. Proper attention to the courtesies and considerations due patients will do much to relieve their anxiety and our preoccupation with consent procedures and malpractice suits.

PROCEDURES FOR MODIFIED ECT

Pretreatment Examinations

Medical Concerns

A detailed medical history and examination should focus on the cardiovascular and neurologic systems (Table 16.5). The principal risk in ECT is cardiovascular, both from the anesthesia and the seizure. Special attention should be paid to evidence of recent myocardial infarction, arrhythmia, or hypertension. Neurologic examination should record the results of tests of orientation and memory and a funduscopic examination to exclude papilledema. Note should be made of the presence of diabetes, renal disease, glaucoma, porphyria, and pulmonary

TABLE 16.5. Medical check-list

History
Cardiovascular
Myocardial damage
Arrhythmia
Hypertension
Neurologic
Seizures
Headache
Memory difficulty
Illnesses
Glaucoma
Diabetes
Porphyria
Renal disease
Bone disease
Examination
Memory tests
Funduscopic
Cardiovascular status
EKG
Blood pressure
Spine X-ray
Dental status
Succinycholine sensitivity

disease, as these conditions or their treatment may increase the anesthetic risk.

No laboratory tests are required prior to ECT, although many should be considered and obtained where indicated. An electrocardiogram is advisable, since cardiac complications may occur. X-rays should be considered, particularly of the dorsal and lumbodorsal spine, in patients with a history of prior ECT, bone pathology, severe osteoarthritis, or bone injury.

In elderly patients, a dental examination is helpful, with special attention to loose teeth and complex bridgework, particularly if these may need special protection during treatment.

An examination by the anesthesiologist prior to the first treatment is also advisable. Succinylcholine blocks neural transmission at the myoneural junction by combining with acetylcholine receptors to produce a transient depolarization and paralysis. Metabolism of acetylcholine is based on its enzymatic hydrolysis through pseudocholinesterase. Persistent neuromuscular blockade may occur in patients deficient in pseudocholinesterase, an uncommon inherited metabolic deficiency. A family history of complications of anesthesia should be sought. Some anesthesiologists may give the patient a test dose of succinylcholine (2 to 4 mg) prior to the first treatment to determine undue sensitivity. A laboratory test is also available to estimate the hydrolyzing capacity of plasma pseudocholinesterase in patients suspected by family history of the deficiency or who may be particular anesthetic risks (Swift and LaDu, 1966). The anesthetic history should also consider the possibility of concurrent treatment for glaucoma or myasthenia gravis (anticholinesterases may prolong the effects of succinylcholine) and any evidence of porphyria.

The administration of other medications during ECT presents problems. There is no evidence that the concurrent use of psychotropic drugs enhances the efficacy of ECT. Indeed, for some compounds, particularly the tricyclic antidepressants, reserpine, monoamine oxidase inhibitors, lithium, and some antipsychotic drugs (e.g., thioridazine), there is evidence of their cardiovascular toxicity, and their use should be precluded during ECT.[1] Where practical, psychotropic drugs should be discontinued during a course of ECT and reinstituted, when indicated, after the last treatment. With drugs recommended for medical conditions, the issues are more complex. The medical consultant should clearly indicate which medication needs to be continued during the course of treatment. Dosage schedules should be defined, noting that oral tablets should not be given immediately prior to anesthesia.

Pretreatment Procedures

For morning treatment, patients should have no solid foods after 10 P.M. If treatment is to be given in the afternoon, then a light, nonsolid breakfast may

---

[1] An assessment of the combination of anesthesia modified ECT and sustained tricyclic drug treatment was reported by Porot et al (1975). They found a slightly higher incidence of interrupted treatment for complications in the combined treatment group (3.6% vs. 2.2%).

be given, with no foods for at least 4 hr prior to treatment. Monitoring of food intake is particularly important in confused and elderly patients.

For anxious patients, sedation to assure a night's sleep is useful; if the patient is particularly anxious, some therapists give intramuscular amobarbital (50 mg), diazepam (5 mg), or chlordiazepoxide (10 mg) from 1 to 2 hr before treatment. Some recommend intravenous diazepam (10 to 20 mg) before anesthesia (Gomez and Dally, 1975).

Atropine or other anticholinergic drugs are usually prescribed to reduce both oral secretions and vagal irritability. To be effective, intramuscular or subcutaneous atropine (0.4 to 1.2 mg) or methscopolamine (0.5 to 1.0 mg) is given 30 to 60 min before anesthesia. An alternate procedure is to give these drugs intravenously as soon as a needle is fixed in the vein in the treatment room. Some authors use intramuscular glycopyrrolate (Robinul) (2 mg) or propantheline (Pro-Banthine) (30 mg) as alternatives.

Patients should void before treatment and should leave all hair pins, ornaments, and removable dentures in their room.

In the treatment room, treatment is usually given on an insulated cart or stretcher, so that electrical grounding cannot occur.

FACILITIES FOR ECT

The risks of ECT are predominantly pulmonary (loss of spontaneous respiration, impaired airway) and cardiovascular (arrhythmia, hypertension, hypotension). Personnel trained to handle such emergencies should be available, as should medical supplies and the necessary equipment in operating condition for emergency use (Table 16.6).

ECT may be given wherever facilities are adequate and personnel are trained for emergency as well as routine care. While ECT is normally given in treatment

TABLE 16.6.

Equipment for ECT
    Anesthesia machine with oxygen tanks
    Intubation set with assorted airways
    Electrocardiograph and defibrillator
    Suction apparatus
    Infusion sets: glucose in water, glucose in saline, and
        sodium bicarbonate solution
    Assorted syringes, needles

Medical supplies for ECT
    Atropine sulfate: 0.4 mg/ml, 10 ml vial
    Calcium chloride: 10% solution, 10 ml ampule or prefilled syringe
    Diazepam: 5 mg/ml, 10 ml
    Epinephrine: 1:10,000 solution, 10 ml
    Lidocaine (xylocaine): 2% solution for cardiac use
    Levophed (norepinephrine): 2 mg/ml, 4 ml ampoules
    Metaraminol (Aramine): 1% solution, 10 ml

rooms in hospital units, treatments may be given in outpatient and office settings and in private rooms in hospitals. The determining factor is the adequacy and immediate availability of emergency support procedures.

In the absence of certification standards in ECT, it may be prudent for administrators and medical boards establishing criteria for privileges of physicians for the institutional use of ECT to consider preceptorship before accreditation. Privileges to give ECT should be determined by criteria similar to those used to accredit physicians for anesthesia or surgery. Trained therapists should exhibit knowledge of (a) selection and common exclusions of patients for ECT, (b) medical and laboratory examinations required before and during ECT, and (c) experience in the administration of ECT, including unilateral and bilateral ECT, monitoring of seizures, administration of anesthesia, and identification of the principal complications. The physician should be skilled in emergency resuscitation of patients in respiratory and cardiac distress. He should have intimate knowledge of psychoactive drugs and the drugs likely to be used in the medical conditions of the patient, and be acquainted with their effects when given concurrently and sequentially with ECT. Electrotherapists should understand the community guidelines for consent and the need to obtain independent consultation in special cases referred for ECT, such as children and adolescents, incompetent and uncooperative patients, special medical risks, and those who may receive more than 30 treatments in any one year. Some consideration should be given to periodic recertification or reexamination, again with guidelines similar to the procedures used at each institution for the continuing certification of those physicians who must maintain similar skills.

Whether ECT should be given by a psychiatrist-electrotherapist alone, or whether an anesthesiologist is necessary to assist in the procedure, is a complex question. For the safety of the patient, the therapist must be skilled in the techniques of anesthesia and in the possible complicating cardiac and respiratory emergencies. The average anesthesiologist—or the average psychiatrist—does not necessarily have training that would preferentially encourage his selection for the administration of the light anesthesia necessary for a successful ECT treatment. Perhaps the question is best answered by requiring the services of personnel, of whatever discipline, trained to administer ECT and anesthesia safely, including the relief of the potential adverse reactions.

TREATMENT PROCEDURES

Anesthesia

There are two common procedures for anesthesia: the use of multiple injections of fixed amounts of anesthetic agents (bolus method) and the multiple drip method. The latter is usually used when a number of patients are to be treated in a session. For both, a butterfly needle, preferably of an 18 or 19 gauge, or an intravenous catheter is put in place, to remain until the patient leaves the treatment room. If an anticholinergic medication has not been given, increments of atropine (0.5 mg) or methscopolamine (0.25 mg) may be given until a noticeable (10%) increase in heart rate is measured. Total doses rarely exceed 1.0 mg atropine or 0.75 mg methscopolamine.

In the drip method, solutions of methohexital (Brevital) (2 mg/cc) and succinylcholine (Anectine) (2 mg/cc) are connected to a three-way stopcock. Methohexital is administered while the patient is asked to count. With slurring of speech, the rate is slowed and continued until the patient does not respond to spoken commands or to tactile stimuli (eyelash reflex), yawns, or respiration becomes noisy (snoring). The dose given is usually 40 to 80 mg methohexital. (If tourniquet-monitoring is used, the blood pressure cuff is now inflated; see below.)

Succinylcholine is administered until spontaneous fasciculations occur in the chest, calf, or small muscles of the feet. A sufficient depth of relaxation can be guaged by the loss of the patellar reflex (its presence should be tested before the infusion begins) or pronounced flaccidity of the lower jaw. The dose needed is usually 20 to 60 mg succinylcholine.

In the bolus method, the procedures are the same, except that stated amounts of the drugs are usually given rapidly, and, to assure anesthesia and relaxation, dosages may be large (60 to 100 mg methohexital, equal to 0.75 to 1.0 mg/kg, and 75 to 125 mg succinylcholine, equal to 1.0 to 1.25 mg/kg). Maximum relaxation is usually measured 40 to 60 sec after the bolus injection of succinylcholine (Buckman et al., 1960).

Oxygenation

The principal complaint of patients after ECT is amnesia. Hypoxia probably contributes to the confusion and amnesia that accompanies treatments. The studies of Holmberg (1953) and the experience with multiple seizures indicate that the risk to short-term memory may be reduced by forced ventilation with high-concentration oxygen. Oxygenation also increases the length of the seizure, which seems to bear a positive correlation with outcome, and reduces postseizure headache and nausea (Holovachka, 1943). Present regimens include (a) voluntary breathing with pure oxygen as soon as the patient is asleep and before succinylcholine is effective, (b) continued forced ventilation with oxygen after the insertion of an oral airway before the treatment, and (c) continued ventilation as soon as practicable after the seizure until the patient breathes fully unaided. Maintenance of an adequate airway and active ventilation with oxygen is an important feature of modified ECT.

Monitoring the Seizure

A probable reason for the belief in the lesser efficacy of unilateral ECT is the occurrence of missed or incomplete seizures. When patients are anesthetized deeply, seizure thresholds rise, and it becomes necessary to increase the current density to elicit a full bilateral seizure. With full muscular paralysis, it is particularly difficult to be certain that a seizure has occurred. Furthermore, the duration of the seizure may be a measure of adequate dosage in ECT. For these reasons, monitoring the seizure and its duration is an integral part of treatment.

Monitoring can be achieved in a number of ways: (a) a tourniquet to block arterial flow to an extremity, (b) EEG, or (c) EMG.

The tourniquet method is the simplest (Addersley and Hamilton, 1953). Before succinylcholine is injected, a tourniquet is inflated over the opposite arm, tight enough to compress the artery, and inflation is sustained until the convulsive movements in that extremity have been timed at longer than 25 sec. (If a seizure is incomplete, the cuff should be released to allow circulation to return).

The EEG requires the application of three EEG electrodes (two active and one ground) to the scalp in areas away from the stimulating electrodes. In nondominant unilateral ECT, one recording electrode is placed over the frontal or temporal area, and the second over the occipital area. If more than a single EEG channel is available, symmetric pairs of electrodes are applied. Recording is done before the treatment for about 1 min; the electrode–machine connection is disrupted before and during application of the ECT currents and reinstituted immediately after the ECT current has ceased. A successful seizure should exhibit spontaneous high voltage, high frequency activity for 15 to 20 sec followed by slow wave activity for 10 to 20 sec, for a total seizure time of 30 sec or more.

EMG monitoring is described by Ives et al. (1976), who developed a small, portable, battery-operated device with an auditory circuit for this purpose. Electrodes are applied to an ipsilateral calf muscle prior to unilateral ECT. When succinylcholine is administered, the normal muscular "sound" first intensifies and then becomes silent. When the stimulating current is followed by a convulsion, even minimal muscular activity may be heard and timed, again to assure a seizure duration greater than 20 sec.

Electrodes and Electrode Placement

Much of the current delivered to the electrodes is dissipated through the skin, galea, and skull, and only small amounts reach the brain. Electrode-skin contact is an important interface; as in electroencephalography, the resistance between the electrode and the skin should be at a minimum. To achieve this, a number of cautions should be considered. Skin areas should be carefully cleansed with a detergent or an organic solvent, or both. Electrodes should be about 1 to 1.5 inches in diameter, and contact should be made using a commercial electrode jelly for metal electrodes or a 25% sodium bicarbonate solution to which a few drops of detergent have been added for soft electrode pads. (If pads are used, these should be replaced frequently so that salt corrosion of the metal contacts does not accumulate and raise electrode resistance).

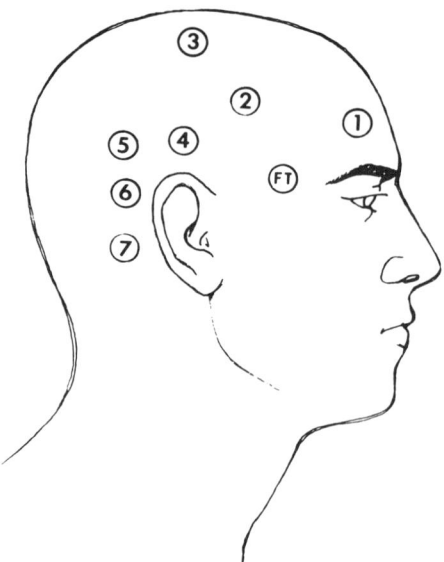

FIG. 16.2. Electrode positions for unilateral ECT. Common frontotemporal electrode **(FT)** is located 1.5 inches on the perpendicular above the imaginary line connecting the outer canthus and the external auditory meatus. Second electrode position varies according to Muller (1971) **(1)**, Lancaster et al. (1958) **(2)**, d'Elia (1970) **(3)**, Zinkin and Birtchnell (1968) **(4)**, McAndrew et al. (1967) **(5)**, Impastato and Karliner (1966) **(6)**, and Halliday et al. (1968) **(7)**. (Redrawn after d'Elia and Raotma, 1975.)

Electrode placement is another important variable. The optimal electrode placement is unilateral nondominant. Although it requires more attention to treatment details to achieve a satisfactory seizure through unilateral electrodes, the benefit in reduced amnesia is clearly worth the effort.

Although no optimal spacing of electrodes has been defined, various devices have been built which space electrodes between 8 and 10 cm apart. The electrodes should be placed over the scalp so that one electrode is between 3 and 5 cm above a point midway between the outer canthus and the external auditory meatus, and the second is at a 70° angle with this imaginary line (Fig. 16.2). Considering the wide range of recommendations reported in the literature, it is unlikely that exact placement is critical, as long as a bilateral seizure is induced. Since higher minimum currents are necessary to induce a generalized seizure with unilateral electrodes, it is especially important to have optimal electrode-skin contact.

Cerebral dominance is determined by asking a patient to indicate the preferred hand, to peer through a rolled-up paper tube, and to walk up to and kick a crumpled piece of paper.[2]

---

[2] If every patient is given right unilateral ECT, about 10% may be misplaced, i.e., be on the effective dominant side. More detailed tests to measure cerebral dominance are described by Clyma (1975) and Fleminger and Bunce (1975).

The individual holding the electrodes in unilateral placement should exert contralateral pressure on the other side of the head to insure good contact; otherwise the head may rotate with the passage of the currents. The electrode handle should be insulated.

If bilateral electrode placement is preferred, the electrodes are placed bilaterally between 3 and 5 cm above the midway point in an imaginary line between the outer canthus and the external auditory meatus. If available, forcep electrodes are useful.

Currents

The intensity of the currents contributes to the degree of amnesia and confusion, and the minimal current necessary to elicit a full grand mal seizure is recommended. Instruments for ECT vary in the type of current and the controls available to the therapist. At present, the principal instruments used in the United States are the Medcraft B-24 (alternating current), Reiter Mol-AC II (unidirectional), and MECTA (rectangular, alternating); in Great Britain, the instruments are produced by Ectron, Ltd. Recommended initial settings for the three instruments are set forth in Table 16.7.

Recent assessments of currents and instruments suggest that brief stimuli may yet provide the optimal currents for treatment. Such instruments produced by Siemens AG and Ectron, Ltd. are in use in Europe. When similar instruments are available in the United States, their use should be carefully assessed.

If a full seizure fails to develop, a second stimulus at a higher intensity or duration of current may be applied after 60 to 90 sec and repeated until a seizure develops. A seizure occasionally fails to develop at maximum instrument settings. The electrode contact should be checked. Some therapists reduce the instrumental controls to 60 to 75% of maximal value and give two applications of current with a momentary delay. If a seizure still fails to develop, pretreatment with pentylenetetrazol may be considered.

Other Concerns

Before a seizure is induced, attention to the mouth and teeth is required. Some therapists use a commercial bite-block, a plastic device similar to that

TABLE 16.7. Current settings

Instrument	Electrodes	
	Unilateral	Bilateral
Medcraft B-24	160–170 V, 1.0 sec	150 V, 0.6 sec
Reiter Mol-AC II	Medium or high, 1.0 sec	Medium, 1.0 sec
MECTA	50–70 Hz, 800 mAmp, 1.0–1.5 msec	50–70 Hz, 0.2–1.0 msec

used by boxers. Others use a sponge-rubber block wrapped in gauze, which is inserted between the teeth just prior to the seizure, particularly in patients with unopposed or poorly aligned teeth. Immediately after the seizure, the bite block is removed, the teeth should be checked, and excessive secretions should be removed by suction.

Forced ventilation should be maintained by the anesthesiologist until the patient breathes spontaneously, regularly, and deeply.

Emergence delirium and excitement may occur in the immediate postictal period; this is best treated by resumption of the infusion of methohexital or amobarbital (Amytal sodium) in a 5% solution, with 200 to 500 mg usually sufficient. Such excitement may recur in subsequent treatments and should be prevented by instituting the methohexital or amobarbital infusion as soon as the seizure is terminated.

Patients are often confused, ataxic, and amnesic after a treatment. They should be transferred from the treatment room to a recovery room where trained nursing personnel can protect them from falling out of bed and, when half-roused, from getting out of bed and falling. Particular attention must be paid also to adequate ventilation, absence of cyanosis, and regularity of pulse rate during the recovery period.

Patients require repeated reassurance and reorientation during their awakening; and this should be done patiently and repeatedly, preferably by someone who knows the patient and whom the patient knows. If family members are available, they are particularly helpful at this time.

Frequency and Number of Seizures

In patients with depressive psychosis, treatments are given either three times or twice weekly. Usually, patients report an elevation in mood and improvement in sleep and appetite after the third or fourth seizure. Treatments are continued until symptoms are well relieved, usually after six to eight treatments. In more severely ill patients, the first few treatments may be given daily; and up to 12 treatments are often prescribed. Similar courses are prescribed for patients with catatonia.

For patients with mania and acute schizophrenia, the frequency of the first treatments may be daily and, in the second and subsequent weeks, three times weekly. A course often requires more seizures, usually between 12 and 20.

The principal criteria for the treatment endpoint are behavioral: a marked alteration in mood and changes in vegetative symptoms. Some therapists, using rating scales, stop when the score has been reduced by half. In some instances, persistent confusion and amnesia may occur early; these warrant termination.

While behavioral criteria are used principally to determine the number of treatments, a therapeutic window may yet be developed, based on the number of seconds of total seizure time. One author suggests that between 210 and 600 sec of total seizure time may be optimal for a course in patients with depressive psychosis (Maletzky, 1978).

Multiple seizures have been recommended by some therapists. Multiple monitored seizures (up to six in one sitting) were suggested by Blachly and Gowing (1966). The initial confirmation studies failed to document increased efficacy, particularly a reduction in total time needed for a course. In addition, a severe confusional syndrome developed in some patients (Chapter 15). At present, such courses should be still considered an investigational use.

Regressive ECT for chronic schizophrenia has recently been recommended again. This regimen, which requires two treatments daily for 10 to 15 days, should also be considered an investigational use (Chapter 15).

FOLLOW-UP CONSIDERATIONS

Medication

After a course of ECT, depressed patients should be given adequate doses of an active antidepressant, preferably one of the tricyclic or newer tetracyclic compounds. Dosage should be equivalent to that given a severely depressed patient (i.e., more than 150 mg/day imipramine, preferably 200 to 250 mg/day) and maintained for 4 to 8 weeks, when the dosage may be reduced to maintenance levels, preferably for 3 months. Ongoing studies of lithium therapy in depression find the need for maintenance ECT to be reduced; reports of these studies should be examined for evidence of the efficacy of lithium maintenance, which may be a useful prophylactic. For patients with catatonia or schizophrenia, the usefulness of maintenance drug therapy is not documented, but the continued treatment of such patients with clinical doses of antipsychotic drugs for 1 to 3 months seems warranted.

Some therapists recommend maintenance ECT treatments spaced at monthly intervals. The evidence for the efficacy of such treatments is slim; for some patients, however, such as those elderly who suffer recurrent depression, such regimens are less compromising than the anticholinergic effects of maintenance tricyclic drug therapy.

For therapists with neurologic experience, follow-up EEG records may demonstrate the development of a well-synchronized, alpha-dominant record within 4 weeks of the last treatment. For patients who suffer a relapse, these patterns are often replaced by increasing amounts of fast activity and EEG desynchronization. When such records are examined as part of follow-up care, the change in the EEG may provide an early indication of relapse.

Laboratory Tests

No routine laboratory tests are indicated after a course of ECT. If anesthesia was protracted, liver function tests are examined to assure integrity after exposure to anesthesia. If convulsions were unusually severe, X-rays of the spine may be retaken, especially if the patient has some symptoms.

Return to Work

With properly administered treatments, the degree of confusion and amnesia associated with the treatment should not interfere with the patient's return to work. Some consideration should be given to a reasonable period of convalescence, as ordinarily accepted after any major illness; but where an early return to work is important to the patient, this should be encouraged. If work involves the handling of mechanical equipment, some limitations may be placed on the patient's activity, as much a response to the effects of maintenance drug therapy as to the effects of ECT.

Except in patients with schizophrenia who may have been given large numbers of treatments, there is no reason to prevent patients exercising their normal responsibilities. In patients receiving regressive ECT, there may be reason to limit activities requiring judgment, but this issue is unclear.

Relapse

The first symptoms of relapse are usually vegetative: anorexia, insomnia, and a loss of interest in work or friends. Depression and withdrawal provide sufficient indication for a psychiatric reassessment and, if medication has been discontinued, for reinstituting drug therapy.

If ECT is reinstituted, it is useful to indicate that subsequent courses of ECT may require more treatments than the first course.

OTHER INDUCTIONS OF SEIZURES

Flurothyl

Procedures for flurothyl (Indoklon) are similar to those for ECT, except that the seizure is induced with three to four forced inhalations of vapor derived from 0.5 cc liquid flurothyl injected into a vaporization chamber attached to the oxygen breathing bag. There are initial myoclonic jerks, followed by the customary tonic and clonic seizure. If only myoclonic jerks follow inhalation, the treatment is incomplete and should be repeated. When anesthesia and succinylcholine are used, the latter is given so that the patient may maintain some respiration. In other respects, indications and cautions are the same as for ECT.

Multiple ECT

Multiple ECT (MECT) is defined as four to eight seizures during a single treatment session. Treatments are monitored with an oscilloscope display or ink-writer record of the EEG obtained from occipitovertex leads. Anesthesia is the same as for ECT, except that an infusion is maintained so that additional doses of succinylcholine can be given, usually after the third or fourth seizure. A useful criterion is the return of the patellar reflex.

Seizures are induced through unilateral or bilateral electrodes at 2-min intervals. The end of a seizure is determined from the EEG. Usually, an EEG period of silence marks the end of the seizure; occasionally, the end is marked by the loss of slow waves and a recurrence of alpha-like activity. Forced ventilation with 100% oxygen throughout the procedure is essential if a severe organic mental syndrome is to be avoided.

The indications for the use of MMECT are unclear, and further study is necessary before its role in treatment is defined.

Special ECT Inductions

Many modifications of ECT have been described over the decades. Few have been adequately studied, and thus their role in treatment is poorly defined.

Petit Mal and Grand Mal

In patients in whom barbiturate anesthesia is contraindicated, amnesia and loss of awareness may be produced by eliciting a petit mal or incomplete seizure before inducing a grand mal seizure with a second application of current. The patient is prepared in the usual way, and succinylcholine is given. Just before the patient experiences the paralysis of respiration, the petit mal stimulus is given (80 V at 0.2 sec with Medcraft B-24; two short, 1/4 sec each, presses of the treatment button, low setting for Mol-AC). Following the petit mal, the succinylcholine infusion continues until full relaxation (loss of patellar reflex) is achieved, when the grand mal seizure is given.

This procedure is quite complex, often leading to pain and panic on the part of the patient and full seizures without adequate muscle relaxation. There is little justification for its use.

Glissando ECT

In glissando ECT, current is increased at a varying rate, as a spring allows a commutator to rapidly pass over coils of a rheostat. There is no evidence that glissando ECT is either helpful or dangerous in an anesthetized patient; nor is there any evidence that it reduces risk of fracture or amnesia. Its continued use seems more a matter of style and adherence to local opinion than a contribution to the efficacy or safety of the treatment.

Electronarcosis

Some authors continue the administration of subconvulsive currents after a grand mal seizure to reduce the depth of anesthesia and postconvulsive stupor. A grand mal seizure is induced, and the electric currents continue through bitemporoparietal electrodes for 5 to 15 min. Currents from a machine that delivers variable milliamperage currents (Reiter CW-47, SOS; Medcraft TC-1,

NC-4) are increased until the patient shows respiratory stridor from spasm of the vocal chords. At this intensity of current, the patient remains unconscious, and respiration is usually adequate. It is clear that only low doses of succinylcholine should be given if this technique is to be employed. Electronarcosis has no defined indication today. The evidence for efficacy is based on uncontrolled studies in severely ill schizophrenic patients, and it is unconvincing.

Shock-Countershock

In some early reports, the passage of low milliamperage, nonconvulsive stimulation following a standard bilateral ECT was reported to reduce memory loss (Alexander, 1953). The initial grand mal seizure is induced by any method; and as soon as the clonic phase is ended, a unidirectional current of 1.0 to 1.5 mAmp is passed through bitemporoparietal leads for 2 min and then discontinued.

Systematic study finds the procedure not only not helpful in reducing amnesia, but the memory changes are worse and the procedure should be discarded (Cronholm and Ottosson, 1961b).

Regressive ECT

Regressive ECT induces an organic mental syndrome, often severe, by the administration of one to three ECT daily for 7 to 14 days. The endpoint is the development of a dementia characterized by incontinence, disorientation, dysarthria, and helplessness. No special techniques for the seizures are described, although each requires anesthesia. Bilateral ECT is usually used.

This technique fell into disuse for a number of decades until some recent studies suggested that the treatment was useful in cases of recurrent, nonresponsive schizophrenia. It is considered an experimental technique and is not recommended for routine clinical use.

Pentylenetetrazol

There are few occasions when pentylenetetrazol (Metrazol) may yet be considered. When used as a convulsant, a 10% solution is prepared, and the initial dose is 5 cc i.v. (0.5 g). If no seizure occurs, additional amounts are given at 40- to 60-sec intervals. In general, this treatment should not be given without the prior administration of a short-acting anesthetic. One use for pentylenetetrazol is in patients in whom a seizure is difficult to elicit with standard ECT instruments. A bolus of 8 to 12 ml pentylenetetrazol (10%) 30 to 60 sec before ECT may reduce the threshold to the seizure sufficiently to induce a seizure. In addition, seizure time will be lengthened (Holmberg et al., 1956).

Chapter 17

L'Envoi

> O Freunde, nicht diese Töne,
> sondern lasst uns angenehmere
> anstimmen, und freudenvollere.
>
> F. Schiller

The changes in brain functions following the repeated induction of seizures are evident in all aspects of behavior—motor activity, speech, memory, orientation, perception, thought processes, vegetative functions—but also in mood and affect. It is the latter changes which are the focus of convulsive *therapy,* and many of the other effects, particularly on memory, orientation, and perception, contribute little to the therapeutic benefits and may be considered side-effects.

The therapeutic efficacy is focused in one population of the mentally ill: those with endogenous depression. Some patients with other conditions also respond well, notably, patients in stupor and catatonia and those refusing to eat. These conditions may have some pathogenic features in common with endogenous depression.

At one time, it was thought that the efficacy of ECT was through psychologic mechanisms, such as amnesia for traumatic events, repression, and punishment. It is more likely, however, that biochemical mechanisms in the brain are brought into play by repeated seizures, and the biochemical changes are the means to alleviate the depressed mood, decreased psychomotor activity, and inhibited vegetative functions which are so responsive. While consideration has been given to many biochemical mechanisms, the present analysis focuses on the role of neurohumors, particularly norepinephrine and acetylcholine, not as direct mediators of mood but as stimulators of changes in neuroendocrine functions. Although the present data are fragmentary and suggestive, it is the changes in the hypothalamic-pituitary and brainstem modulators that elicit the changes in mood and vegetative dysfunctions so responsive to ECT.

RESEARCH

The effects of convulsive therapy in patients with psychotic depression, catatonia, withdrawal, and mania are similar. This finding encourages two conclusions. ECT may be a nonspecific therapy, affecting different mechanisms in each of these conditions, or these syndromes may be manifestations of a common pathogenesis, responsive to a single mechanism called into play with equal facility by repeated seizures.

A psychopathology classification scheme based on the response to stressors has been proposed and tested before, as in amobarbital (sedation threshold) and pentothal tests and autonomic measures. These classifications, which had some heuristic merit, were generally not applicable, possibly because the stressor had little to do with either the pathogenesis of the disorders studied or the mechanism of action of the treatments. It is the merit of ECT in endogenous depression that it is specific for the syndrome, with a rapid and high response rate. It is difficult to escape the conclusion that ECT must be affecting mechanisms that are central to the pathogenesis of depression. Given the present analyses (Chapter 14), measures of neuroendocrine functions probably will provide better predictors and classifiers to identify homogeneous populations of the mentally ill than the earlier stressors. The measures of neuroendocrine function that are abnormal in some mental states and that recover with ECT are the ones most likely to provide useful indices for prediction, classification, and understanding of the mechanism of action of ECT. Such studies provide a better strategy to identify index cases with a common pathogenesis for the genetic and family studies of the pathogenesis of the endogenous depressions.

The recent reviews of neuroendocrine relationships identify changes in hormone functions that are important in patients with endogenous depression (Michael and Gibbons, 1963; Rubin and Mandell, 1966; Fawcett and Bunney, 1967; Carpenter and Bunney, 1971; Carroll, 1975, 1977; Carroll and Mendels, 1976; Ettigi and Brown, 1977). Classification tests are provided by the dexamethasone suppression of cortisol excretion (Carroll et al., 1976 b, c) and the growth hormone response to amphetamine (Langer et al., 1976), insulin (Sachar et al., 1971a), and levodopa (Sachar et al., 1973a), among others (Carroll and Mendels, 1976).

Clinical trials with hypothalamic peptides are particularly compelling. The antidepressant effect of TRH was transient, but one would hope that stereoisomers or analogs of TRH could increase its duration of activity and yet retain its central activity. It is also probable that the dose of TRH that has been given has been inadequate, particularly as to the duration of the treatment. From the experience with ECT and tricyclic drugs in the treatment of psychotic depression, we know that the response usually requires treatment for 7 to 12 days. Few, if any of the studies of TRH have simulated this regimen. Before the final chapter of experience with TRH in the treatment of depression is written, trials of parenteral infusions on a daily basis for 8 to 12 days should be carefully done.

Fractions of ACTH have been identified which separate adrenocorticotrophic and cerebral effects, the latter being focused on memory and attention (de Wied, 1969; van Riezen et al., 1977; Miller et al., 1977). There is some evidence that MIF-1 may have antidepressant activity (Ehrensing and Kastin, 1974, 1978; Kastin et al., 1976a). Others have sought to assess the central and behavioral effects of peptide fragments of β-lipotropin (Kline et al., 1977; de Wied et al., 1978).

A reassessment of the classification and pathogenesis of catatonia and mania is also of interest. Catatonia that is rapidly responsive to ECT seems to be related more to primary depression than to schizophrenia. The same may be said for mania responsive to ECT, although the response to lithium is such that it already provides a meaningful diagnostic and classificatory device for this subgroup of patients with mood disorders.

Anorexia nervosa is a puzzling clinical syndrome in which hypothalamic dysfunction has been implicated (Sheldon, 1939; Reiss, 1943; Bliss and Migeon, 1957; Marks and Bannister, 1963). Recent reviews suggest that evidence of hypothalamic dysfunction is secondary to starvation and is not the cause of the anorexia (Russell et al., 1965; Katz et al., 1976; Vigersky and Loriaux, 1977; Katz and Walsh, 1978). Many remedies have been tried, including ECT, but the reports are not constructive (Gallinek, 1952a; Laboucarie and Barres, 1954; Balduzzi, 1955; Bernstein, 1964). In a recent letter, Katz and Walsh (1978) note an intimate relationship between anorexia nervosa and depression, and they cite a report of the success of amitriptyline in anorexia nervosa as evidence of this association. The indecisive nature of the efficacy of ECT in this condition precludes judgment, but a clinical trial with monitoring of the neuroendocrine relationships may give further evidence about the relationships between hypothalamic functions and mood.

TREATMENT AND TRAINING

Although ECT has undergone a progressive development, surveys of practice find that the usage has not kept pace with the clinical and laboratory findings. There is room, as suggested by the report of the American Psychiatric Association Task Force on Convulsive Therapy (Frankel, 1978), for improvements in clinical practice: in the selection of patients, monitoring of seizures, administration of anesthesia, selection of electrode placements, and use of medications. The available equipment for ECT is inadequate, and instruments are needed that will deliver the minimum amounts of currents, probably brief square wave in type, under the present clinical conditions of anesthesia.

Some attention must also be paid to reimbursement mechanisms which seem to favor the usage of ECT in middle- and upper-class patients treated in private centers and to the insurance and legal problems facing community physicians working in federal, state, and municipal institutions who may be capable of administering ECT but are precluded from doing so because of adverse legal and financial risks.

The educational programs to remedy some of the deficiencies high-lighted in the survey are already underway, but these require additional attention, particularly in medical centers not now using ECT.

There is also a need for the research community, particularly the administration and the advisory committee of the National Institute of Mental Health, to encourage studies of ECT in their programs dedicated to the study of depression. There is much to be gained from the study of depressed patients receiving ECT, perhaps as much as from the collaborative studies focused on antidepressant drugs.

The issues of consent, and the attitudes of the community to the patients who have received ECT and the therapists who administer it, also require some attention. There is little *a priori* reason to apply special rules for consent in the treatment of patients receiving ECT, which are not applied to the same patients when they receive antidepressant drug therapies. Special rules for ECT serve to limit its study and to preclude its inclusion in well-designed, comparative trials or treatments.

CONCLUSION

ECT remains an accepted treatment of primary depression after more than 40 years of experience. It is a long time for a medical regimen to survive the clinical marketplace, particularly a regimen whose mechanism is said to be unknown and whose application is fraught with controversy. It was once thought that this complex treatment would be replaced by antidepressant drugs; and to a large extent this has been true for certain subpopulations of the mentally ill. For the severely depressed, however, ECT remains a principal recourse and satisfies a need not fulfilled by other treatments.

Our present views of the action of ECT and the rapid progress in our knowledge of brain chemistry provide optimism that ECT will soon be replaced by a more specific pharmacologic or physiologic therapy. When that time comes, and the history of ECT is written, it is hoped that the neuroscientists and psychiatrists will respect the intrepid nature of the physicians from central Europe who introduced this remarkable treatment. ECT has provided not only a treatment of unequaled efficacy but a means to study more directly the interactions of brain functions and behavior in man. Its continued study is to be encouraged. It will provide more information about the physiology, psychology, and chemistry of the brain under experimental conditions not likely to be duplicated by any other means, not only for our understanding of ECT, but for our understanding of brain function as well.

References

Abely, P., Loine, B., and Asailly, A. Une hypothese sur le mode d'action de l'electro-choc. *Ann. Med.-psychol.,* 106:453–456, 1948.
Abiuso, P., Dunkelman, R, and Proper, M. Electroconvulsive therapy in patients with pacemakers. *JAMA* 240:2459–2460, 1978.
Abrams, R. Daily administration of unilateral ECT. *Am. J. Psychiatry,* 124:384–386, 1967.
Abrams, R. Multiple ECT: What have we learned? In: M. Fink, S. Kety, J. McGaugh, and T. Williams (Eds.): *Psychobiology of Convulsive Therapy.* V. H. Winston & Sons, Washington, D.C., pp. 79–84, 1974.
Abrams, R. Drugs in combination with ECT. In: M. Greenblatt (Ed.): *Drugs in Combination with Other Therapies.* Grune & Stratton, New York, pp. 157–164, 1975a.
Abrams, R. ECT and psychotropic drugs. In: F. J. Ayd, Jr. (Ed.): *Rational Psychopharmacotherapy and the Right to Treatment.* Ayd Medical Communications, Baltimore, pp. 151–160, 1975b.
Abrams, R., and deVito, R. A. Clinical efficacy of unilateral ECT. *Dis. Nerv. Syst.,* 30:262–263, 1969.
Abrams, R., Essman, W. B., Taylor, M. A., and Fink, M. Concentration of 5-hydroxyindoleacetic acid, homovanillic acid, and tryptophan in the cerebrospinal fluid of depressed patients before and after ECT. *Biol. Psychiatry,* 11:85–90, 1976.
Abrams, R., and Fink, M. *Convulsive Therapy: Methods and Applications.* New York Medical College, New York, 65 pp., 1969.
Abrams, R., and Fink, M. Clinical experience with multiple electroconvulsive treatments. *Compr. Psychiatry,* 13:115–121, 1972.
Abrams, R., Fink, M., Dornbush, R. L., Feldstein, S., Volavka, J., and Roubicek, J. Unilateral and bilateral ECT: Effects on depression, memory, and the electroencephalogram. *Arch. Gen. Psychiatry,* 27:88–91, 1972.
Abrams, R., Fink, M., and Feldstein, S. Prediction of clinical response to ECT. *Br. J. Psychiatry,* 122:457–460, 1973a.
Abrams, R., and Taylor, M. A. Anterior bifrontal ECT: A clinical trial. *Br. J. Psychiatry,* 122:587–590, 1973.
Abrams, R., and Taylor, M. A. Electroconvulsive therapy and the diencephalon: A preliminary report. *Compr. Psychiatry,* 15:233–236, 1974.
Abrams, R., and Taylor, M. A. Catatonia. *Arch. Gen. Psychiatry,* 33:579–584, 1976a.
Abrams, R., and Taylor, M. A. Diencephalic stimulation and the effects of ECT in endogenous depression. *Br. J. Psychiatry,* 129:482–485, 1976b.
Abrams, R., and Taylor, M. A. Catatonia: Prediction of response to somatic treatments. *Am. J. Psychiatry,* 134:78–80, 1977.
Abrams, R., Volavka, J., and Fink, M. EEG seizure patterns during multiple unilateral and bilateral ECT. *Compr. Psychiatry,* 14:25–28, 1973b.
Abrams, R., Volavka, J., Roubicek, J., Dornbush, R., and Fink, M. Lateralized EEG changes after unilateral and bilateral electroconvulsive therapy. *Dis. Nerv. Syst. [Suppl.],* 31:28–33, 1970.
Abse, W. Theory of the rationale of convulsive therapy. *Br. J. Med. Psychol.,* 20:33–50, 1944.
Achte, K. A., and Apo, M. Schizophrenic patients in 1950–1952 and 1957–1959. A comparative study. *Psychiatr. Q.,* 41:422–441, 1967.
Ackner, B., and Grant, Q. A. F. R. The prognostic significance of depersonalization in depressive illnesses treated with electroconvulsive therapy. *J. Neurol. Neurosurg. Psychiatry,* 23:242–246, 1960.
Ackner, B., Harris, A., and Oldham, A. J. Insulin treatment of schizophrenia: Controlled study. *Lancet,* 2:607–611, 1957.
Ackner, B., and Pampiglione, G. An evaluation of the sedation threshold test. *J. Psychosom. Res.,* 3:271–281, 1959.
Addersley, D. J., and Hamilton, M. Use of succinylcholine in E.C.T. *Br. Med. J.,* 1:195–197, 1953.

Aden, G. C. Lithium carbonate versus E.C.T. in the treatment of the manic state of identical twins with bipolar affective disease. *Dis. Nerv. Syst.,* 37:393–397, 1976.
Adler, M. W. Pharmacology of flurothyl: Laboratory and clinical applications. In: W. B. Essman and L. Valzelli (Eds.): *Current Developments in Psychopharmacology.* Spectrum Publications, New York, vol. 2, pp. 29–62, 1975.
Adler, M. W., Reidenberg, M. M., Harakal, C., Rusy, B. F., and Papcostas, C. A. Cardiovascular effects of hexafluorodiethyl ether. *Int. J. Neuropsychiatry,* 1:511–512, 1965.
Adorno, T. W., Frenkel-Brunswik, E., Levinson, D. J., and Sanford, R. N. *The Authoritarian Personality.* Harper and Brothers, New York, 990 pp., 1950.
Adrian, E. D. The spread of activity in the cerebral cortex. *J. Physiol.,* 88:127–161, 1936.
Aird, R. B. Clinical correlates of electroshock therapy. *Arch. Neurol. Psychiatry,* 79:633–639, 1958.
Aird, R. B., and Strait, L. Protective barriers of the central nervous system: An experimental study with trypan red. *Arch. Neurol. Psychiatry,* 51:54–66, 1945.
Aird, R. B., Strait, L. A., Pace, J. W., Hrenoff, M. K., and Bowditch, S. C. Neurophysiologic effects of electrically induced convulsions. *Arch. Neurol. Psychiatry,* 75:371–378, 1956a.
Aird, R. B., Strait, L. A., Pace, J. W., Hrenoff, M. K., and Bowditch, S. C. Current pathway and neurophysiologic effects of electrically induced convulsions. *J. Nerv. Ment. Dis.,* 123:505–512, 1956b.
Alexander, F. G., and Selesnick, S. T. *The History of Psychiatry.* Harper & Row, New York, 471 pp., 1966.
Alexander, L. *Treatment of Mental Disorder.* W. B. Saunders, Philadelphia, 507 pp., 1953.
Alexander, L., and Löwenbach, H. Experimental studies on electro-shock treatment: 1. The intracerebral vascular reaction as an indicator of the path of the current and the threshold of early changes within the brain tissue. *J. Neuropathol. Exp. Neurol.,* 2:139–171, 1944.
Alexander, S. P., Gahagan, L. H., and Lewis, W. H. Deaths following electrotherapy. *JAMA,* 161:577–580, 1956.
Allen, J. P., Denney, D., Kendwall, J. W., and Blachly, P. H. Corticotropin release during ECT in man. *Am. J. Psychiatry,* 131:1225–1228, 1974.
Allen, R. E., and Pitts, F. N. ECT for depressed patients with lupus erythematosus. *Am. J. Psychiatry,* 135:367–368, 1978.
Alpern, H. P., and Kimble, D. P. Retrograde amnesic effects of diethyl ether and bis (trifluoroethyl) ether. *J. Comp. Physiol. Psychol.,* 63:168–171, 1967.
Alpers, B. J. Personality and emotional disorders associated with hypothalamic lesions. In: J. F. Fulton, S. W. Ranson, and A. M. Frantz (Eds.): *The Hypothalamus and Central Levels of Autonomic Function.* Williams & Wilkins, Baltimore, vol. 20, pp. 725–752, 1939.
Alpers, B. J. Brain changes associated with electrical shock treatment: A critical review. *Lancet,* 66:363–369, 1946.
Alpers, B. J., and Hughes, J. The brain changes in electrically induced convulsions in the human. *J. Neuropathol. Exp. Neurol.,* 1:173–180, 1942.
Altman, L. L., Pratt, D., and Cotton, J. M. Cardio-vascular response to acetyl-beta-methylcholine (Mecholyl) in mental disorders. *J. Nerv. Ment. Dis.,* 97:296–309, 1943.
Altschule, M. D. Further observations on vagal influences on the heart during electroshock therapy for mental disease. *Am. Heart J.,* 39:88–91, 1950.
Altschule, M. D., Cline, J. E., and Tillotson, K. J. Fall in plasma protein level associated with rapid gain in weight during course of electroshock therapy. *Arch. Neurol. Psychiatry,* 59:476–480, 1948a.
Altschule, M. D., Cram, J. E., and Tillotson, K. J. Hemoconcentration after electrically induced convulsions in man. *Arch. Neurol. Psychiatry,* 59:29–38, 1948b.
Altschule, M. D., Parkhurst, B. H., and Tillotson, K. J. Decreases in blood eosinophilic leucocytes after electrically induced convulsions in man. *J. Clin. Endocrinol.,* 9:440–445, 1949.
Altschule, M. D., Promisel, E., Parkhurst, B. H., and Grunebaum, H. Effects of ACTH in patients with mental disease. *Arch. Neurol. Psychiatry,* 64:641–649, 1950.
Altschule, M. D., Sulzbach, W. M. and Tillotson, K. J. Effect of electrically induced convulsions on peripheral venous pressure in man. *Arch. Neurol. Psychiatry,* 58:193–199, 1947a.
Altschule, M. D., Sulzbach, W. M., and Tillotson, K. J. Significance of change in the electrocardiogram after electrically induced convulsions in man. *Arch. Neurol. Psychiatry,* 58:716–720, 1947b.
Anderson, E. Earlier ideas of hypothalamic function, including irrelevant concepts. In: W. Haymaker, E. Anderson, and W. J. H. Nauta (Eds.): *The Hypothalamus.* Charles C Thomas, Springfield, Ill., pp. 1–12, 1969.

Androp, S. Electric shock therapy in the psychoses: Convulsive and subconvulsive methods. *Psychiatr. Q.,* 16:730–749, 1941.

Angel, C., Hartman, A. M., Burkett, M. L., and Roberts, A. J. Effects of electroshock and trypan red on the blood-brain barrier and response retention in the rat. *J. Nerv. Ment. Dis.,* 140:405–411, 1965.

Angel, C., and Roberts, A. J. Effect of electroshock and antidepressant drugs on cerebrovascular permeability to cocaine in the rat. *J. Nerv. Ment. Dis.,* 142:376–380, 1966.

Anton, A. H., Uy, D. S., and Redderson, C. L. Autonomic blockade and the cardiovascular and catecholamine response to electroshock. *Anesth. Analg.,* 56:46–54, 1977.

Apo, M., and Achte, K. A. A comparative study of schizophrenia in 1950–52 and 1957–59. *Nord. Psykiatic Tidsskr.,* 20:125–140, 1966.

Appel, K. E., Myers, J. M., and Scheflen, A. E. Prognosis in psychiatry: Results of psychiatric treatment. *Arch. Neurol. Psychiatry,* 70:459–468, 1953.

Arajarvi, T., Alanen, Y. O., and Viitamaki, O. Psychoses in childhood. *Acta Psychiatr. Scand. [Suppl. 174],* 40:1–93, 1964.

Arfwidsson, L., Arn, L., Beskow, J., d'Elia, G., Laurell, B., Ottosson, J.-O., Perris, C., Persson, G., and Wistedt, B. Chlorpromazine and the antidepressive efficacy of electroconvulsive therapy. *Acta Psychiatr. Scand.,* 49:580–587, 1973.

Arneson, G. A., and Butler, T. Cardiac arrest and electroshock therapy. *Am. J. Psychiatry,* 117:1020–1022, 1961.

Arneson, G. A., and Ourso, R. Bromide intoxication and electroshock therapy. *Am. J. Psychiatry,* 121:1115–1116, 1965.

Arnold, O. H. Results and efficacy of insulin shock therapy. In: M. Rinkel (Ed.): *Insulin Treatment in Psychiatry.* Philosophical Library, New York, pp. 199–221, 1959.

Arnold, O. H., and Böck-Greissau, W. Elektroschock und Muskelrelaxantien. *Wien. Ztschr. Nervenheilk. Grenzgeb.,* 4:326–349, 1952.

Ashby, W. R. The effects of convulsive therapy on the excretion of cortins and ketosteroids. *J. Ment. Sci.,* 95:275–324, 1949.

Ashby, W. R. The mode of action of electro-convulsive therapy. *J. Ment. Sci.,* 99:202–215, 1953.

Ashton, R., and Hess, N. Amnesia for random shapes following unilateral and bilateral electroconvulsive shock therapy. *Percept. Mot. Skills,* 42:669–670, 1976.

Asnis, G. Parkinson's disease, depression, and ECT: A review and case study. *Am. J. Psychiatry,* 134:191–195, 1977.

Asnis, G., Fink, M., and Saferstein, S. ECT in metropolitan New York hospitals: A survey of practice, 1975–1976. *Am. J. Psychiatry,* 135:479–482, 1978.

Assael, M. I., Halpern, B., and Alpern, S. Centrencephalic epilepsy induced by electrical convulsive treatment. *Electroencephalogr. Clin. Neurophysiol.,* 23:195, 1967.

Avery, D., and Winokur, G. Mortality in depressed patients treated with electroconvulsive therapy and antidepressants. *Arch. Gen. Psychiatry,* 33:1029–1037, 1976.

Avery, D., and Winokur, G. The efficacy of electroconvulsive therapy and antidepressants in depression. *Biol. Psychiatry,* 12:507–524, 1977.

Ayd, F. Guidelines for treating cardiac patients with tricyclic and tetracyclic antidepressants. *Int. Drug Ther. Newsletter,* 13:9–12, 1978.

Ayd, F., and Blackwell, B. *Discoveries in Biological Psychiatry.* J. B. Lippincott, Philadelphia, 254 pp., 1970.

Ayres, C. M. The relative value of various somatic therapies in schizophrenia. *J. Neuropsychiatry,* 1:154–162, 1960.

Babington, R. G., and Wedeking, P. W. The pharmacology of seizures induced by sensitization with low-intensity brain stimulation. *Pharmacol. Biochem. Behav.,* 1:461–467, 1973.

Babington, R. G., and Wedeking, P. W. Blockade of tardive seizures in rats by electroconvulsive shock. *Brain Res.,* 88:141–144, 1975.

Baker, A. A., Bird, G., Lavin, N. I., and Thorpe, J. G. ECT in schizophrenia. *J. Ment. Sci.,* 106:1506–1511, 1960a.

Baker, A. A., Game, J. A., and Thorpe, J. G. Some research into the treatment of schizophrenia in the mental hospital. *J. Ment. Sci.,* 106:203–213, 1960b.

Baldessarini, R. J. The basis for amine hypothesis in affective disorders. *Arch. Gen. Psychiatry,* 32:1087–1093, 1975a.

Baldessarini, R. J. Biogenic amine hypotheses in affective disorders. In: F. F. Flach, and S. S.

Draghi (Eds.): *The Nature and Treatment of Depression.* John Wiley & Sons, New York, pp. 347–385, 1975*b.*

Baldessarini, R. J. Schizophrenia. *N. Engl. J. Med.,* 297:988–995, 1977.

Balduzzi, E. In tema di terapia dell'anoressia mentale: Considerazioni a proposito dell'insorgenza di reazioni bulimiche dopo elettroshock. *Note Riv. Psichiatr.,* 47:64–72, 1955.

Bankhead, A. J., Torrens, J. K., and Harris, T. H. Anticipation and prevention of cardiac complications in electroconvulsive therapy. *Am. J. Psychiatry,* 106:911–917, 1950.

Banta, H. D. ECT: A cost-benefit analysis. Conference: *ECT: Efficacy and Impact.* New Orleans, February 25, 1978.

Barker, J. C., and Baker, A. A. Deaths associated with electroplexy. *J. Ment. Sci.,* 105:339–348, 1959.

Barnacle, C. H. Grief reactions and their treatment. *Dis. Nerv. Syst.,* 10:173–176, 1949.

Barrera, S. E., Lewis, N. D. C., Pacella, B. L., and Kalinowsky, L. Brain changes associated with electrically induced seizures. *Trans. Am. Neurol. Assoc.,* 68:31–35, 1942.

Barron, S. P., and Sullivan, T. M. The use of the cardiac pacemaker in an ECT-induced cardiac arrest. *Am. J. Psychiatry,* 124:395–396, 1967.

Barton, J. L. ECT in depression: The evidence of controlled studies. *Biol. Psychiatry,* 12:687–695, 1977.

Barton, J. L., Mehta, S., and Snaith, R. P. The prophylactic value of extra ECT in depressive illness. *Acta Psychiatr. Scand.,* 49:386–392, 1973.

Bassett, M., and Ashby, W. R. The effect of electro-convulsive therapy on the psycho-galvanic response. *J. Ment. Sci.,* 100:632–642, 1954.

Battie, W. *Treatise on Madness.* Whiston & White, London, pp. 84–85, 1758.

Bayles, S., Busse, E. W., and Ebaugh, F. G. Square waves (BST) versus sine waves in electroconvulsive therapy. *Am. J. Psychiatry,* 107:34–41, 1950.

Beck, P. J., and Reis, D. J. A toxic interaction between lithium and some psychotropic agents in rat. *Res. Commun. Psychol. Psychiatr. Behav.,* 1:269–282, 1976.

Beck, S. J. Effects of shock therapy on personality, as shown by the Rorschach test. *Arch. Neurophysiol.,* 50:483–484, 1943.

Bellet, S., Kershbaum, A., and Furst, W. The electrocardiogram during electric shock treatment of mental disorders. *Am. J. Med. Sci.,* 201:167–177, 1941.

Bender, L. The life course of children with schizophrenia. *Am. J. Psychiatry,* 130:783–786, 1973.

Bender, M. B. *Disorders in Perception.* Charles C Thomas, Springfield, Ill., 109 pp., 1952.

Bennett, A. E. Convulsive (pentamethylenetetrazol) shock therapy in depressive psychoses. *Am. J. Ment. Sci.,* 196:420–429, 1938.

Bennett, A. E. Metrazol convulsive shock therapy in affective psychoses. A follow-up of results obtained in 61 depressive and 9 manic cases. *Am. J. Ment. Sci.,* 198:695–701, 1939.

Bennett, A. E. Preventing traumatic complications in convulsive shock therapy by curare. *JAMA,* 114:322–324, 1940.

Bennett, A. E. Curare: A preventive of traumatic complications in convulsive shock therapy. Including a report on a synthetic curare-like drug. *Am. J. Psychiatry,* 97:1040–1060, 1941.

Bennett, A. E. Convulsive shock therapy in involutional states after complete failure with previous estrogenic treatment. *Am. J. Med. Sci.,* 208:170–176, 1944.

Bennett, A. E. The introduction of curare into clinical medicine. Present and potential usefulness. *Am. Sci.,* 34:424–431, 1946.

Bennett, A. E. The history of the introduction of curare into medicine. *Anesth. Analg. (Cleve.),* 47:484–492, 1968.

Bennett, A. E. *Fifty Years in Neurology and Psychiatry.* Intercontinental Book, New York, 166 pp., 1972.

Bennett, A. E., and Wilbur, C. B. Convulsive shock therapy in involutional states after complete failure with previous estrogenic treatment. *Am. J. Med. Sci.,* 208:170–176, 1944.

Bennie, E. H. ECT and lithium. *Br. Med. J.,* 1:578–579, 1978.

Bente, D., Itil, T., and Schmid, E. E. Elektroencephalographische Studien zur Wirkungsweise des LSD-25. *Psychiatr. Neurol.,* 135:273–284, 1958.

Berent, S., Cohen, B. D., and Silverman, A. J. Changes in verbal and non-verbal learning following a single left or right unilateral electroconvulsive treatment. *Biol. Psychiatry,* 10:95–100, 1975.

Beresford, H. R. Legal issues relating to ECT. *Arch. Gen. Psychiatry,* 25:100–102, 1971.

Beresford, H. R. Electroconvulsive therapy: Neurological side effects. Conference: *ECT: Efficacy and Impact.* New Orleans, February 23, 1978.

Beresford, H. R., Posner, J. B., and Plum, F. Changes in brain lactate during induced cerebral seizures. *Arch. Neurol.*, 20:243–248, 1969.
Berg, S., Gabriel, A. R., and Impastato, D. J. Comparative evaluation of the safety of chlorpromazine and reserpine used in conjunction with ECT. *J. Neuropsychiatry*, 1:104–107, 1959.
Berger, H. Über das Elecktroencephalogramm des Menschen. *Arch. f. Psychiat. u. Nervenkrank.* 87:527–570, 1929.
Bergman, P. S., Impastato, D. J., Berg, S., and Feinstein, R. Electroencephalographic changes following electrically induced focal seizures. *Confin. Neurol.*, 13:271–277, 1953.
Berkwitz, N. J. Non-convulsive electric (faradic) shock therapy of psychoses associated with alcoholism, drug intoxications and syphilis. Am. J. Psychiatry, 99:364–373, 1942.
Bernstein, I. C. Anorexia nervosa treated successfully with electroshock therapy and subsequently followed by pregnancy. *Am. J. Psychiatry*, 120:1023–1024, 1964.
Bernstein, I. C., Bernstein, D. M., and Adzick, G. R. Electrotherapy and renal transplantation—Impediment to treatment. *Minn. Med.*, 60:410–411, 1977.
Berson, S., and Yalow, R. Radioimmunoassay of ACTH in plasma. *J. Clin. Invest.*, 47:2725–2751, 1968.
Beuret, L., and Swanson, D. W. Endocrine effects of electroconvulsive therapy: A review. *Psychiatr. Q.*, 43:650–661, 1969.
Bianchi, J. A., and Chiarello, C. J. Shock therapy in the involutional and manic-depressive psychoses. *Psychiatr. Q.*, 18:118–126, 1944.
Bianchi, J. A., and Chiarello, C. J. Comparative results of electric shock and metrazol convulsive treatment in dementia praecox. *Psychiatr. Q.*, 21:304–311, 1947.
Bidder, T. G., and Strain, J. J. Modifications of electroconvulsive therapy. *Compr. Psychiatry*, 2:507–517, 1970.
Bidder, T. G., Strain, J. J., and Brunschwig, L. Bilateral and unilateral ECT: Follow-up study and critique. *Am. J. Psychiatry*, 127:737–745, 1970.
Biggs, J. T. Clinical pharmacology and toxicology of antidepressants. *Hosp. Practice*, 13:79–84, 1978.
Bilikiewicz, A., and Krzyzowski, J. Application of unilateral electric shock in psychiatry. *Neurol. Neurochir. Psychiatr. Pol.*, 14:663–669, 1964.
Bini, L. Ricerche sperimentali sull'accesso epilettico da corrente elettrica. *Schweiz. Arch. Neurol. Psychiatr.*, 39:121–122, 1937.
Bini, L., and Bazzi, T. L'elettroshockterapia col metodo dell'annihilimento nelle forme gravi di psiconneurosi. *Rassegna Neuropsichiatr.*, 1:59–70, 1947.
Bjerner, B., Broman, T., and Swensson, Å. Tierexperimentelle Untersuchungen über Schädigungen der Gefässe mit Permeabilitätsstorungen und Blutungen im Gehirn bei Insulin-, Cardiazol- und Electroshock-behandlung. *Acta Psychiatr. Neurol.*, 19:431–452, 1944.
Björum, N., Plenge, P., and Rafaelson, O. J. Electrolytes in CSF in endogenous depression. *Acta Psychiatr. Scand.*, 48:533–539, 1972.
Blachly, P. H. New developments in electroconvulsive therapy. *Dis. Nerv. Syst.*, 37:356–358, 1976.
Blachly, P., and Gowing, D. Multiple monitored electroconvulsive treatment. *Compr. Psychiatry*, 7:100–109, 1966.
Black, F. W., Williams, A. V., and Bowen, C. D. Electroconvulsive treatment (ECT) in illicit drug-related psychosis: Case reports. *Milit. Med.*, 139:887–888, 1974.
Blackman, L. *Clonotherapy: A Manual for Convulsive Therapies.* Private printing, 102 pp., 1974.
Blaurock, M. F., Lorimer, F. M., Segal, M. M., and Gibbs, F. A. Focal electroencephalographic changes in unilateral electric convulsive therapy. *Arch. Neurol. Psychiatry*, 64:220–226, 1950.
Bliss, E. L., and Migeon, C. J. Endocrinology of anorexia nervosa. *J. Clin. Endocrinol. Metab.*, 17:766–776, 1957.
Bliss, E. L., Migeon, C. J., Nelson, D. H., Samuels, L. T., and Branch, C. H. H. Influence of E.C.T. and insulin coma on level of adrenocortical steroids in peripheral circulation. *Arch. Neurol. Psychiatry*, 72:352–361, 1954.
Blum, J. D. On changes in psychiatric diagnosis over time. *Am. Psychol.* 33:1017–1031, 1978.
Blumberg, A. G., Cohen, L., and Miller, J. S. A. The relation of mecholyl induced hypotension to the classification of psychiatric patients and its prognostic significance with electroshock therapy. *J. Hillside Hosp.*, 5:216–231, 1956.
Blumenthal, I. J. Spontaneous seizures and related electroencephalographic findings following shock therapy. *J. Nerv. Ment. Dis.*, 122:581–588, 1955.

Boardman, R. H., Lomas, J., and Markowe, M. Insulin and chlorpromazine in schizophrenia: Comparative study in previously untreated cases. *Lancet,* 2:487–494, 1956.

Bodlander, F. M. S. Deaths associated with anesthesia. *Br. J. Anaesth.,* 47:36–40, 1975.

Bolwig, T. G., Hertz, M. M., and Holm-Jensen, J. Blood-brain barrier permeability during electroshock seizures in the rat. *Eur. J. Clin. Invest.,* 7:95–100, 1977a.

Bolwig, T. G., Hertz, M. M., Paulson, O. B., Spotoft, H., and Rafaelson, O. J. The permeability of the blood-brain barrier during electrically induced seizures in man. *Eur. J. Clin. Invest.,* 7:87–93, 1977b.

Bond, E. D. Results of treatment in psychoses—with a control series. (Involutional psychotic reaction.) *Am. J. Psychiatry,* 110/12:881–883, 1954.

Bonner, C. A., and Kent, G. H. Overlapping symptoms in catatonic excitement and manic excitement. *Am. J. Psychiatry,* 92:1311–1322, 1936.

Borowitz, A. H. An investigation into combined electroconvulsive and chlorpromazine therapy in the treatment of schizophrenia. *S. Afr. Med. J.,* 33:836–840, 1959.

Bourne, H. Convulsion dependence. *Lancet,* 2:1193–1196, 1954.

Bourne, H. Convulsion dependence and rational convulsion therapy. *J. Indian Med. Profession* 3:1–6, 1956.

Bourne, P. *Men, Stress and Vietnam.* Little, Brown & Co., Boston, 193 pp, 1970.

Bowman, K. M. Sakel and biological treatment of schizophrenia. In: M. Rinkel (Ed.): *Biological Treatment of Mental Illness.* Farrar, Straus and Giroux, New York, pp. 54–61, 1966.

Bowman-Barany, M. On the treatment of mania with electrically-induced convulsions. *Nord. Med.,* 15:2535–2536, 1942.

Boyd, D. A., Jr. Electroshock therapy in atypical pain syndromes. *Lancet,* 76:22–25, 1956.

Boyd, D. A., and Brown, D. W. Electroconvulsive therapy in mental disorders associated with childbearing. *J. Missouri Med.,* 45:573–579, 1948.

Bradley, P., and Fink, M. (Eds.): *Anticholinergic Drugs and Brain Functions in Animals and Man. Progress in Brain Research, 28.* Elsevier, Amsterdam, 184 pp., 1968.

Brambilla, F., Smeraldi, E., Sacchetti, E., Negri, F., Cocchi, D. and Müller, E. E. Deranged anterior pituitary responsiveness to hypothalamic hormones in depressed patients. *Arch. Gen. Psychiat.* 35:1231–1238, 1978.

Bratfos, O., and Haug, J. O. Electroconvulsive therapy and antidepressant drugs in manic-depressive disease. *Acta Psychiatr. Scand.,* 41:588–596, 1965.

Brazier, M. A. B. *Bibliography of Electroencephalography.* Int. Fed. EEG Clin. Neurophysiol., Montreal, 178 pp., 1950.

Breakey, W. R., and Kala, A. K. Typhoid catatonia responsive to ECT. *Br. Med. J.,* 2:357–359, 1977.

Breitner, C. Localized electric stimulation of the diencephalon in the treatment of mental disorders. *Dis. Nerv. Syst. [Suppl.],* 18:14–20, 1957.

Brengelmann, J. C. The effect of repeated electroshock on learning in depressives. *Monogr. Gesamtgeb. Neurol. Psychiatr.,* 84:1–52, 1959.

Brewer, C. Risks of tricyclic antidepressants. *Br. J. Psychiatry,* 132:107–108, 1978.

Bridenbaugh, R. H., Drake, F. R., and O'Regan, T. J. Multiple monitored electroconvulsive treatment of schizophrenia. *Compr. Psychiatry,* 13:9–17, 1972.

Bridges, P. K., and Bartlett, J. R. Psychosurgery: Yesterday and today. *Br. J. Psychiatry,* 131: 249–260, 1977.

Brill, H. Contributions of biological treatments to psychiatry. In: Rinkel, M. (Ed.): *Biological Treatment of Mental Illness.* Farrar, Straus and Giroux, New York, pp. 62–70, 1966.

Brill, N. Q., Crumpton, E., Eiduson, S., Grayson, H. M., Hellman L. I., Richards, R. A., Strassman, H. D., and Unger, A. A. Investigation of the therapeutic components and various factors associated with improvement with electroconvulsive treatment: A preliminary report. *Am. J. Psychiatry,* 113:997–1008, 1957.

Brill, N. Q., Crumpton, E., Eiduson, S., Grayson, H. M., and Hellman, L. I. Predictive and concomitant variables related to improvement with actual and simulated ECT. *Arch. Gen. Psychiatry,* 1:263–272, 1959a.

Brill, N. Q., Crumpton, E., Eiduson, S., Grayson, H. M., Hellman, L. I., and Richards, R. A. Relative effectiveness of various components of electroconvulsive therapy. *Arch. Neurol. Psychiatry,* 81:627–635, 1959b.

Brockman, R. J., Brockman, J. C., Jacobsohn, N., Gleser, G. C., and Ulett, G. A. Changes in convulsive threshold as related to type of treatment. *Confin. Neurol.,* 16:97–104, 1956.

Brody, M. B. Prolonged memory defects following electro-therapy. *J. Ment. Sci.,* 90:777–779, 1944.

Brooks, B. R., and Adams, R. D. Cerebrospinal fluid acid-base and lactate changes after seizures in unanesthetized man. I. Idiopathic seizures. *Neurology,* 25:935–942, 1975.
Bross, R. Near fatality with combined ECT and reserpine. *Am. J. Psychiatry,* 113:933, 1957.
Brown, D. G., Hullin, R. P., and Roberts, J. M. Fluid distribution and the response of depression to E.C.T. and imipramine. *Br. J. Psychiatry,* 109:395–398, 1963.
Brown, G. L. Parkinsonism, depression, and ECT. *Am. J. Psychiatry,* 132:1084, 1975.
Brown, M. L., Brown, G. W., and Hines, H. M. Changes in blood flow, blood pressure and cardiac rate associated with electroconvulsive shock. *Am. J. Psychiatry,* 109:27–31, 1952.
Brown, M. L., Huston, P. E., Hines, H. M., and Brown, G. W. Cardiovascular changes associated with electroconvulsive therapy in man. *Arch. Neurol. Psychiatry,* 69:601–608, 1953a.
Brown, M. L., Huston, P. E., Hines, H. M., and Brown, G. W. Cardiovascular changes associated with electroconvulsive shock in monkeys. *Arch. Neurol. Psychiatry,* 69:609–614, 1953b.
Bruce, E. M., Crone, N., Fitzpatrick, G., Frewin, S. J., Gillis, A., Lascelles, C. F., Levene, L. J., and Mersky, H. A comparative trial of ECT and Tofranil. *Am. J. Psychiatry,* 117:76, 1960.
Brune, G. G., and Himwich, H. E. Biogenic amines and behavior in schizophrenic patients. *Recent Adv. Biol. Psychiatry,* 5:144–160, 1963.
Brunschwig, L., Strain, J., and Bidder, T. G. Issues in the assessment of post-ECT memory changes. *Br. J. Psychiatry,* 119:73–74, 1971.
Brussel, J. A., and Schneider, J. The B.E.S.T. in the treatment and control of chronically disturbed mental patients. *Psychiatr. Q.,* 25:55–64, 1951.
Buckingham, J. C., and Hodges, J. R. Production of corticotrophin releasing hormone by the isolated hypothalamus of the rat. *J. Physiol.,* 272:469–479, 1977.
Buckman, C., Krell, A., Pinsley, I., Impastato, A. S., and Impastato, D. J. The "adequate relaxation interim" following succinylcholine administration in electroshock therapy. *Am. J. Psychiatry,* 117:342–345, 1960.
Cade, J. A significant elevation of plasma magnesium levels in schizophrenia and depressive states. *Med. J. Aust.,* 1:195–196, 1964.
Callaway, E., and Boucher, F. Slow wave phenomena in intensive electroshock. *Electroencephalogr. Clin. Neurophysiol.,* 2:157–162, 1950.
Cameron, D. E. Production of differential amnesia as a factor in the treatment of schizophrenia. *Compr. Psychiatry,* 1:26–34, 1960.
Cameron, D. E., Lohrenz, J. H., and Handcock, K. A. The depatterning treatment of schizophrenia. *Compr. Psychiatry,* 3:65–76, 1962.
Cammer, L. *Up from Depression.* Simon and Schuster, New York, 254 pp., 1969.
Campbell, J. E., Weiss, W. A., and Rieder F. Evaluation of deaths associated with anesthesia. *Anesth. Analg. (Cleve.),* 40:54–68, 1961.
Campbell, M. Biological interventions in psychoses of childhood. *J. Autism Child. Schizo.,* 3:347–373. 1973.
Campbell, M. Introduction. Clinical trials of TRH. *Psychopharmacol. Bull.,* 11: 19–20, 1975.
Cannicott, S. M. Unilateral electro-convulsive therapy. *Postgrad. Med. J.,* 38:451–459, 1962.
Cannicott, S. M. Order out of confusion. Discussion: E. Miller: Psychological theories of ECT: A review. *Int. J. Psychiatry,* 5:165–168, 1969.
Cannicott, S. M., and Waggoner, R. W. Unilateral and bilateral electroconvulsive therapy. *Arch. Gen. Psychiatry,* 16:229–232, 1967.
Caplan, G. Electrical convulsion therapy in the treatment of epilepsy. *J. Ment. Sci.,* 92:784, 1946.
Carman, J. S., Post, R. M., Goodwin, F. K., and Bunney, W. E. Calcium and electroconvulsive therapy of severe depressive illness. *Biol. Psychiatry,* 12:5–17, 1977.
Carman, J. S., and Wyatt, R. J. Alterations in cerebrospinal fluid and serum total calcium with changes in psychiatric state. In: E. Usdin, D. A. Hamburg, and J. Barchas (Eds.): *Neuroregulators and Psychiatric Disorders.* Oxford University Press, New York, pp. 488–494, 1977.
Carney, M. W. P., Roth, M., and Garside, R. F. The diagnosis of depressive syndromes and the prediction of E.C.T. response. *Br. J. Psychiatry,* 111:659–674, 1965.
Carney, M. W. P., and Sheffield, B. F. Electroconvulsive therapy and the diencephalon. *Lancet,* 1:1505–1506, 1973.
Carney, M. W. P., and Sheffield, B. F. The effects of pulse ECT in neurotic and endogenous depression. *Br. J. Psychiatry,* 125:91–94, 1974.
Carney, M. W. P., Sheffield, B. F., and Sebastian, J. Serum magnesium, diagnosis, ECT and season. *Br. J. Psychiatry,* 122:427–429, 1973.
Carpenter, W., and Bunney, W. E. Adrenal cortical activity in depressive illness. *Am. J. Psychiatry,* 123:387–400, 1971.

Carroll, B. Review of clinical research strategies in affective illness. In J. Mendels (Ed.): *Psychobiology of Depression.* Spectrum, New York, pp. 143–159, 1975.
Carroll, B. J. Psychiatric disorders and steroids. In: E. Usdin, D. A. Hamburg, and J. D. Barchas (Eds.): *Neuroregulators and Psychiatric Disorders.* Oxford University Press, New York, pp. 276–283, 1977.
Carroll, B. J. Neuroendocrine function in psychiatric disorders. In: M. A. Lipton, A. DiMascio, and K. F. Killam (Eds.): *Psychopharmacology: A Generation of Progress.* Raven Press, New York, pp. 487–497, 1978.
Carroll, B. J., Curtis, G. C., Davies, B. M., Mendels, J., and Sugerman, A. A. Urinary free cortisol excretion in depression. *Psychol. Med.,* 6:43–50, 1976a.
Carroll, B. J., Curtis, G. C., and Mendels, J. Neuroendocrine regulation in depression. I. Limbic system-adrenocortical dysfunction. *Arch. Gen. Psychiatry,* 33:1039–1044, 1976b.
Carroll, B. J., Curtis, G. C., and Mendels, J., Neuroendocrine regulation in depression. II. Discrimination of depressed from nondepressed patients. *Arch. Gen. Psychiatry,* 33:1051–1058, 1976c.
Carroll, B. J., Curtis, G. C., and Mendels, J. Cerebrospinal fluid and plasma free cortisol concentrations in depression. *Psychol. Med.,* 6:235–244, 1976d.
Carroll, B. J., and Mendels, J. Neuroendocrine regulation in affective disorders. In: E. J. Sachar (Ed.): *Hormones, Behavior and Psychopathology.* Raven Press, New York, pp. 193–224, 1976.
Carse, J., and Slater, E. Lymphocytosis after electric convulsion. *J. Neurol. Neurosurg. Psychiatry,* 9:1–4, 1946.
Cash, P. T., and Hoekstra, C. S. Preliminary curarization in electric convulsive shock therapy. *Psychiatr. Q.,* 17:20–34, 1943.
Catalano-Nobili, C., and Cerquetelli, G. *L'Elettroshock. Trent'Anni di Espierienza.* Il Pensiero Scientifico, Rome, 239 pp., 1972.
Cerletti, U. Old and new information about electroshock. *Am. J. Psychiatry,* 107:87–94, 1950.
Cerletti, U. Electroshock therapy. In: F. Marti-Ibanez, A. M. Sackler, M. D. Sackler, and R. R. Sackler (Eds.): *The Great Physiodynamic Therapies in Psychiatry.* Hoeber-Harper, New York, pp. 91–120, 1956.
Cerletti, U., and Bini, L. Un nuevo metodo di shockterapie "L'elettro-shock" *Boll. Acad. Med. Roma,* 64:136–138, 1938.
Chafetz, M. E. An active treatment for chronically ill patients. *J. Nerv. Ment. Dis.,* 98:464–473, 1943.
Chase, L. S., and Silverman, S. Prognostic criteria in schizophrenia. *Am. J. Psychiatry,* 98:360–368, 1941.
Chatrian, G. E., and Petersen, M. C. The convulsive patterns provoked by Indoklon, Metrazol and electroshock: Some depth electrographic observations in human patients. *Electroencephalogr. Clin. Neurophysiol.,* 12:715–725, 1960.
Checkley, S. A., and Crammer, J. L. Hormone responses to methylamphetamine in depression: A new approach to the noradrenaline depletion hypothesis. *Br. J. Psychiatry,* 131:582–586, 1977.
Cheney, C. O., and Drewry, P. H. Results of nonspecific treatment in dementia praecox. *Am. J. Psychiatry,* 95:203–217, 1938.
Cherkin, A. Effects of flurothyl (Indoklon) upon memory in the chick, In: M. Fink, S. Kety, J. McGaugh, and T. A. Williams (Eds.): *Psychobiology of Convulsive Therapy.* V. H. Winston & Sons, Washington, D.C., pp. 129–141, 1974.
Chessen, D. H., Geha, D. G., and Salzman, C. ECT, glaucoma, and prolonged apnea. *Dis. Nerv. Syst.,* 35:152–153, 1974.
Childers, R. T. Comparison of four regimens in newly admitted female schizophrenics. *Am. J. Psychiatry,* 120:1010–1011, 1964.
Choi, S. J., Taylor, M. A., and Abrams, R. Depression, ECT, and erythrocyte adenosinetriphosphatase activity. *Biol. Psychiatry,* 12:75–81, 1977.
Churchill-Davidson, H. C., and Griffiths, W. J. A simple test-paper method for clinical determination of plasma pseudocholinesterase. *Br. Med. J.,* 2:994–995, 1961.
Chusid, J. G., and Pacella, B. L. The electroencephalogram in the electric shock therapies. *J. Nerv. Ment. Dis.,* 116:95–107, 1952.
Cicardo, V. H. Physiochemical mechanisms in experimental epilepsy. *J. Nerv. Ment. Dis.,* 101:527–536, 1945.
Clare, A. *Psychiatry in Dissent.* Tavistock Publications, London, 438 pp., 1976.
Clark, G., and Sarkaria, D. S. Acid fuschin convulsions and electroshock in the mouse. *J. Neuropathol. Exp. Neurol.,* 17:612–619, 1958.

Cleghorn, R. A., Graham, B. F., Saffran, M., and Cameron, D. E. A study of the effect of pituitary ACTH in depressed patients. *Can. Med. Assoc. J.*, 63:329–331, 1950.

Clemedson, C. J., Hartelius, H., and Holmberg, G. The influence of carbon dioxide inhalation on the cerebral vascular permeability to trypan blue (the blood brain barrier). *Acta Pathol. Microbiol. Scand.*, 42:137–149, 1958.

Clower, C. G., and Migeon, C. J. Psychoendocrine aspects of depression and ECT. *Johns Hopkins Med. J.*, 121:227–233, 1967.

Clyma, E. A. Unilateral electroconvulsive therapy: How to determine which hemisphere is dominant. *Br. J. Psychiatry*, 126:372–379, 1975.

Coble, P., Foster, F. G., and Kupfer, D. J. Electroencephalographic sleep diagnosis of primary depression. *Arch. Gen. Psychiatry*, 33:1124–1127, 1976.

Cohen, B. D., Noblin, C. D., and Silverman, A. J. On the functional asymmetry of the human brain. *Science*, 162:475–477, 1968.

Cohen, H. B., and Dement, W. C. Sleep: Suppression of rapid eye movement phase in the cat after electroconvulsive shock. *Science*, 154:396–398, 1966.

Cohen, H. B., Duncan, R. F., and Dement, W. C. Sleep: The effect of electroconvulsive shock in cats deprived of REM sleep. *Science*, 156:1646–1648, 1967.

Cohen, M. B., Baker, G., Cohen, R. A., Fromm-Reichmann, F., and Weigert, E. An intensive study of twelve cases of manic-depressive psychosis. *Psychiatry*, 17:103–137, 1954.

Cohen, W. J., and Cohen, N. H. Lithium carbonate, haloperidol and irreversible brain damage. *JAMA*, 230:1283–1287, 1974.

Cole, J. O., and Davis, J. M. Antidepressant drugs. In: A. M. Freedman and H. I. Kaplan (Eds.): *Comprehensive Textbook of Psychiatry*. Williams & Wilkins, Baltimore, pp. 1263–1275, 1967.

Collins, R. C., Posner, J. B., and Plum, F. Cerebral energy metabolism during electroshock seizures in mice. *Am. J. Physiol.*, 218:943–950, 1970.

Collins, V. J. *Principles of Anesthesiology*. Lea & Febiger, Philadelphia, pp. 184–188, 1976.

Colon, E. J., and Notermans, J. L. H. A long term study of the effects of electro-convulsions on the structure of the cerebral cortex. *Acta Neuropathol.*, 32:21–25, 1975.

Colville, K. I., Schroeder, J. C., de Beer, E. J., and Gahagan, L. H. Response of the coronary arterial bed to electroshock: An experimental study in dogs. *Am. Heart J.*, 60:237–243, 1960.

Conrad, J. *A Personal Record*. Harper & Brothers, New York, 219 pp., 1912.

Coppen, A. J. Abnormality of the blood-cerebrospinal fluid barrier of patients suffering from a depressive illness. *J. Neurol. Neurosurg. Psychiatry*, 23:156–161, 1960.

Coppen, A., Noguera, R., and Bailey, J. Prophylactic lithium in affective disorders. Controlled trial. *Lancet*, 2:275–279, 1971.

Coppen, A., and Shaw, D. M. Mineral metabolism in melancholia *Br. Med. J.*, 1:1439–1444, 1963.

Coppen, A., Shaw, D. M., Malleson, A., and Costain, R. Mineral metabolism in mania. *Br. Med. J.*, 1:71–75, 1966.

Corsellis, J. A. N., and Meyer, A. Histological changes in the brain after uncomplicated electroconvulsant treatment. *J. Ment. Sci.*, 100:375–383, 1954.

Costain, D. W., Green, A. R., and Grahame-Smith, D. G. Enhanced 5-hydroxytryptamine-mediated behavioural responses in rats following repeated electroconvulsive shock: Relevance to the mechanism of the antidepressive effect of electroconvulsive therapy. *Psychopharmacology (in press)*.

Costello, C. G., Belton, G. P., Abra, J. C., and Dunn, B. E. The amnesic and therapeutic effects of bilateral and unilateral ECT. *Br. J. Psychiatry*, 116:69–78, 1970.

Cotter, L. H. Operant conditioning in a Vietnamese mental hospital. *Am. J. Psychiatry*, 124:24–25, 1967.

Craddock, W. L., and Gilbert, H. P. Transient auricular fibrillation complicating electric shock therapy. *Am. J. Psychiatry*, 104:744–745, 1948.

Cremerius, J., and Jung, R. Über die Veränderungen des Elektroencephalograms nach Elektroschockbehandlung. *Nervenarzt*, 18:193–205, 1947.

Crome, P., Braithwaite, R., Newman, B., and Montgomery, S. Choosing an antidepressant. *Br. Med. J.*, 1:859, 1978.

Cronholm, B., and Blomquist, C. Memory disturbances after electroconvulsive therapy: II. Conditions one week after a series of treatments. *Acta Psychiatr. Scand.*, 34:18–25, 1959.

Cronholm, B., and Molander, L. Memory disturbances after electroconvulsive therapy. I. Conditions six hours after electroshock treatment. *Acta Psychiatr. Scand.*, 32:280–306, 1957.

Cronholm, B., and Molander, L. Memory disturbances after electroconvulsive therapy. IV. Influence

of an interpolated electroconvulsive shock on retention of memory material. *Acta Psychiatr. Scand.,* 36:83–90, 1961.
Cronholm, B., and Molander, L. Memory disturbances after electroconvulsive therapy. V. Conditions one month after a series of treatments. *Acta Psychiatr. Scand.,* 40:212–216, 1964.
Cronholm, B., and Ottosson, J.-O. Experimental studies of the therapeutic action of electroconvulsive therapy in endogenous depression. *Acta Psychiatr. Neurol. Scand. [Suppl.],* 35:69–102, 1960.
Cronholm, B., and Ottosson, J.-O. Memory functions in endogenous depression before and after electroconvulsive therapy. *Arch. Gen. Psychiatry,* 5:193–199, 1961a.
Cronholm, B., and Ottosson, J.-O. "Countershock" in electroconvulsive therapy. Influence on retrograde amnesia. *Arch. Gen. Psychiatry,* 4:254–258, 1961b.
Cronholm, B., and Ottosson, J.-O. The experience of memory function after electroconvulsive therapy. *Br. J. Psychiatry,* 109:251–258, 1963a.
Cronholm, B., and Ottosson, J.-O. Ultrabrief stimulus technique in electroconvulsive therapy. I. Influence on retrograde amnesia of treatments with the Elther ES electroshock apparatus, Siemens Konvulsator III and of lidocaine-modified treatment. *J. Nerv. Ment. Dis.,* 137:117–123, 1963b.
Cronholm, B., and Ottosson, J.-O. Ultrabrief stimulus technique in electroconvulsive therapy. II. Comparative studies of therapeutic effects and memory disturbances in treatment of endogenous depression with the Elther ES electroshock apparatus and Siemens Konvulsator III. *J. Nerv. Ment. Dis.,* 137:268–276, 1963c.
Cronholm, B., Ottosson, J.-O., and Schalling, D. A study of memory in aged people. In H. Zippel (Ed.): *Memory and Transfer of Information.* Plenum Press, New York, pp. 23–42, 1973.
Cronick, C. H., Scherb, R. F., and Karnosh, L. J. Modification of the manic-depressive cycle by Metrazol. *Dis. Nerv. Syst.,* 1:10–15, 1940.
Cronin, D., Bodley, P., Potts, L., Mather, M. D., Gardner, R. K., and Tobin, J. C. Unilateral and bilateral ECT: A study of memory disturbance and relief from depression. *J. Neurol. Neurosurg. Psychiatry,* 33:705–713, 1970.
Cropper, C. F. J., and Hughes, M. Cardiac arrest (with apnoea) after E.C.T. *Br. J. Psychiatry,* 110:222–225, 1964.
Cumming, J., and Kort, K. Apparent reversal by cortisone of an electroconvulsive refractory state in a psychotic patient with Addison's disease. *Can. Med. Assoc. J.,* 74:291–292, 1956.
Currier, G. E., Cullinan, C., and Rothschild, C. Results of treatment of schizophrenia in a state hospital. *Arch. Neurol. Psychiatry,* 67:80–88, 1952.
D'Agostino, A. M. Depression: Schism in contemporary psychiatry. *Am. J. Psychiatry,* 132:629–632, 1975.
Danziger, L., and Kindwall, J. A. Prediction of the immediate outcome of shock therapy in dementia praecox. *Dis. Nerv. Syst.,* 7:299–303, 1946.
Darling, H. F. Shock treatment in psychopathic personality. *J. Nerv. Ment. Dis.,* 101:247–250, 1945.
Dattner, B. *The Management of Neurosyphilis.* Grune & Stratton, New York, 398 pp., 1944.
Davidson, J. R. T., McLeod, M., Kurland, A. A., and White, H. L. Antidepressant drug therapy in psychotic depression. *Brit. J. Psychiatry,* 131:493–496, 1977.
Davidson, J., McLeod, M., Law-Yone, B., and Linnoila, M. Comparison of electroconvulsive therapy and combined phenelzine-amitriptyline in refractory depression. *Arch. Gen. Psychiatry,* 35:639–644, 1978.
Davies, R. K., Detre, T. P., Egger, M. D., Tucker, G. J., and Wyman, R. J. Electroconvulsive therapy instruments. *Arch. Gen. Psychiatry,* 25:97–99, 1971.
Davis, E., Halpern, L., Laszlo, L., and Heim, O. Effect of electric convulsive shock on human capillaries. *Confin. Neurol.,* 15:84–90, 1955.
Davis, J. Clinical efficacy of ECT in depressive states. Conference: *ECT: Efficacy and Impact.* New Orleans, February 22, 1978.
Davis, R. A., Abrams, R., and Taylor, M. A. Failure of bromide psychosis to respond to ECT. *Br. J. Psychiatr.,* 133:94, 1978.
Dawson, M. E., Schell, A. M., and Catania, J. J. Autonomic correlates of depression and clinical improvement following electroconvulsive shock therapy. *Psychophysiology,* 14:569–578, 1977.
Delay, J. *L'Electrochoc et la Psycho-Physiologie.* Masson & Cie, Paris, 169 pp., 1946.
Delgado, H. Treatment of schizophrenia with cardiazol in convulsant doses. *J. Nerv. Ment. Dis.,* 89:810–824, 1939.
Delgado, J. M. R., Hamlin, H., and Chapman, W. P. Technique of intracranial electrode implacement for recording and stimulation and its possible therapeutic value in psychotic patients. *Confin. Neurol.,* 12:315–319, 1952.

d'Elia, G. Unilateral electroconvulsive therapy. *Acta Psychiatr. Scand. [Suppl.],* 215:5–98, 1970a.
d'Elia, G. Elettroshockterapia unilaterale e turbe della memoria. *Psychiatr. Gen. Evol.,* 8:177–193, 1970b.
d'Elia, G. Unilateral electroconvulsive therapy. In: M. Fink, S. Kety, J. McGaugh, and T. Williams (Eds.): *Psychobiology of Convulsive Therapy.* V. H. Winston & Sons, Washington, D.C., pp. 21–34, 1974.
d'Elia, G. Memory changes after unilateral electroconvulsive therapy with different electrode positions. *Cortex,* 12:280–289, 1976.
d'Elia, G., Frederikson, S.-O., Raotma, H., and Widepalm, K. Comparison of fronto-frontal and temporo-parietal unilateral ECT. *Acta Psychiatr. Scand.,* 56:233–239, 1977a.
d'Elia, G., Laurell, B., and Perris, C. EEG photically elicited alpha blocking responses in depressive patients before and after convulsive therapy. *Acta Psychiatr. Scand. [Suppl.],* 255:159–172, 1974.
d'Elia, G., Lehmann, J., and Raotma, H. Evaluation of the combination of tryptophan and ECT in the treatment of depression. I. Clinical analysis. *Acta Psychiatr. Scand.,* 56:303–318, 1977b.
d'Elia, G., Lehmann, J., and Raotma, H. Evaluation of the combination of tryptophan and ECT in the treatment of depression. II. Biochemical analysis. *Acta Psychiatr. Scand.,* 56:319–334, 1977c.
d'Elia, G., Lehmann, J., and Raotma, H. Influence of tryptophan on memory functions in depressive patients treated with unilateral ECT. *Acta Psychiatr. Scand.,* 57:259–268, 1978.
d'Elia, G., Lorentzson, S., Raotma, H., and Widepalm, K. Comparison of unilateral dominant and non-dominant ECT on verbal and non-verbal memory. *Acta Psychiatr. Scand.,* 53:85–94, 1976.
d'Elia, G., and Perris, C. Seizure and post-seizure electroencephalographic pattern. *Acta Psychiatr. Scand. [Suppl.],* 215:9–29, 1970.
d'Elia, G., and Perris, C. Cerebral functional dominance and depression. An analysis of EEG amplitude in depressed patients. *Acta Psychiatr. Scand.,* 49:191–197, 1973.
d'Elia, G., and Raotma, H. Is unilateral ECT less effective than bilateral ECT? *Br. J. Psychiatry,* 126:83–89, 1975.
d'Elia, G., and Raotma, H. Memory impairment after convulsive therapy. *Arch. Psychiatr. Nervenkr.,* 223:219–226, 1977.
d'Elia, G., and Widepalm, K. Comparison of frontoparietal and temporoparietal unilateral electroconvulsive therapy. *Acta Psychiatr. Scand.,* 50:225–232, 1974.
Delitala, G., Masala, A., Rosati, G., Aiello, I., and Agnetti, V. Effect of electroconvulsive therapy (electroshock) on plasma ACTH, GH, LH, FSH, TSH and 11-OH-CS in patients with mental disorders. *Panminerva Medica* 19:237–243, 1977.
Deliyiannis, S., Eliakim, M., and Bellet, S. The electrocardiogram during electroconvulsive therapy as studied by radioelectrocardiography. *Am. J. Cardiol.,* 10:187–192, 1962.
Delmas-Marsalet, P. L'électro-choc par courant continu. *Ann. Med. Psychol.,* 100:70–74, 1942.
Delmas-Marsalet, P. *Electro-choc et Therapeutiques Nouvelles en Neuropsychiatrie.* J. B. Bailliere et fils, Paris, 377 pp., 1946.
Demars, J. P. C. A. Neuromuscular effects of long-term phenothiazine medication, electroconvulsive therapy and leucotomy. *J. Nerv. Ment. Dis.,* 143:73–79, 1966.
Denber, H. C. B. Studies on mescaline: III. Action in epileptics. *Psychiat. Quart.,* 29:433–438, 1955.
Denber, H. C. B. Chlorpromazine in the treatment of mental illness. *Am. J. Psychiatry,* 113:972–978, 1957.
De Robertis, E., Alberici, M., and Delores, A. Astroglial swelling and phosphohydrolases in cerebral cortex of metrazol convulsant rats. *Brain Res.,* 12:461–466, 1969.
Desclin, L. Hypothalamic control of lactation. In: W. Haymaker, E. Anderson, and W. J. H. Nauta (Eds.): *The Hypothalamus.* Charles C Thomas, Springfield, Ill., pp. 431–462, 1969.
Deshaies, G., and Pellier, S. Les accidents de l'électrochocthérapie. *Ann. Med. Psychol.,* 108:606–626, 1950.
Deshaies, G., and Renard, E. La tension cephalo-rachidienne dans l'electro-choc. *Ann. Med. Psychol.,* 106:18–28, 1948.
Detre, T., and Jarecki, H. C. Convulsive Therapies. In: *Modern Psychiatric Treatment,* J. B. Lippincott, Philadelphia, pp. 635–655, 1971.
de Wet, J. S. Evaluation of a common method of convulsive therapy in bantu schizophrenics. *J. Ment. Sci.,* 103:739–757, 1957.
Dewhurst, K. Treatment of neurosyphilitic psychoses. *Acta Psychiatr. Scand.,* 45:63–74, 1969.

de Wied, D. Effects of peptide hormones on behavior. In: W. F. Ganong and L. Martini (Eds.): *Frontiers in Neuroendocrinology.* Oxford University Press, New York, pp. 97–140, 1969.

de Wied, D., and Bohus, B. Long term and short term effects on retention of a conditioned avoidance response in rats by treatment with long acting pitressin and α-MSH. *Nature,* 212:1484–1486, 1966.

de Wied, D., Bohus, B., van Ree, J. M., Kovacs, G. L., and Greven, H. M. Neuroleptic-like activity of [Des-Tyr¹]-γ-endorphin in rats. *Lancet,* 1:1046, 1978.

Diaz-Guerrero, R., Feinstein, R., and Gottlieb, J. S. EEG findings following intravenous injection of diphenhydramine hydrochloride (Benadryl). *Electroencephalogr. Clin. Neurophysiol.,* 8:299–306, 1956.

Dietz, P. E., Rappeport, J. R., Lion, J. R., Cowen, J. R., and Turek, I. S. The Maryland psychiatric treatments survey: Prevalence of treatments. Presented at the American Psychiatric Association, Toronto, May, 1977.

Dimsdale, J. E. Emotional causes of sudden death. *Am. J. Psychiatry,* 134:1361–1366, 1977.

Di Perri, R., Meduri, M., and Messina, C. L'attivita elettrica cerebrale da sonno notturno in soggetti sottoposti ad elettroshock uni o bilaterale. *Sist. Nerv.,* 21:199–201, 1969.

Doan, D. I., and Huston, P. E. Electric shock during pregnancy. *Psychiatr. Q.,* 22:1–5, 1948.

Dolenz, B. J. Unilateral ECT. *Am. J. Psychiatry,* 120:1133, 1964.

Dolenz, B. J. Indoklon: A clinical review. *Psychosomatics,* 6:200–205, 1965.

Donovan, B. T. The behavioural actions of the hypothalamic peptides: A review. *Psychol. Med.,* 8:305–316, 1978.

Doongaji, D. R., Jeste, D. V., Saoji, N. J., Kane, P. V., and Ravindranath, S. Unilateral versus bilateral ECT in schizophrenia. *Br. J. Psychiatry,* 123:73–79, 1973.

Dornbush, R. L. Memory and induced ECT convulsions. *Semin. Psychiatry,* 4:47–54, 1972.

Dornbush, R., Abrams, R., and Fink, M. Memory changes after unilateral and bilateral convulsive therapy. *Br. J. Psychiatry,* 119:75–78, 1971.

Dornbush, R. L., and Williams, M. Memory and ECT. In: M. Fink, S. Kety, J. McGaugh, and T. Williams (Eds.): *Psychobiology of Convulsive Therapy.* V. H. Winston & Sons, Washington, D.C., pp. 199–205, 1974.

Doust, J. W. L., Barcha, R., Lee, R. S. Y., Little, M. H., and Watkinson, J. S. Acute effects of ECT on the cerebral circulation in man: A computerized study by cerebral impedance plethysmography. *Eur. Neurol.,* 12:47–62, 1974.

Doust, J. W. L., and Raschka, L. B. Enduring effects of modified ECT on the cerebral circulation in man: A computerized study by cerebral impedance plethysmography. *Psychiatr. Clin.,* 8:293–303, 1975.

Dressler, D. M., and Folk, J. The treatment of depression with ECT in the presence of brain tumor. *Am. J. Psychiatry.,* 132:1320–1321, 1975.

Driver, M. V., and Edenberg, M. D. Photoconvulsive threshold in depressive illness and the effect of ECT. *J. Ment. Sci.,* 106:611–617, 1960.

Drooby, A. S. Electroconvulsive therapy and schizophrenia. *Leb. Med. J.,* 25:325–335, 1972.

Dudley, W. H., Jr., and Williams, J. G. Electroconvulsive therapy in delirium tremens. *Compr. Psychiatry.,* 13:357–360, 1972.

Dunn, A. J., and Bondy, S. C. *Functional Chemistry of the Brain.* Spectrum Publications, New York, 272 pp., 1974.

Dunn, A., Giuditta, A., and Pagliuca, N. The effect of electroconvulsive shock on protein synthesis in mouse brain. *J. Neurochem.,* 18:2093–2099, 1971.

Dunn, A., Giuditta, A., Wilson, J. E., and Glassman, E. The effect of electroshock on brain RNA and protein synthesis and its possible relationship to behavioral effects. In: M. Fink, S. Kety, J. McGaugh, and T. Williams (Eds.): *Psychobiology of Convulsive Therapy.* V. H. Winston & Sons, Washington, D.C., pp. 185–197, 1974.

Dysken, M., Evans, H. M., Chan, C. H., and Davis, J. M. Improvement of depression and parkinsonism during ECT: A case study. *Neuropsychobiology,* 2:81–86, 1976.

Eastwood, M. R., and Peacocke, J. E. Diagnosis and evaluation of ECT. *Can. Psychiatr. Assoc. J.,* 21:55–90, 1976a.

Eastwood M. R., and Peacocke, J. Seasonal patterns of suicide, depression and electroconvulsive therapy. *Br. J. Psychiatry,* 129:472–475, 1976b.

Eastwood, M. R., and Peacocke, J. Antipsychiatrists and ECT: Response. *Br. Med. J.,* 1:280, 1976c.

Eastwood, M. R., and Stiasny, S. The use of electroconvulsive therapy. *Can. Psychiatr. Assoc, J.,* 23:29–34, 1978.

REFERENCES

Ebaugh, F. G., Barnacle, C. H., and Neuberger, K. T. Fatalities following electric convulsive therapy: Report of two cases, with autopsy. *Arch. Neurol. Psychiatry,* 49:107–117, 1943.
Ebaugh, F. G., and Shanahan, W. M. Status of chemotherapy in schizophrenic and affective reactions. *Am. J. Med. Sci.,* 197:862–873, 1939.
Ebert, M. H., Baldessarini, R. J., Lipinski, J. F., and Berv, K. Effects of electroconvulsive seizures on amine metabolism in the rat brain. *Arch. Gen. Psychiatry,* 29:397–401, 1973.
Editor. Antipsychiatrists and ECT. *Br. Med. J.,* 1:1, 1975.
Editor. Electroconvulsive therapy. *Lancet,* 1:593–594, 1977a.
Editor. Treatment of depression. *Br. Med. J.,* 1:1105, 1977b.
Editor. Special Section: Electroconvulsive therapy—Current perspectives. *Am. J. Psychiatry,* 134:991–1019, 1977c.
Edwalds, R. M. Experimental studies with PM 1090. *Int. Rec. Med. & G. P. Clin.* (Wash.) 169:469–472, 1956.
Ehrensing, R. H., and Kastin, A. J. Melanocyte-stimulating hormone-releasing inhibiting hormone as an anti-depressant: A pilot study. *Arch. Gen. Psychiatry,* 30:63–65, 1974.
Ehrensing, R. H., and Kastin, A. J. Dose-related biphasic effect of prolyl-leucyl-glycinamide (MIF-1) in depression. *Am. J. Psychiatry,* 135:562–566, 1978.
Ehrensing, R. H., Kastin, A. J., Schalch, D. S., Friesen, H. G., Vargas, J. R., and Schally, A. V. Affective state and thyrotropin and prolactin response after repeated injections of thyrotropin releasing hormone in depressed patients. *Am. J. Psychiatry,* 131:714–718, 1974.
Eiduson, S., Brill, N. Q., and Crumpton, E. The effect of electroconvulsive therapy on spinal fluid constituents. *J. Ment. Sci.,* 106:692–698, 1960.
El-Islam, M. F., Ahmed, S. A., and Erfan, M. E. The effect of unilateral ECT on schizophrenic delusions and hallucinations. *Br. J. Psychiatry,* 117:447–448, 1970.
Elithorn, A., Bridges, P. K., and Hodge, J. R. Adrenocortical responsiveness during courses of electro-convulsive therapy. *Br. J. Psychiatry,* 114:575–580, 1968.
Ellison, E. A., and Hamilton, D. M. The hospital treatment of dementia praecox. *Am. J. Psychiatry,* 106:454–461, 1949.
Ellison, G. D. Animal models of psychopathology: The low-norepinephrine and low-serotonin rat. *Am. Psychol.,* 32:1036–1045, 1977.
Elmore, J. I., and Sugerman, A. A. Precipitation of psychosis during electroshock therapy. *Dis. Nerv. Syst.,* 36:115–117, 1975.
Emrich, H. M. and Höllt, V. Studies on a possible pathological significance of endorphin. Conference, CINP, Vienna, Austria, July 13, 1978.
Ende, M., Klauber, B., and Gendel, B. R. Electric shock therapy of acute psychosis associated with pernicious anemia. *Arch. Neurol. Psychiatry,* 63:110–112, 1950.
Engel, G. L. Psychologic factors in instantaneous cardiac death. *N. Engl. J. Med.,* 294:664–665, 1976.
Epstein, J. Electric shock therapy in the psychoses: A study of 100 cases. *J. Nerv. Ment. Dis.,* 98:115–129, 1943.
Epstein, J. Monopolar electro-shock therapy. *Dis. Nerv. Syst.,* 16:3–8, 1955.
Epstein, J., and Wender, L. Alternating current vs. unidirectional current for electroconvulsive therapy: Comparative studies. *Confin. Neurol.,* 16:137–146, 1956.
Esecover, H., Jaffe, J., and Kahn, R. L. Psychotherapeutic techniques with electroshock patients. *J. Hillside Hosp.,* 7:17–25, 1958.
Esquibel, A., Krantz, J. C., Truitt, E. B., Ling, A. S. C., and Kurland, A. A. Hexafluorodiethyl ether (Indoklon)—Its use as a convulsant in psychiatric treatment. *J. Nerv. Ment. Dis.,* 126:530–534, 1958.
Essig, C. F. Frequency of repeated electroconvulsions and the acquisition rate of a tolerance-like response. *Exp. Neurol.,* 25:571–574, 1969.
Essman, W. B. *Neurochemistry of Cerebral Electroshock.* Spectrum Publications, New York, 181 pp., 1973.
Essman, W. B. Effects of electroconvulsive shock on cerebral protein synthesis. In: M. Fink, S. Kety, J. McGaugh, and T. A. Williams (Eds.): *Psychobiology of Convulsive Therapy.* V. H. Winston & Sons, Washington, D.C., pp. 237–250, 1974.
Essman, W. B. Antidepressant action of electroconvulsive therapy. *Lancet,* 1:935, 1978.
Ettigi, P. G., and Brown, G. M. Psychoneuroendocrinology of affective disorder: An overview. *Am. J. Psychiatry,* 134:493–501, 1977.
Evans, J. P. M., Grahame-Smith, D. G., Green, A. R., and Tordoff, A. F. C. Electroconvulsive

shock increases the behavioural responses of rats to brain 5-hydroxytryptamine accumulation and central nervous system stimulant drugs. *J. Pharmacol.*, 56:193–199, 1976.

Ewald, G. Zur Theorie der Schizophrenie und der Insulinschockbehandlung. *Allg. Z. Psychiatr.*, 110, 1939.

Ewald, G., and Haddenbrock, S. Die Elektrokrampftherapie. Ihre Grundlagen und ihre Erfolge. *Z. Gesamte. Neurol. Psychiatr.*, 174:635–669, 1942.

Exner, J. E., and Murillo, L. G. A long term follow-up of schizophrenics treated with regressive ECT. *Dis. Nerv. Syst.*, 38:162–168, 1977.

Fahy, P., Imlah, N., and Harrington, J. A controlled comparison of electroconvulsive therapy, imipramine and thiopentone sleep in depression. *J. Neuropsychiatry*, 4:310–314, 1963.

Faragalla, F. F., and Flach, F. F. Studies of mineral metabolism in mental depression. I: The effects of imipramine and electric convulsive therapy on calcium balance and kinetics. *J. Nerv. Ment. Dis.*, 151:120–129, 1970.

Fawcett, J. A., and Bunney, W. E. Pituitary adrenal function and depression: An outline for research. *Arch. Gen. Psychiatry*, 16:517–535, 1967.

Feinberg, I. Current status of the Funkenstein test. *Arch. Neurol. Psychiatry*, 80:488–501, 1958.

Ferguson, H. C., Bartram, A. C. G., Fowlie, H. C., Cathro, D. M., Birchall, K., and Mitchell, F. L. A preliminary investigation of steroid excretion in depressed patients before and after electroconvulsive therapy. *Acta Endocrin. (Kbh.)*, 47/1:58–68, 1964.

Ferraro, A., and Roizin, L. Cerebral morphologic changes in monkeys subjected to a large number of electrically induced convulsions. *Am. J. Psychiatry*, 106:278–284, 1949.

Ferraro, A., Roizin, L., and Helfand, M. Morphologic changes in the brain of monkeys following convulsions electrically induced. *J. Neuropathol. Exp. Neurol.*, 5:285–308, 1946.

Feuillet, C. Electroshock and prolonged melancholia. *Arch. Int. Neurol.*, 67:110–114, 1948.

Fieschi, C., Rizzo, M., Delmonte, P., and Rossi, R. Disturbi della memoria da terapia electroconvulsivante mono-e bilaterale e da Terapie Chemiconvulsivante con flurotil (Indoklon). *Riv Sper. Freniat. Med. Leg. Alienz. Ment.* 94:916–926, 1970.

Fink, M. A unified theory of the action of physiodynamic therapies. *J. Hillside Hosp.*, 6:197–206, 1957.

Fink, M. Effect of anticholinergic agent, Diethazine, on EEG and behavior: Significance for theory of convulsive therapy. *Arch. Neurol. Psychiatry*, 80:380–387, 1958a.

Fink, M. Lateral gaze nystagmus as an index of the sedation threshold. *Electroencephalogr. Clin. Neurophysiol.*, 10:162–163, 1958b.

Fink, M. Effect of an anticholinergic agent, Diethazine, on EEG and behavior. Significance for theory of convulsive therapy. In: J. Masserman (Ed.): *Biological Psychiatry I:* Grune & Stratton, New York, pp. 184–194, 1959a.

Fink, M. Alteration of brain function in therapy. In: N. Kline (Ed.): *Psychopharmacology Frontiers.* Little, Brown & Co. Boston, pp. 325–332, 1959b.

Fink, M. Effect of anticholinergic compounds on post-convulsive EEG and behavior of psychiatric patients. *Electroencephalogr. Clin. Neurophysiol.*, 12:359–369, 1960.

Fink, M. Prediction of individual patient response to convulsive therapy. *VA Coop. Chemother. Studies Psychiatry*, 6:317–324, 1961.

Fink, M. The mode of action of convulsive therapy: The neurophysiologic-adaptive view. *J. Neuropsychiatry*, 3:231–233, 1962.

Fink, M. Quantitative electroencephalography in human psychopharmacology. II. Drug patterns. In: G. Glaser (Ed.): *EEG and Behavior.* Basic Books, New York, pp. 177–197, 1963.

Fink, M. Cholinergic aspects of convulsive therapy. *J. Nerv. Ment. Dis.*, 142:475–484, 1966.

Fink, M. Neurophysiological response strategies in the classification of mental illness. In: M. M. Katz, J. O. Cole, and W. E. Barton (Eds.): *The Role of Methodology of Classification in Psychiatry and Psychopathology.* Govt. Printing Office, Washington, D.C., pp. 535–540, 1968.

Fink, M. EEG and human psychopharmacology. *Ann. Rev. Pharmacol.*, 9:241–258, 1969.

Fink, M. CNS effects of convulsive therapy: Significance for a theory of depressive psychosis. In: J. Zubin, and F. Freyhan (Eds.): *Disorders of Mood.* Johns Hopkins Press, Baltimore, pp. 93–112, 1972a.

Fink, M. (Ed.): Convulsive therapy. *Semin. Psychiatry.*, 4:1–79, 1972b.

Fink, M. The therapeutic process in ECT. *Semin. Psychiatry*, 4:39–46, 1972c.

Fink, M. How shocking is shock therapy? *Biol. Psychiatry*, 7:79–80, 1973.

Fink, M. Brain function, verbal behavior, and psychotherapy. *Compr. Psychiatry*, 15:257–266, 1974a.

Fink, M. Clinical progress in convulsive therapy. In: M. Fink. S. Kety, J. McGaugh, and T. Williams (Eds.): *Psychobiology of Convulsive Therapy.* V. H. Winston & Sons, Washington, D.C., pp. 271–278, 1974*b.*
Fink, M. Induced seizures and human behavior. In: M. Fink, S. Kety, J. McGaugh, and T. A. Williams (Eds.): *Psychobiology of Convulsive Therapy.,* V. H. Winston & Sons, Washington, D.C., pp. 1–18, 1974*c.*
Fink, M. Psychiatric diagnosis—phenotypic or pathophysiologic? Editorial. *Biol. Psychiatry,* 9:227–229, 1974*d.*
Fink, M. EEG profiles and bioavailability measures of psychoactive drugs. In: T. Itil (Ed.): *Psychotropic Drugs and the Human EEG.* S. Karger, Basel, pp. 76–98, 1974*e.*
Fink, M. Antipsychiatrists and ECT. *Br. Med. J.,* 1:280, 1976.
Fink, M. CNS sequellae of EST: Risks of therapy and their prophylaxis, In: C. Shagass and A. Friedhoff (Eds.): *Psychopathology and Brain Dysfunction.* Raven Press, New York, pp. 223–239, 1977*a.*
Fink, M. EST. A special case in pharmacotherapy. In: W. E. Fann, I. Karacen, A. D. Pokorny, and R. C. Williams (Eds.): *Phenomenology and Treatment of Depression.* Spectrum Publications, New York, pp. 285–294, 1977*b.*
Fink, M. Myths of "shock therapy". *Am. J. Psychiatry,* 134:991–996, 1977*c.*
Fink, M. EEG response strategies in psychiatric diagnosis. In: R. Spitzer and D. F. Klein (Eds.): *Critical Issues in Psychiatric Diagnosis.* Raven Press, New York, 253–263, 1978*a.*
Fink, M. Efficacy and safety of induced seizures (EST) in man. *Compr. Psychiatry,* 19:1–18, 1978*b.*
Fink, M. Is ECT a useful therapy of schizophrenia? In: J. P. Brady and H. K. H. Brodie (Eds.): *Controversy in Psychiatry.* W. B. Saunders, Philadelphia, pp. 183–193, 1978*c.*
Fink, M. Mania and electroseizure therapy (EST). In: B. Shopsin (Ed.): *A Profile of Psychobiological Research: Manic Illness.* Raven Press, New York, pp. 221–230, 1978*d.*
Fink, M. EST and other somatic therapies of schizophrenia. In: L. Bellak (Ed.): *Disorders of the Schizophrenic Syndrome.* Basic Books, New York, *in press.*
Fink, M., and Abrams, R. Answers to questions about ECT. *Semin. Psychiatry,* 4:33–38, 1972.
Fink, M., and Green, M. Electroencephalographic correlates of the electroshock process. *Dis. Nerv. Syst.,* 19:227, 1958.
Fink, M., Jaffe, J., and Kahn, R. L. Drug induced changes in interview patterns: Linguistic and neurophysiologic indices. In: G. J. Sarwer-Foner (Ed.): *The Dynamics of Psychiatric Drug Therapy.* Charles C Thomas, Springfield, Ill., pp. 29–44, 1960.
Fink, M., and Kahn, R. L. Relation of EEG delta activity to behavioral response in electroshock: Quantitative serial studies. *Arch. Neurol. Psychiatry,* 78:516–525, 1957.
Fink, M., and Kahn. R. L. Behavioral patterns in convulsive therapy. *Arch. Gen. Psychiatry,* 5:30–36, 1961.
Fink, M., Kahn, R. L., and Green, M. A. Experimental studies of convulsive and drug therapies in psychiatry: Theoretical implications. *Arch. Neurol. Psychiatry,* 80:733–734, 1958*a.*
Fink, M., Kahn, R. L., and Green, M. Experimental studies of the electroshock process. *Dis. Nerv. Syst.,* 19:113–118, 1958*b.*
Fink, M., Kahn, R. L., Karp, E., Pollack, M., Green, M., Alan, B., and Lefkowits, H. J. Inhalant-induced convulsions: Significance for the theory of the convulsive therapy process. *Arch. Gen. Psychiatry,* 4:259–266, 1961.
Fink, M., Kahn, R. L., and Korin, H. Relation of tests of altered brain function to behavioral change following induced convulsions. In: L. van Bogaert and J. Radermaker (Eds.): *First International Congress of Neurological Sciences.* Pergamon Press, London, pp. 613–619, 1959*a.*
Fink, M., Kahn, R. L., and Pollack, M. Psychological factors affecting individual differences in behavioral response to convulsive therapy. *J. Nerv. Ment. Dis.,* 128:243–248, 1959*b.*
Fink, M., Kety, S., McGaugh, J., and Williams, T. (Eds.): *Psychobiology of Convulsive Therapy.* V. H. Winston & Sons, Washington, D.C., 312 pp., 1974.
Fink, M., Shapiro, D., Hickman, C., and Itil, T. Quantitative analysis of the electroencephalogram by digital computer methods. In: N. S. Kline and E. Laska (Eds.): *Computers and Electronic Devices in Psychiatry.* Grune & Stratton, New York, pp. 109–123, 1968.
Fink, M., Shaw, R., Gross, G., and Coleman, F. S. Comparative study of chlorpromazine and insulin coma in therapy of psychosis. *JAMA,* 166:1846–1850, 1958.
Finner, R. W. Duration of convulsion in electric shock therapy. *J. Nerv. Ment. Dis.,* 119:530–537, 1954.

Fishbein, I. L. Involutional melancholia and convulsive therapy. *Am. J. Psychiatry,* 106:128–135, 1949.

Fish, B. Psychiatric treatment of children: Organic therapies. In: A. M. Freedman and H. I. Kaplan (Eds.): *Comprehensive Textbook of Psychiatry.* Williams & Wilkins, Baltimore, pp. 1468–1472, 1967.

Fisher, H., and Bannister, A. K. Suxethonium bromide in E.C.T. *J. Ment. Sci.,* 99:796–799, 1953.

Fisher, K. A. Changes in test performance of ambulatory depressed patients undergoing electroshock therapy. *J. Gen. Psychol.,* 41:195–232, 1949.

Flach, F. F. Calcium metabolism in states of depression. *Br. J. Psychiatry,* 110:588–593, 1964.

Flach, F. F., Liang, E., and Stokes, P. E. Effects of electric convulsive treatments on nitrogen, calcium, and phosphorus metabolism in psychiatric patients. *J. Ment. Sci.,* 106:638–647, 1960.

Fleming, T. C. An inquiry into the mechanism of action of electric shock treatments. *J. Nerv. Ment. Dis.,* 124:440–450, 1956.

Fleminger, J. J., and Bunce, L. Investigation of cerebral dominance in 'left-handers' and 'right-handers' using unilateral electroconvulsive therapy. *J. Neurol. Neurosurg. Psychiatry,* 38:541–545, 1975.

Fleminger, J. J., Horne, D. J. de L., Nair, N. P. V., and Nott, P. N. Differential effect of unilateral and bilateral ECT. Am. J. Psychiatry, 127:430–436, 1970.

Folstein, M., Folstein, S., and McHugh, P. R. Clinical predictors of improvement after electroconvulsive therapy of patients with schizophrenia, neurotic reactions, and affective disorders. *Biol. Psychiatry,* 7:147–152, 1973.

Ford, H., and Jameson, G. K. Chlorpromazine in conjunction with other psychiatric therapies. *Dis. Nerv. Syst.,* 16:179–185, 1955.

Forssman, H. Follow-up study of 16 children whose mothers were given electric convulsive therapy during gestation. *Acta Psychiatr. Neurol. Scand.,* 30:437–441, 1955.

Foster, M. W., Jr., and Gayle, R. F., III. Chlorpromazine and reserpine as adjuncts in electroshock treatment. *South. Med. J.,* 49:731–735, 1956.

Foulon, L. Electrochoc bilateral ou unilateral? *Acta Psychiatr. Belg.,* 73:356–378, 1973.

Fox, B. The investigation of the effects of psychiatric treatment. *J. Ment. Sci.,* 107:493–502, 1961.

Frankel, F. H. Electro-convulsive therapy in Massachusetts: A task force report. *Mass. J. Ment. Health,* 3:3–29, 1973.

Frankel, F. Current perspectives on ECT: A discussion. *Am. J. Psychiatry,* 134:1014–1019, 1977.

Frankel, F. H. (Ed.): Report No. 14 of the American Psychiatric Association Task Force on Convulsive Therapy. APA, Washington, D.C. 200 pp., 1978.

Freeman, C. P. L., Basson, J. V., and Crighton, A. Double-blind controlled trial of electroconvulsive therapy (E.C.T.) and simulated E.C.T. in depressive illness. *Lancet,* 1:738–740, 1978.

Freeman, T., and Cameron, J. L. Anxiety after electroshock therapy in involuntional melancholia. *Br. J. Psychol.,* 26:245–262, 1953.

Freeman, W. Multiple lobotomies. *Am. J. Psychiatry,* 123:1450–1452, 1967.

Freeman, W., and Watts, J. W. *Psychosurgery.* Charles C Thomas, Springfield, Ill. 337 pp., 1942.

French, O. Electroshock therapy and inadequate ventilation. *Chest,* 66:468, 1974.

Freund, J. D., and Warren, F. Z. A clinical impression of hexaflurodiethyl ether (Indoklon) following more than 800 treatments. *Dis. Nerv. Syst.,* 25:56–57, 1965.

Friedberg, J. *Shock Treatment is Not Good for Your Brain.* Glide Publications, San Francisco, 176 pp., 1976.

Friedberg, J. Shock treatment, brain damage and memory loss: A neurological perspective. *Am. J. Psychiatry,* 134:1010–1014, 1977.

Friedman, E. Unidirectional electrostimulated convulsive therapy. I: The effect of wave form and stimulus characteristics on the convulsive dose. *Am. J. Psychiatry,* 99:218–223, 1942.

Friedman, E. New convulsant anesthetic agents. Further studies of compounds #22451 and #31777 (Lilly). *Dis. Nerv. Syst.,* 21:398–404, 1960.

Friedman, E., and Wilcox, P. H. Electrostimulated convulsive doses in intact humans by means of unidirectional currents. *J. Nerv. Ment. Dis.,* 96:56–63, 1942.

Frizel, D., Coppen, A., and Marks, V. Plasma magnesium and calcium. *Br. J. Psychiatry,* 115:1375–1377, 1969.

Fromholt, P., Christensen, A., and Strömgren, L. S. The effects of unilateral and bilateral electroconvulsive therapy on memory. *Acta Psychiatr. Scand.,* 49:466–478, 1973.

Frosch, J., and Impastato, D. The effects of shock treatment on the ego. *Psychoanal. Q.,* 17:226–239, 1948.

Frost, I. Unilateral electro-shock. *Lancet,* 1:157–158, 1957.
Frostig, J. P., Van Harreveld, A., Resnick, S., Tyler, D. P., and Wiersma, C. A. G. Electronarcosis in animals and in man. *Arch. Neurol. Psychiatry,* 51:232–242, 1944.
Fukuda, T., and Matsuda, Y. Comparative characteristics of slow wave EEG, autonomic function and clinical picture in typical and atypical schizophrenia during and following electroconvulsive shock treatment. *Int. Pharmacopsychiatry,* 3:13–41, 1969.
Fulton, J. F., Ranson, S. W., and Frantz, A. M. *The Hypothalamus and Central Levels of Autonomic Function.* Williams & Wilkins, Baltimore, 980 pp., 1940.
Funk, I. C., Shatin, L., Freed, E. X., and Rockmore, L. Somato-psychotherapeutic approach to long-term schizophrenic patients. *J. Nerv. Ment. Dis.,* 121:423–437, 1955.
Funkenstein, D. H., Greenblatt, M., and Solomon, H. C. Autonomic nervous system changes following electric shock treatment. *J. Nerv. Ment. Dis.,* 108:409–422, 1948.
Funkenstein, D. H., Greenblatt, M., and Solomon, H. C. A test which predicts the clinical effects of electroshock treatment on schizophrenic patients. *Am. J. Psychiatry,* 106:889–901, 1950.
Funkenstein, D. H., Greenblatt, M., and Solomon, H. C. An autonomic nervous system test of prognostic significance in relation to electroshock treatment. *Psychosom. Med.,* 14:347–362, 1952.
Funkhouser, J. B. The symptomatic use of ECT for acute psychosis of military personnel. *Psychiatr. Quart.* 22:204–212, 1948.
Gaitz, C. M., Pokorny, A. D., and Mills, M., Jr. Death following electroconvulsive therapy. *Arch. Neurol. Psychiatry,* 75:493–499, 1956.
Galaburda, A. M., LeMay, M., Kemper, T. L., and Geschwind, N. Right-left asymmetries in the brain. *Science,* 199:852–856, 1978.
Gallagher, E. B., Levinson, D. J., and Erlich, I. Some sociopsychological characteristics of patients and their relevance for psychiatric treatment. In: M. Greenblatt, D. J. Levinson, and R. H. Williams (Eds.): *The Patient and the Mental Hospital,* Free Press, Chicago, 1957.
Gallinek, A. Controversial indications for electric convulsive therapy. *Am. J. Psychiatry,* 109:361–366, 1952 a.
Gallinek, A. Organic sequelae of electric convulsive therapy including facial and body dysgnosias. *J. Nerv. Ment. Dis.,* 115:377–393, 1952 b.
Gambill, J. M., and Wilson, I. C. Activation of chronic withdrawn schizophrenics. *Dis. Nerv. Syst.,* 27:615–617, 1966.
Gander, D. R., Bennett, P. J., and Kelly, D. H. W. Hexaflurodiethyl ether (Indoklon) convulsive therapy: A pilot study. *Br. J. Psychiatry,* 113:1413–1418, 1967.
GAP (Group for the Advancement of Psychiatry). Letter. *Shock Therapy,* September 15, 1947.
Garcia, J. H., and Cervos-Navarro, J. Electro-convulsive therapy (ECT): Its effects on the brain and other tissues (A review). Conference: *ECT: Efficacy and Impact,* New Orleans, February 23, 1978.
Garratini, S., Kato, R., and Valzelli, L. Biochemical and pharmacological effects induced by electroshock. *Psychiatr. Neurol.,* 140:190–206, 1960.
Garrett, E. S., and Mockbee, C. W. New hope for far advanced schizophrenia: Intensive regressive electroconvulsive therapy in treatment of severely regressed schizophrenics. *Ohio State Med. J.,* 48:505–508, 1952.
Gastaut, H., and Cossa, P. Le choc cardiazolique facilite par la stimulation lumineuse intermittente ou "photo-choc". *Sem. Hop. Paris,* 25:2738, 1949.
Gayle, R. F., Jr., and Josephs, D. Brief stimulus therapy. *South. Med. J.,* 41:245–251, 1948.
Gelenberg, A. J., and Mandel, M. R. Catatonic reactions to high-potency neuroleptic drugs. *Arch. Gen. Psychiatry,* 34:947–950, 1977.
Geller, M. R. Studies on electroconvulsive therapy 1939–1963. Supt. Documents, Washington, D.C., PHS 1447, 413 pp., 1965.
Gellhorn, E. The effects of hypoglycemia and anoxia on the central nervous system: A basis for a rational therapy of schizophrenia. *Arch. Neurol. Psychiatry,* 40:125–146, 1938.
Gellhorn, E. *Physiological Foundations of Neurology and Psychiatry.* University of Minnesota Press, Minneapolis, 556 pp., 1953.
Gellhorn, E. Analysis of autonomic hypothalamic functions in the intact organism. *Neurology,* 6:335–343, 1956.
Gellhorn, E., and Ballin, H. M. Further investigations on effect of anoxia on convulsions. *Am. J. Physiol.,* 162:503–506, 1950.
Gellhorn, E., and Safford, H. Influence of repeated anoxia, electroshock, and insulin hypoglycemia on the reactivity of the sympatheticoadrenal system. *Proc. Soc. Exp. Biol. Med.,* 68:74–79, 1948.

Geoghegan, J. J. Manic phase and electroshock. *Can. Med. Assoc. J.,* 55:54, 1946.
Geoghegan, J. J., and Stevenson, G. H. Prophylactic electroshock. *Am. J. Psychiatry,* 105:494–496, 1949.
Gerbino, L., Oleshansky, M., and Gershon, S. Clinical use and mode of action of lithium. In: M. A. Lipton, A. DiMascio, and K. F. Killam (Eds.): *Psychopharmacology: A Generation of Progress.* Raven Press, New York, pp. 1261–1275, 1978.
Gershon, S., and Shopsin, B. *Lithium: Its Role in Psychiatric Research and Treatment.* Plenum Press, New York, 358 pp., 1975.
Gerstmann, J. Problems of imperception of disease and of impaired body territories with organic lesions: Relation to body scheme and its disorders. *Arch. Neurol. Psychiatry,* 48:890–913, 1942.
Gibbons, J. L. Total body sodium and potassium in depressive illness. *Clin. Sci.,* 19:133–138, 1960.
Giberti, F. Aspetti comparativi degli effetti dell'-elettroshock (bi- o monopolare), dell'-elettronarcosi e del trattamento chemioconvulsivante (fluoretil) in pazienti psichiatrici. *Sist. Nerv.,* 21:210–216, 1969.
Gibson, A. C. How ECT works. *Br. Med. J.,* 1:169, 1975.
Gillin, J. C., Duncan, W. C., Pettigrew, K. D., Frankel, B. L., and Snyder, F. Diagnosis of depression and insomnia by EEG sleep. Presented at the American Psychiatric Association, May 8, 1978.
Gillis, A. A case of schizophrenia in childhood. *J. Nerv. Ment. Dis.,* 121:471–472, 1955.
Glassman, A. H. Patient response, drug response and drop-outs: A study of 140 consecutive endogenous depressives. Presented at the American Psychiatric Association, May 8, 1978.
Glassman, A., Kantor, S. J., and Shostak, M. Depression, delusions and drug response. *Am. J. Psychiatry,* 132:716–719, 1975.
Globus, J. H., van Harreveld, A., and Wiersma, C. A. G. The influence of electric application on the structure of the brain of dogs. *J. Neuropathol. Exp. Neurol.,* 2:263–276, 1943.
Glueck, B. C. Psychopathologic reactions and electric-shock therapy. *NY State J. Med.,* 42:1553–1557, 1942.
Glueck, B. C., Reiss, H., and Bernard, L. E. Regressive electric shock therapy. *Psychiatr. Q.,* 31:117–136, 1957.
Goddard, G., McIntyre, D., and Leech, C. A permanent change in brain function resulting from daily electrical stimulation. *Exp. Neurol.,* 25:295–330, 1969.
Gold, L. Autonomic balance in patients treated with insulin shock as measured by mecholyl chloride. *Arch. Neurol. Psychiatry,* 50:311–317, 1943.
Gold, L., and Chiarello, C. J. The prognostic value of clinical findings in cases treated with electric shock. *J. Nerv. Ment. Dis.,* 100:577–583, 1944.
Gold, P. W. Quoted in meeting report, Eighth International Conference, Society of Psychoneuroendocrinology. *Psychoneuroendocrinology,* 2:417–426, 1977.
Gold, P. W., Goodwin, F. K. and Reus, V. I. Vasopressin in affective illness. Lancet 1:1233–1236, 1978.
Goldfarb, W., and Kieve, H. The treatment of psychotic like regressions of combat soldiers. *Psychiatr. Q.,* 19:555–565, 1945.
Goldman, D. Brief stimulus electric shock therapy. *J. Nerv. Ment. Dis.,* 110:36–45, 1949.
Goldman, D. Historical aspects of electroshock therapy, electrical current modifications, treatment techniques and some electroencephalographic observations. *J. Neuropsychiatry,* 3:210–215, 1962.
Goldman, H., Gomer, F. E., and Templer, D. L. Long-term effects of electroconvulsive therapy upon memory and perceptual-motor performance. *J. Clin. Psychol.,* 28:32–34, 1972.
Goldstein, K. *The Organism.* American Book, New York, 553 pp., 1939.
Golla, E., Walter, W. G., and Fleming, G. W. Electrically induced convulsions. *Proc. R. Soc. Med.,* 33:261–267, 1940.
Goller, E. S. A controlled trial of reserpine in chronic schizophrenia. *J. Ment. Sci.,* 106:1408–1412, 1960.
Gomez, J. Death after E.C.T. *Br. Med. J.,* 1:45, 1974.
Gomez, J. Subjective side-effects of ECT. Br. J. Psychiatry, 127:609–611, 1975.
Gomez, J., and Dally, P. Intravenous tranquillization with ECT. *Br. J. Psychiatry,* 127:604–608, 1975.
Gonzalez, J. R., and Imahara, J. K. Electroshock therapy with the phenothiazines and reserpine. *Am. J. Psychiatry,* 121:253–256, 1964.
Gorden, A. E. Results of European clinical trials of therapeutic use of thyrotropin releasing hormone (TRH) in psychiatry. *Psychopharmacol. Bull.,* 11:20–21, 1975.
Gordh, T., and Silfverskiöld, B. P. Disturbance of circulation in convulsions of epileptic type: I.

Intrathoracic and intra-abdominal pressure during electroshock. *Acta Med. Scand.,* 113:183–190, 1943.
Gordon, H. L. Objectors to electric shock treatment are refractory to its therapy. *NY State J. Med.,* 46:407–410, 1946.
Gordon, H. L. Fifty shock therapy theories. *Milit. Surg.,* 103:397–401, 1948.
Gottlieb, G., and Wilson, I. Cerebral dominance: Temporary disruption of verbal memory by unilateral electroconvulsive shock therapy. *J. Comp. Physiol. Psychol.,* 60:368–372, 1965.
Gottlieb, J. S., and Huston, P. E. Treatment of schizophrenia. A comparison of three methods: Brief psychotherapy, insulin coma and electric shock. *J. Nerv. Ment. Dis.,* 113:237–246, 1951.
Graber, H. K., and McHugh, R. B. Regressive electroshock therapy in chronic schizophrenia, a controlled study. *Lancet,* 80:24–27, 1960.
Graham, B. F., and Cleghorn, R. A. Changes in the circulating leucocytes following electrically induced convulsions in man. *J. Clin. Endocrinol.,* 11:1469–1480, 1951.
Grahame-Smith, D. G. Cerebral mechanisms of mood and behaviour. *Psychol. Med.,* 6:523–528, 1976.
Grahame-Smith, D. G., Green, A. R., and Costain, D. W. Mechanism of the antidepressant action of electroconvulsive therapy. *Lancet,* 1:254–256, 1978.
Gralnick, A. Fatalities associated with electric shock treatment of psychoses. *Arch. Neurol. Psychiatry,* 51:397–402, 1944.
Gralnick, A. Shock therapy in psychoses complicated by pregnancy. *Am. J. Psychiatry,* 102:780–782, 1946.
Granville-Grossman, K. *Recent Advances in Clinical Psychiatry.* J. A. Churchill, London, pp. 1–17, 1971.
Gravenstein, J. S., Anton, A. H., Weiner, S. M., and Tetlow, A. G. Catecholamine and cardiovascular response to electroconvulsion therapy in man. *Br. J. Anaesth.,* 37:833–839, 1965.
Green, A. R. Repeated exposure of rats to the convulsant agent flurothyl enhances 5-hydroxytryptamine- and dopamine-mediated behavioural responses. *Br. J. Pharmacol.,* 62:325–331, 1978.
Green, A. R., Heal, D. J., and Grahame-Smith, D. G. Further observations on the effect of repeated electroconvulsive shock on the behavioural responses of rats produced by increases in the functional activity of brain 5-hydroxytryptamine and dopamine. *Psychopharmacology,* 52:195–200, 1977.
Green, A. R., Peralta, E., Hong, J. S., Mao, C. C., Atterwill, C. K. and Costa, E. Alterations in GABA metabolism and met-enkephalin content in rat brain following repeated electroconvulsive shocks. *J. Neurochem. (in press).*
Green, J. D. Neural pathways to the hypophysis: Anatomical and functional. In: W. Haymaker, E. Anderson, and W. J. H. Nauta (Eds.): *The Hypothalamus.* Charles C Thomas, Springfield, Ill., pp. 276–310, 1969.
Green, M. A. Significance of individual variability in EEG response to electroshock. *J. Hillside Hosp.,* 6:229–240, 1957.
Green, M. A. Relation between threshold and duration of seizures and electrographic change during convulsive therapy. *J. Nerv. Ment. Dis.,* 131:117–120, 1960.
Green, M. A., and Fink, M. Clinical and electroencephalographic effects of megimide in patients without cerebral disease. *Neurology,* 8:682–685, 1958.
Green, W. J., and Stajduhar, P. P. The effect of ECT on the sleep dream cycle in a psychotic depression. *J. Nerv. Ment. Dis.,* 143:123–134, 1966.
Greenblatt, M. Efficacy of ECT in affective and schizophrenic illness. *Am. J. Psychiatry,* 134:1001–1005, 1977.
Greenblatt, M., Freeman, H., Meshorer, E., and Sharp, M. Comparative efficacy of antidepressant drugs and placebo in relation to electric shock treatment. In: M. Rinkel (Ed.): *Biological Treatment of Mental Illness,* L. C. Page, New York, pp. 574–594, 1966.
Greenblatt, M., Grosser, G. H., and Wechsler, H. A comparative study of selected antidepressant medications and ECT. *Am. J. Psychiatry,* 119:144–153, 1962.
Greenblatt, M., Grosser, G. H., and Wechsler, H. Differential response of hospitalized depressed patients in somatic therapy. *Am. J. Psychiatry,* 120:935–943, 1964.
Gregoire, F., Brauman, H., De Buck, R., and Corvilain, J. Hormone release in depressed patients before and after recovery. *Psychoneuroendocrinology,* 2:303–312, 1977.
Grinker, R. R., and MacLean, H. V. The courses of depression treated by psychotherapy and metrazol. *Psychosom. Med.,* 2:119–138, 1940.
Grinker, R., and Spiegel, J. *War Neuroses in North Africa.* Josiah Macy, New York, 300 pp., 1943.

Grinspoon, L., and Greenblatt, M. Pharmacotherapy combined with other treatment methods. *Compr. Psychiatry,* 4:256–262, 1963.

Grosser, G. H., Pearsall, D. T., Fisher, C. L., and Geremonte, L. The regulation of electroconvulsive treatment in Massachusetts: A follow-up. *Mass. J. Ment. Health,* 5:12–25, 1975.

Gunn, D. R., Blazic, C., Thomas, E., Eng, P., and Britt, B. A. Cerebrospinal fluid pressure during flurothyl convulsive and electro-convulsive therapies. *Can. Psychiatr. Assoc. J. [Suppl.],* 11:78–85, 1966.

Guttmann, E., Mayer-Gross, W., and Slater, E. T. O. Short-distance prognosis of schizophrenia. *J. Neurol. Psychiatry,* 2:25–34, 1939.

Guze, S. B. The occurrence of psychiatric illness in systemic lupus erythematosus. *Am. J. Psychiatry,* 123:1562–1570, 1967.

Guze, S. B., Winokur, G., and Levin, M. E. The effect of electroshock therapy in the absence of both adrenal glands. *J. Nerv. Ment. Dis.,* 124:195–198, 1956.

Haard, G., Holmberg, G., and Ramqvist, N. Experiments in the prolongation of convulsions induced by electric shock treatment. *Acta Psychiatr. Neurol. Scand.,* 311:61–70, 1956.

Haase, H. J., and Janssen, P. A. J. *The Action of Neuroleptic Drugs.* Year Book Medical Publishers, Chicago, 174 pp., 1965.

Halliday, A. M., Davison, K., Browne, M. W., and Kreeger, L. C. A comparison of the effects on depression and memory of bilateral ECT and unilateral ECT to the dominant and non-dominant hemispheres. *Br. J. Psychiatry,* 114:997–1012, 1968.

Halpern, F. Rorschach interpretations of the personality structure of schizophrenics who benefit from insulin therapy. *Psychiatr. Q.,* 14:826–833, 1940.

Hamadah, K., Holmes, H., Barker, G. B., Hartman, G. C., and Parke, D. V. W. Effects of electric convulsion therapy on urinary excretion of $3'$, $5'$ cyclic adenosine monophosphate. *Br. Med. J.,* 3:439–441, 1972.

Hamilton, D. M. and Wall, J. H.: Hospital treatment of dementia praecox. *Am. J. Psychiatr.* 105:346–352, 1948.

Hamilton, D. M., and Ward, G. M. The hospital treatment of involutional psychosis. *Am. J. Psychiatry,* 104:801–804, 1948.

Hamilton, M. Prediction of response to E.C.T. in depressive illness. In: J. Angst (Ed.): *Classification and Prediction of Outcome in Depression.* F. K. Schattauer Verlag, Stuttgart, pp. 273–280, 1974.

Hamilton, M. *Fish's Schizophrenia.* John Wright & Sons, Bristol, 212 pp., 1976.

Hamilton, M., and White, J. M. Factors related to the outcome of depression treated with ECT. *J. Ment. Sci.,* 106:1031–1041, 1960.

Harper, R. G., and Wiens, A. N. Electroconvulsive therapy and memory. *J. Nerv. Ment. Dis.,* 161:245–254, 1975.

Harris, G. W. *Neural Control of the Pituitary Gland.* Arnold, London, 298 pp., 1955.

Harris, G. W., and George, R. Neurohumoral control of the adenohypophysis and the regulation of the secretion of TSH, ACTH and growth hormone. In: W. Haymaker, E. Anderson, and W. J. H. Nauta (Eds.): *The Hypothalamus.* Charles C Thomas, Springfield, Ill., pp. 326–388, 1969.

Harris, J. A., and Robin, A. A. A controlled trial of phenelzine in depressive reactions. *J. Ment. Sci.,* 106:1432–1437, 1960.

Hartelius, H. Cerebral changes following electrically induced convulsions. An experimental study on cats. *Acta Psychiatr. Scand.,* 77:1–128, 1952.

Hartshorn, E. A. Interactions of CNS drugs—antidepressants. *Drug Intell. Clin. Pharm.,* 8:591–606, 1974.

Hastings, D. W. Circular manic-depressive reaction modified by "prophylactic electroshock." *Am. J. Psychiatry,* 118:258–260, 1961.

Havens, L. L. A comparative study of modified and unmodified electric shock treatment. *Dis. Nerv. Syst.,* 19:29–34, 1958.

Havens, L. L., Zileli, M. S., DiMascio, A., Boling, L., and Goldfien, A. Changes in catecholamine response to successive electric convulsive treatments. *J. Ment. Sci.,* 105:821–829, 1959.

Hayes, K. J. The current path in electric convulsion shock. *Arch. Neurol. Psychiatry,* 63:102–109, 1950.

Haymaker, W., Anderson, E., and Nauta, W. J. H. *The Hypothalamus.* Charles C Thomas, Springfield, Ill., 805 pp., 1969.

Head, H. *Aphasia and Kindred Disorders of Speech.* Cambridge University Press, Cambridge, 979 pp., 1926.

Heath, E. S., Adams, A., and Wakeling, P. L. G. Short courses of ECT and simulated ECT in chronic schizophrenia. *Br. J. Psychiatry,* 110:800–807, 1964.

Heath, R. G., and Norman, E. C. Electroshock therapy by stimulation of discrete cortical sites with small electrodes. *Proc. Soc. Exp. Biol. Med.,* 63:496–502, 1946.

Heggtveit, H. A. Coronary occlusion during EST. *Am. J. Psychiatry,* 120:78–79, 1963.

Heilbrunn, G., and Feldman, P. Electric shock treatment in general paresis. *Am. J. Psychiatry,* 99:702–705, 1943.

Heilbrunn, G, and Liebert, E. Biopsies on the brain following artificially produced convulsions. *Arch. Neurol. Psychiatry,* 46:548–550, 1941.

Heilbrunn, G., and Weil, A. Pathologic changes in the central nervous system in experimental electric shock. *Arch. Neurol. Psychiatry,* 47:918–930, 1942.

Hemphill, R. E., MacLeod, L. D., and Reiss, M. Changes in output of 17-ketosteroids after shock treatment, pre-frontal leucotomy and other procedures. *J. Ment. Sci.,* 88:554–558, 1942.

Hemphill, R. E., and Reiss, M. Corticotrophic hormone in treatment of involutional melancholia with hypopituitarism and pituitary cachexia. *J. Ment. Sci.,* 88:559–565, 1942.

Hemphill, R. E., and Walter, W. G. The treatment of mental disorders by electrically induced convulsions. *J. Ment. Sci.,* 87:256–275, 1941.

Henry, G. M., Weingartner, H., and Murphy, D. L. The influence of affective states and psychoactive drugs on verbal learning and memory. *Am. J. Psychiatry,* 130:966–971, 1973.

Herrington, R. N., Bruce, A., Johnstone, E. C., and Lader, M. H. Comparative trial of L-tryptophan and E.C.T. in severe depressive illness. *Lancet,* 2:731–734, 1974.

Heshe, A. J., and Roeder, E. Elektroshock i Denmark. *Ugeskr. Laeger.,* 137:939–941, 1975.

Heshe, A. J., and Roeder, E. Electroconvulsive therapy in Denmark. *Br. J. Psychiatry,* 128:241–245, 1976.

Hess, W. R. *Diencephalon, Autonomic and Extrapyramidal Function.* Grune & Stratton, New York, 1954.

Heuyer, G., Dauphin, M., and Lebovici, S. Electroshock therapy in children. *Z. Kinderpsychiatr.,* 14:60–64, 1947.

Hift, E., Hift, S., and Spiel, W. Results of shock therapy on schizophrenics in childhood. *Schweiz. Arch. Neurol. Psychiatr.,* 86:256–272, 1960.

Hill, D., Loe, P. St. J., Theobald, J., and Waddell, M. A central homeostatic mechanism in schizophrenia. *J. Ment. Sci.,* 97:111–131, 1951.

Hill, D., and Parr, G. (Eds.): *Electroencephalography.* Macmillan, New York, 509 pp., 1963.

Hill, L. B., and Patton, J. D. When physical therapy (shock) facilitates psychotherapy. *Am. J. Psychiatry,* 113:60–66, 1956.

Hillard, J. R., and Folger, R. Patients' attitudes and attributions to electroconvulsive shock therapy. *J. Clin. Psychol.,* 33:855–861, 1977.

Hinterhuber, H., and Nowak, H. Erfahrungen mit unilateraler Elektrokonvulsionstherapie. *Arch. Psychiatr. Nervenkr.,* 217:149–156, 1973.

Hirano, A., Becker, N. H., and Zimmerman, H. M. The use of peroxidase as a tracer in studies of alterations in the blood brain barrier. *J. Neurol. Sci.,* 10:205–213, 1970.

Hoagland, H., Callaway, E., Elmadjian, F. and Pincus, G. Adrenal cortical responsivity of psychotic patients in relation to electroshock treatment. *Psychosom. Med.,* 12:73–77, 1950.

Hoagland, H., Malamud, W., Kaufman, I. C., and Pincus, G. Changes in electroencephalogram and in the execretion of 17-ketosteroids accompanying electroshock therapy of agitated depression. *Psychosom. Med.,* 8:246–251, 1946.

Hoagland, H., and Pincus, G. Pituitary-adrenocortical function in patients with severe personality disorders. *Clin. ACTH Conference.* Blackiston, Philadelphia, 1950.

Hobson, R. F. Prognostic factors in electric convulsive therapy. *J. Neurol. Neurosurg. Psychiatry,* 16:275–281, 1953.

Hoenig, J., Leiberman, D. M., and Auerbach, I. The effect of insulin coma and ECT on the short term prognosis of schizophrenia. *J. Neurol. Neurosurg. Psychiatry,* 19:130–136, 1956.

Hohman, L. B., and Wilkinson, W. E. Pain equivalents treated with electroshock. *US Armed Forces Med. J.,* 4:1025, 1953.

Hökfeldt, T., Elde, R., Fuxe, K., Johansson, O., Ljungdahl, H., Goldstein, M., Luft, R., Efendic, S., Nilsson, G., Terenius, L., Ganten, D., Jeffcoate, S. L., Rehfeld, J., Said, S., Perex da la Mora, M., Passani, L., Tapia, R., Teran, L., and Palacios, R. Aminergic and peptidergic pathways in the nervous system with special reference to the hypothalamus. In: S. Reichlin, R. Baldessarini, and J. B. Martin (Eds.): *The Hypothalamus.* Raven Press, New York, pp. 69–136, 1978.

Hollender, M. H., and Steckler, P. P. Multiple sclerosis and schizophrenia: A case report. *Psychiatr. Med.*, 3:251–257, 1972.

Hollingshead, A. B., and Redlich, F. C. *Social Class and Mental Illness: A Community Study.* John Wiley & Sons, New York, 442 pp., 1958.

Hollister, L. E., Davis, K. L., and Berger, P. A. Thyrotropin-releasing hormone and psychiatric disorders. In: E. Usdin, A. Hamburg, and J. D. Barchas (Eds.): *Neuroregulators and Psychiatric Disorders,* Oxford University Press, New York, pp. 242–249, 1977.

Holmberg, G. The influence of oxygen administration on electrically induced convulsions in man. *Acta Psychiatr. Neurol.,* 28:365–386, 1953 a.

Holmberg, G. The factor of hypoxemia in electroshock therapy. *Am J. Psychiatry,* 110:115–118, 1953 b.

Holmberg, G. Effect on electrically induced convulsions of the number of previous treatments in a series. *Arch. Neurol. Psychiatry,* 71:619–623, 1954 a.

Holmberg, G. Influence of sex and age on convulsions induced by electric shock treatment. *Arch. Neurol. Psychiatry,* 71:473–476, 1954 b.

Holmberg, G. The effect of certain factors on the convulsions in electric shock treatment. *Acta Psychiatr. Neurol. Scand. [Suppl.],* 98:1–19, 1955.

Holmberg, G. Biological aspects of electroconvulsive therapy. *Int. Rev. Neurobiol.,* 5:389–412, 1963.

Holmberg, G., Haard, G., and Ramqvist, N. Experiments in the prolongation of convulsions induced by electric shock treatment. *Acta Psychiatr. Neurol. Scand.,* 31:61–70, 1956.

Holmberg, G., and Thesleff, S. Succinyl-choline-iodide as a muscular relaxant in electroshock therapy. *Am. J. Psychiatry,* 108:842–846, 1952.

Holmberg, G., Thesleff, S., von Dardel, O., Hard, G., Ramqvist, N., and Pettersson, H. Circulatory conditions in electroshock therapy with and without a muscle relaxant. *Arch. Neurol. Psychiatry,* 72:73–79, 1954.

Holovachka, A. Oxygen in electro-shock therapy. *J. Nerv. Ment. Dis.,* 98:485–487, 1943.

Holt, W. L. Intensive maintenance EST. A clinical note concerning two unusual cases. *Int. J. Neuropsychiatry,* 1:391–394, 1965.

Holt, W. L., and Borkowski, W. Drug-modified electric shock therapy. *Psychiatr. Q.,* 25:581–558, 1951.

Holt, W. L., Jr., McCandless, F. D., Yacoubian, J., and Mebed, A. A. K. A comparison of "anectine" (succinylcholine) and "flaxedil" effects on blood pressure, pulse and respiration in 30 cardiac and 49 other patients given convulsive therapy. *Confin. Neurol.,* 13:313–319, 1953.

Hordern, A., Holt, H. F., Burt, C. G., and Gordon, W. F. Amitriptyline in depressive cases. *Br. J. Psychiatry,* 109:815–825, 1963.

Hoyt, R., and Rosvold, H. E. Effect of electroconvulsive shock on body temperature of the rat. *Proc. Soc. Exp. Biol. Med.,* 78:582–583, 1951.

Huddleson, J. H., and Lowinger, L. Note on initial and succeeding voltages to obtain grand mal in electroshock therapy. *J. Nerv. Ment. Dis.,* 102:191–193, 1945.

Huggins, P. K., Sandifer, M. G., and Pearson, W. S. Electroshock with and without barbiturate anesthesia. *J. Nerv. Ment. Dis.,* 138:141–145, 1964.

Hughes, J., Wigton, R., and Jardon, F. Electroencephalographic studies on patients receiving electroshock treatment. *Arch. Neurol. Psychiatry,* 46:748–749, 1941.

Hunt, H. F. Electro-convulsive shock and learning. *Trans. NY Acad. Sci.,* 27:923–945, 1965.

Hunter, J., and Jasper, H. Effects of thalamic stimulation in unanesthetised animals. *Electroencephalogr. Clin. Neurophysiol.,* 1:305–324, 1949.

Hurwitz, T. D. Electroconvulsive therapy: A review. *Compr. Psychiatry,* 15:303–314, 1974.

Hussar, A. E., and Pachter, M. Myocardial infarction and fatal coronary insufficiency during electroconvulsive therapy. *JAMA,* 204:1004–1007, 1968.

Huston, P. E., and Locher, L. M. Manic-depressive psychosis. Course when treated and untreated with electric shock. *Arch. Neurol. Psychiatry,* 60:37–48, 1948 a.

Huston, P. E., and Locher, L. M. Involutional psychosis: Course when untreated and when treated with electric shock. *Arch. Neurol. Psychiatry,* 59:385–394, 1948 b.

Hutchinson, J. T., and Smedberg, D. Treatment of depression: A comparative study of ECT and six drugs. *Br. J. Psychiatry,* 109:536–538, 1963.

Ilaria, R., and Prange, A. J. Convulsive therapy and other biological treatments. In: F. F. Flach and S. S. Draghi (Eds.): *The Nature and Treatment of Depression.* John Wiley & Sons, New York, pp. 271–308, 1975.

Imlah, N. W., Ryan, E., and Harrington, J. A. The influence of antidepressant drugs on the response

to electroconvulsive therapy and on subsequent relapse rates. *Neuropsychopharmacology,* 4:438–442, 1965.
Impastato, D. Prevention of fatalities in electroshock therapy. *Dis. Nerv. Syst. [Suppl.],* 18:34–75, 1957.
Impastato, D. J., Berg, S., and Pacella, B. L. Electroshock therapy: Focal spread technique. A new form of treatment of psychiatric illness. *Confin. Neurol.,* 13:266–270, 1953.
Impastato, D. J., Frosch, J., Robertiello, R. C., and Wortis, S. B. Improved electroconvulsive therapy with low amperage unidirectional currents. *Dis. Nerv. Syst.,* 12:3–7, 1951.
Impastato, D. J., Frosch, J., and Wortis, S. B. Reduction of complications in electro-shock therapy. The Reiter machine. *Comptes. Rendus des Séances* 1171:163–168, Hermann & Cie, Paris, 1952.
Impastato, D. J., Gabriel, A. R., and Lardaro, H. H. Electric and insulin shock therapy during pregnancy. *Dis. Nerv. Syst.,* 25:542–546, 1964.
Impastato, D. J., and Karliner, W. Control of memory impairment in EST by unilateral stimulation of the non-dominant hemisphere. *Dis. Nerv. Syst.,* 27:182–188, 1966.
Impastato, D. J., and Pacella, B. L. Electrically produced unilateral convulsions. *Dis. Nerv. Syst.,* 13:368–369, 1952.
Inglis, J. Electrode placement and the effect of ECT on mood and memory in depression. *Can. Psychiatr. Assoc. J.,* 14:463–471, 1969.
Itil, T. Elektroencephalographische Befunde zur Klassifikation neuro und thymoleptischer Medikamente. *Med. Exp.,* 5:347–363, 1961.
Itil, T. *Elektroencephalographische Studien Bei Psychosen Und Psychotropen Medikamenten.* Ahmet Sait Matbaasi, Istanbul, 128 pp., 1964.
Itil, T. (Ed.): *Psychotropic Drugs and the Human EEG.* S. Karger, Munich, 377 pp., 1974.
Itil, T., and Fink, M. Anticholinergic drug induced delirium (experimental modification, quantitative EEG and behavioral correlations). *J. Nerv. Ment. Dis.,* 143:492–507, 1966.
Ives, J. O., Weaver, L. A., and Williams, R. Portable electromyograph monitoring of unilateral ECT. *Am. J. Psychiatry,* 133:1340–1341, 1976.
Jackson, H. H. *Selected Writings.* Hodder & Stroughton, London, 1932.
Jacoby, M. G., and van Houten, Z. Regressive shock therapy. *Dis. Nerv. Syst.,* 21:582–583, 1960.
Jaffe, J. An objective study of communication in psychiatric interviews. *J. Hillside Hosp.,* 6:207–215, 1957.
Jaffe, J. Language of the dyad. *Psychiatry,* 21:249–258, 1958.
Jaffe, J., Esecover, H., Kahn, R. L., and Fink, M. Modification of psychotherapeutic transactions by altered brain function. *Am. J. Psychother.,* 15:46–55, 1961.
Jaffe, J., Fink, M., and Kahn, R. L. Changes in verbal transaction with induced altered brain function. *J. Nerv. Ment. Dis.,* 130:235–239, 1960.
Janis, I. L. Memory loss following electric convulsive treatments. *J. Pers.,* 17:29–32, 1948.
Janis, I. L. Psychologic effects of electric convulsive treatments (post-treatment amnesias). *J. Nerv. Ment. Dis.,* 111:359–382, 1950a.
Janis, I. L. Psychologic effects of electric convulsive treatments (changes in word association reactions). *J. Nerv. Ment. Dis.,* 111: 383–397, 1950b.
Janis, I. L. Psychologic effects of electric convulsive treatments (changes in affective disturbances). *J. Nerv. Ment. Dis.,* 111:469–489, 1950c.
Janowsky, D. S., Fann, W. E., and Davis, J. M. Monoamines and ovarian hormone-linked sexual and emotional changes. *Arch. Sex. Behav.,* 1:205–218, 1971.
Jasper, H. H. Diffuse projection systems: The integrative action of the thalamic reticular system. *Electroencephalogr. Clin. Neurophysiol.,* 1:405–420, 1949.
Jensen, E. S. Unilateral elektroshockbehandlung. *Nord. Med.,* 22:253–255, 1968.
Jensen, G. D., and Stainbrook, E. Effects of electrogenic convulsions on the estrus cycle and the weight of rats. *J. Comp. Physiol. Psychol.,* 42:502–505, 1949.
Johnson, L. C., Ulett, G. A., Johnson, M., Sineth, K., and Sines, J. O. Electroconvulsive therapy (with and without atropine). *Arch. Gen. Psychiatry,* 2:324–336, 1960a.
Johnson, L. C., Ulett, G. A., Sines, J. O., and Stern, J. A. Cortical activity and cognitive functioning. *Electroencephalogr. Clin. Neurophysiol.,* 12:861–874, 1960b.
Jori, A., Dolfini, E., Casati, C., and Argenta, G. Effect of ECT and imipramine treatment on the concentration of 5-hydroxyindoleacetic acid (5-HIAA) and homovanillic acid (HVA) in the cerebrospinal fluid of depressed patients. *Psychopharmacologia,* 44:87–90, 1975.
Juba, A. Über nach Electroshock auftretende kortikale Funktionsstörungen (Gerstmannsches Syndrom, Gesichts- und Raumagnosien). *Schweiz. Arch. Neurol. Psychiatr.,* 61:217–226, 1948.
Kaelbling, R., Koski, E. G., and Hartwig, C. D. Reduction of rapid eye movement sleep after

electroconvulsions—an experiment in cats on the mode of action of electroconvulsive treatment. *J. Psychiatr. Res.,* 6:153–157, 1968.
Kafi, A., Dennis, M. Advantages of Indoklon convulsive therapy. *Hosp. Community Psychiatry,* 17:297–300, 1966.
Kafi, A., Dennis, M., and Todd R. Indoklon and electric convulsive therapy: A comparative study of their effects on memory. *Behav. Neuropsychiatry,* 1:25–30, 1969.
Kahlbaum, K. L. *Die Katatonie.* Kirschwald, Berlin, 102 pp., 1874.
Kahn, R. L. Staff attitudes toward psychiatric treatment in a voluntary mental hospital. *J. Hillside Hosp.,* 10:97–106, 1961.
Kahn, R. L., and Fink, M. Perception of embedded figures after induced altered brain function. *Am. Psychol.,* 12:361, 1957.
Kahn, R. L., and Fink, M. Changes in language during electroshock therapy. In: P. Hoch and J. Zubin (Eds.): *Psychopathology of Communication.* Grune & Stratton, New York, pp. 126–139, 1958.
Kahn, R. L., and Fink, M. Personality factors in behavioral response to electroshock therapy. *J. Neuropsychiatry,* 1:45–49, 1959.
Kahn, R. L., and Fink, M. Prognostic value of Rorschach criteria in clinical response to convulsive therapy. *J. Neuropsychiatry,* 1:242–245, 1960.
Kahn, R. L., Fink, M., and Siegel, N. Sociopsychological aspects of psychiatric treatment. *Arch. Gen. Psychiatry,* 14:20–25, 1966.
Kahn, R. L., Fink, M., and Weinstein, E. A. The amytal test in patients with mental illness. *J. Hillside Hosp.,* 4:3–13, 1955.
Kahn, R. L., Fink, M., and Weinstein, E. A. Relation of amobarbital test to clinical improvement in electroshock. *Arch. Neurol. Psychiatry,* 76:23–29, 1956.
Kahn, R. L., and Pollack, M. Prognostic application of psychological techniques in convulsive therapy. *Dis. Nerv. Syst.,* 20:180–184, 1959.
Kahn, R. L., and Pollack, M. Sociopsychological factors affecting therapist-patient relationships. In: J. Masserman (Ed.) *Psychoanalysis and Human Values.* Grune & Stratton, New York, pp. 155–168, 1960.
Kahn, R. L., Pollack, M., and Fink, M. Social factors in selection of therapy in a voluntary mental hospital. *J. Hillside Hosp.,* 6:216–228, 1957.
Kahn, R. L., Pollack, M., and Fink, M. Sociopsychologic aspects of psychiatric treatment in a voluntary mental hospital: Duration of hospitalization, discharge ratings and diagnosis. *Arch. Gen. Psychiatry,* 1:565–574, 1959.
Kahn, R. L., Pollack, M., and Fink, M. Figure-ground discrimination after induced altered brain function. *Arch. Neurol.,* 2:547–551, 1960a.
Kahn, R. L., Pollack, M., and Fink, M. Social attitude (California F scale) and convulsive therapy. *J. Nerv. Ment. Dis.,* 130:187–192, 1960b.
Kalinowsky, L. B. Electric convulsive therapy, with emphasis on importance of adequate treatment. *Arch. Neurol. Psychiatry,* 50:652–660, 1943.
Kalinowsky, L. B. Organic psychotic syndromes occurring during electric convulsive therapy. *Arch. Neurol. Psychiatry,* 53:269–273, 1945.
Kalinowsky, L. B. Failures with electric shock therapy. In: Hoch, P. (Ed.): *Failures in Psychiatric Treatment.* Grune & Stratton, New York, pp. 161–169, 1948.
Kalinowsky, L. Some problems in electric convulsive therapy of depressions. In: P. H. Hoch and J. Zubin (Eds.): *Depression.* Grune & Stratton, New York, pp. 190–198, 1954.
Kalinowsky, L. B. Electric convulsive therapy within the framework of other available treatments. In: M. Rinkel (Ed.): *Biological Treatment of Mental Illness.* L. C. Page, New York, pp. 665–673, 1962.
Kalinowsky, L. B. Electric convulsive therapy after ten years of pharmaco-therapy. *Am. J. Psychiatry,* 120:944–949, 1964.
Kalinowsky, L. Biological psychiatric treatments preceding pharmacotherapy. In: F. Ayd and B. Blackwell (Eds.): *Discoveries in Biological Psychiatry.* J. B. Lippincott, Philadelphia, pp. 59–67, 1970.
Kalinowsky, L., Barrera, E. S., and Horwitz, W. A. The "petit-mal" response in electric shock therapy. *Am. J. Psychiatry,* 98:708–711, 1942.
Kalinowsky, L., and Hippius, H. *Pharmacological, Convulsive and Other Treatments in Psychiatry.* Grune & Stratton, New York, 470 pp., 1972.
Kalinowsky, L., and Hoch, P. *Shock Treatment and other Somatic Procedures in Psychiatry.* Grune & Stratton, New York, 294 pp, 1946.

Kalinowsky, L., and Hoch, P. H. *Shock Treatment, Psychosurgery and Other Somatic Treatments in Psychiatry.* Grune & Stratton, New York, 396 pp., 1952.
Kalinowsky, L., and Hoch, P. H. *Somatic Treatment in Psychiatry.* Grune & Stratton, New York, 413 pp., 1961.
Kalinowsky, L. B., and Worthing, H. J. Results with electric convulsive treatment in 200 cases of schizophrenia. *Psychiatr. Q.,* 17:144–153, 1943.
Kallio, I. V. I., and Tala, E. O. J. Changes in the free 17-hydroxycorticosteroid levels in plasma after electroshock therapy. *Acta Endocrinol.,* 30:99–108, 1959.
Kantor, S. J., and Glassman, A. H. Delusional depressions: Natural history and response to treatment. *Br. J. Psychiatry,* 131:351–360, 1977.
Kantor, S. J., Glassman, A. H., Bigger, J. T., Perel, J. M., and Giardina, E. V. The cardiac effects of therapeutic plasma concentrations of imipramine. *Am. J. Psychiatry,* 135:534–538, 1978.
Kaplan, A. I., and Lefkowits, H. J. Influences of staff attitudes and environmental factors on treatment selection. *J. Hillside Hosp.,* 10:84–96, 1961.
Karagulla, S. Evaluation of ECT as compared with conservative methods of treatment in depressive states. *J. Ment. Sci.,* 96:1060–1091, 1950.
Kardiner, A. The bio-analysis of the epileptic reaction. *Psychoanal. Q.,* 1:375–483, 1932.
Karliner, W. Epileptic states following electroshock therapy. *J. Hillside Hosp.,* 5:1–9, 1956.
Karliner, W. Clinical experience with intravenous Indoklon: A new convulsant drug. *J. Neuropsychiatry,* 4:184–189, 1963.
Karliner, W. Further clinical experience with 10% intravenous Indoklon. *Am. J. Psychiatry,* 120:1007–1008, 1964.
Karliner, W., and Padula, L. Improved technique for Indoklon convulsive therapy. *Am. J. Psychiatry,* 116:358, 1959a.
Karliner, W., and Padula, L. Indoklon combined with penthothal and anectine. *Am. J. Psychiatry,* 115:1041–1042, 1959b.
Karliner, W., and Padula L. The use of hexaflurodiethyl ether in psychiatric treatment. *J. Neuropsychiatry,* 2:67–70, 1960.
Karliner, W., and Padula, L. Further clinical studies of hexaflurodiethyl ether convulsive treatments. *J. Neuropsychiatry,* 3:159–162, 1962.
Karliner, W., and Wehrheim, H. K. Maintenance convulsive treatments. *Am. J. Psychiatry,* 121:113–115, 1965.
Kastin, A. J., Ehrensing, R. H., Schalch, D. S., and Anderson, M. S. Improvement in mental depression with decreased thyrotropin response after administration of thyrotropin-releasing hormone. *Lancet,* 2:740–742, 1972.
Kastin, A. J., Plotnikoff, N. P., Schally, A. V., and Sandman, C. A. Endocrine and CNS effects of hypothalamic peptides and MSH. In: S. Ehrenpreis, and I. J. Kopin (Eds.): *Reviews of Neuroscience Vol. 2,* Raven Press, New York, pp. 111–148, 1976a.
Kastin, A. J., Schally, A. V., Gonzalez-Barcena, D., Zarate, A., Besser, M., and Hall, R. Clinical studies with hypothalamic peptides. In: A. L. C. Salgado, R. Fernandez-Duranto, and J. G. Lopez del Campo (Eds.): *Applications and Clinical Uses of Hypothalamic Hormones.* American Elsevier, New York, pp. 235–243, 1976b.
Katz, J. L., Boyar, R. M., Weiner, H., Gorzynski, G., Roffwarg, H., and Hellman, L. Toward an elucidation of the psychoendocrinology of anorexia nervosa. In: E. J. Sachar (Ed.): *Hormones, Behavior, and Psychopathology.* Raven Press, New York, pp. 263–283, 1976.
Katz, J. L., and Walsh, B. T. Depression in anorexia nervosa. *Am. J. Psychiatry,* 135:507, 1978.
Katzenelbogen, S., Brody, M., Hayman, M., and Margolin, E. Metrazol convulsions in man: Clinical and biochemical studies. *Am. J. Psychiatry,* 95:1343–1348, 1939.
Kay, D. W. K., Fahy, T., and Garside, R. F. A seven month double-blind trial of amitriptyline and diazepam in ECT-treated depressed patients. *Br. J. Psychiatry,* 117:667–671, 1970.
Kelly, D. H. W., and Sargant, W. Present treatment of schizophrenia—a controlled follow-up study. *Br. Med. J.,* 1:147–150, 1965.
Kendall, B. S., Mills, W. B., and Thale, T. Comparison of two methods of electroshock in their effect on cognitive functions. *J. Consult. Psychol.,* 20:423–429, 1956.
Kendall, R. E., Pichot, P., and von Cranach, M. Differences in concepts of affective disorders amongst European psychiatrists. In: J. Angst (Ed.): *Classification and Prediction of Outcome of Depression.* F. K. Schattauer Verlag, Stuttgart, pp. 27–38, 1974.
Kendell, R. E. Electroconvulsive therapy. (editorial). *J. Roy. Soc. Med.* 71:319–321, 1978.
Kendler, K. S., and Davis, K. L. Elevated corticosteroids as a possible cause of abnormal neuroendocrine function in depressive illness. *Commun. Psychopharmacol.* 3:183–193, 1977.

Kennard, M. A., and Willner, M. D. Significance of changes in the electroencephalogram which result from shock therapy. *Am. J. Psychiatry,* 105:40–45, 1948.
Kennedy, C. J. C., and Anchel, D. Regressive electric shock in schizophrenics refractory to other shock therapies. *Psychiatr. Q.,* 22:317–320, 1948.
Kerman, E. F. Electric shock with special reference to relapses and effort to prevent them. *J. Nerv. Ment. Dis.* 102:231–242, 1945.
Kerman, E. G. Prevention of recurrence of mental illness with modified prophylactic electroshock therapy. *Dis. Nerv. Syst.,* 18:189–191, 1957.
Kessler, M., and Gellhorn, E. Effect of electrically induced convulsions on the vago-insulin and sympathetico-adrenal system. *Proc. Soc. Exp. Biol. Med.,* 46:64–66, 1941.
Kessler, M., and Gellhorn, E. The effect of electrically and chemically induced convulsions on conditioned reflexes. *Am. J. Psychiatry,* 99:687–691, 1943.
Kety, S. S. Catecholamines in neuropsychiatric states. *Pharmacol. Rev.* 18:787–798, 1966.
Kety, S. Biochemical and neurochemical effects of electroconvulsive shock. In: M. Fink, S. Kety, J. McGaugh, and T. Williams (Eds.): *Psychobiology of Convulsive Therapy.* V. H. Winston & Sons, Washington, D.C., pp. 285–294, 1974.
Kety, S., Javoy, F., Thierry, A. M., Julou, L., and Glowinski, J. A sustained effect of electroconvulsive shock on the turnover of norepinephrine in the central nervous system of the rat. *Proc. Natl. Acad. Sci. USA,* 58:1249–1254, 1967.
Kiersey, D. K., Bickford, R. G., and Faulconer, A. Electro-encephalographic patterns produced by thiopental sodium during surgical operations. *Br. J. Anaesth.,* 23:141–152, 1951.
Kiloh, L. G. The use of electroconvulsive treatment in depressive illness. In: G. D. Burrows (Ed.): *Handbook of Studies on Depression.* Excerpta Medica, Amsterdam, pp. 229–252, 1977.
Kiloh, L. G., Child, J. P., and Latner, G. A controlled trial of iproniazid in the treatment of endogenous depression. *J. Ment. Sci.,* 106:1139–1144, 1960.
Kindwall, E. P. *Manual for Electro-convulsive Therapy.* Massachusetts Mental Health Center, 29 pp., 1966.
King, P. D. Regressive ECT, chlorpromazine, and group therapy in treatment of hospitalized chronic schizophrenics. *Am. J. Psychiatry,* 115:354–357, 1958.
King, P. D. Phenelzine and ECT in the treatment of depression. *Am. J. Psychiatry,* 116:64–68, 1959a.
King, P. D. A comparison of REST and ECT in the treatment of schizophrenics. *Am. J. Psychiatry,* 116:358–359, 1959b.
King, P. D. Chlorpromazine and electroconvulsive therapy in the treatment of newly hospitalized schizophrenics. *J. Clin. Exp. Psychopathol.,* 21:101–105, 1960.
Kino, F. F. Reflex studies in electrical shock procedure. *Brain,* 66:152–161, 1943.
Kino, F. F. Eye movement in electrical shock procedure. *J. Ment. Sci.,* 90:592–594, 1944.
Kino, F. F., and Thorpe, F. T. The occurrence of the grasping reflex in the postconvulsive stage of electrically induced seizures and its behaviour in various mental diseases. *J. Ment. Sci.,* 88:541–544, 1942.
Kino, F. F., and Thorpe, F. T. Electrical convulsion therapy in 500 selected psychotics. *J. Ment. Sci.,* 92:138–145, 1946.
Kinross-Wright, V. Chlorpromazine treatment of mental disorders. *Am. J. Psychiatry,* 111:907–912, 1955.
Kirby, G. H. The catatonic syndrome and its relation to manic-depressive insanity. *J. Nerv. Ment. Dis.,* 40:694–704, 1913.
Kirkegaard, C., Bjørum, N., Cohn, D., and Lauridsen, U. B. Thyrotropin-releasing hormone (TRH) stimulation test in manic-depressive illness. *Arch. Gen. Psychiatr.,* 35:1017–1021, 1978.
Kirkegaard, C., Nørlem, N., Lauridsen, U. B., and Bjørum, N. Prognostic value of thyrotropin-releasing hormone stimulation test in endogenous depression. *Acta Psychiatr. Scand.,* 52:170–177, 1975.
Kirkegaard, C., and Smith, E. Continuation therapy in endogenous depression controlled by changes in the TRH stimulation test. *Psycholog. Med.* 8:501–503, 1978.
Kizer, J. S., and Youngblood, W. W. Neurotransmitter systems and central neuroendocrine regulation. In: M. A. Lipton, A. DiMascio, and K. F. Killam, (Eds.): *Psychopharmacology: A Generation of Progress.* Raven Press, New York, pp. 465–486, 1978.
Klein, D. F., and Davis, J. M. *Diagnosis and Drug Treatment of Psychiatric Disorders.* Williams & Wilkins, Baltimore, 480 pp., 1969.
Klein, D. F., and Fink, M. Psychiatric reaction patterns to imipramine (Tofranil). *Am. J. Psychiatry,* 119:449–459, 1962a.

Klein, D. F., and Fink, M. Behavioral reaction patterns with phenothiazines. *Arch. Gen. Psychiatry,* 7:449–459, 1962b.
Klerman, G. L. Unipolar and bipolar depression. In: J. Angst (Ed.): *Classification and Prediction of Outcome in Depression.* F. K. Schattauer Verlag, Stuttgart, pp. 49–73, 1974.
Kline, N. S., Li, C. H., Lehmann, H. E., Lajtha, A., Laska, E., and Cooper, T. β-Endorphin-induced changes in schizophrenic and depressed patients. *Arch. Gen. Psychiatry,* 34:1111–1115, 1977.
Klotz, M. Serial electroencephalographic changes due to electrotherapy. *Dis. Nerv. Syst.,* 16:120–121, 1955.
Knott, J. R., Gottlieb, J. S., Leet, H. H., and Hadley, H. D. Changes in the electroencephalogram following metrazol shock therapy. *Arch. Neurol. Psychiatry,* 50:529–534, 1943.
Koella, W. P. The central nervous control of sleep. In: W. Haymaker, E. Anderson, and W. J. H. Nauta (Eds.): *The Hypothalamus.* Charles C Thomas, Springfield, Ill., pp. 622–644, 1969.
Koenig, J. H., and Feldman, H. Non-standard method of electric shock therapy. *Psychiatr. Q.,* 25:65–72, 1951.
Kolb, L. C., and Vogel, V. H. The use of shock therapy in 305 mental hospitals. *Am. J. Psychiatry,* 99:90–100, 1942.
Kooi, K. A. *Fundamentals of Electroencephalography.* Harper & Row, New York, 260 pp., 1971.
Kopin, I. J. *Neurotransmitters. Res. Publ. Assoc. Nerv. Ment. Dis., Vol. 50.* Williams & Wilkins, Baltimore, 556 pp., 1972.
Korin, H., and Fink, M. Role of stimulus intensity in perception of simultaneous cutaneous electrical stimuli. *J. Hillside Hosp.,* 6:241–250, 1957.
Korin, H., and Fink, M. The role of set in the perception of simultaneous tactile stimuli. *Am. Psychol.,* 72:384–392, 1959.
Korin, H., Fink, M., and Kwalwasser, S. Relation of changes in memory and learning to improvement in electroshock. *Confin. Neurol.,* 16:88–96, 1956.
Kraicer, J. Mechanism of action of hypothalamic releasing hormones. In: K. Lederis and K. E. Cooper (Eds.): *Recent Studies of Hypothalamic Function.* S. Karger, Basel, pp. 207–215, 1974.
Kramer, J. C., Klein, D. F., and Fink, M. Withdrawal symptoms following discontinuation of imipramine therapy. *Am. J. Psychiatry,* 118:549–550, 1961.
Krantz, J. C., Jr., Carr, C. J., Lu, G., and Bell, F. K. Anesthesia action of trifluroethyl vinyl ether. *J. Pharmacol. Exp. Ther.,* 108:488–495, 1953.
Krantz, J. C., Jr., Esquibel, A., Truitt, E. G., Jr., Ling, A. S. C., and Kurland, A. A. Hexaflurodiethyl ether (Indoklon)—an inhalant convulsant. Its use in psychiatric treatment. *JAMA,* 166:1555–1556, 1958.
Krantz, J. C., Manchey, L. L., Truitt, E. B., Ling, A. S. C., and Kurland, A. The availability of hexafluorodiethyl in psychiatric treatment. *J. Nerv. Ment. Dis.* 129:92–94, 1959.
Krantz, J. C., Jr., Truitt, E. B., Jr., Speers, L., and Ling, A. S. C. New pharmacoconvulsive agent. *Science,* 126:353–354, 1957.
Kriss, A., Blumhardt, L., Halliday, A. M., and Pratt, R. T. C. Electrophysiological and neurological asymmetries immediately following unilateral ECT. *Electroencephalogr. Clin. Neurophysiol.,* 43:773, 1977.
Kriss, A., Halliday, A. M., Halliday, E. and Pratt, R. T. C. EEG immediately after unilateral ECT. *Acta psychiat. scand.* 58:231–244, 1978.
Kristiansen, E. S. A comparison of treatment of endogenous depression with electroshock and with imipramine. *Acta Psychiatr. Scand.,* 37:179–188, 1961.
Kronfol, Z., Hamsher, K. deS., Digre, K., and Waziri, R. Depression and hemispheric functions: Changes associated with unilateral ECT. *Br. J. Psychiatr.,* 132:560–567, 1978.
Kukopulos, A., Reginaldi, D., Tondo, L., Ernabei, A., and Caliari, B. Spontaneous length of depression and response to ECT. *Psychol. Med.,* 7:625–629, 1977.
Kupfer, D. J., and Foster, F. G. The sleep of psychotic patients: Does it all look alike? In: D. X. Freedman (Ed.): *Biology of the Major Psychoses. Res. Publ. Assoc. Nerv. Ment. Dis. Vol. 54,* Raven Press, New York, pp. 143–159, 1975.
Küppers, E. Die Insulin- und Cardiazol-behandlung der Schizophrenie. *Allg. Z. Psychiatr.,* 107:76, 1938.
Küppers, E. Metrazol shock therapy. *Nervenarzt,* 12:449–453, 1939.
Kurland, A. A., Hanlon, T. E., Esquibel, A. J., Krantz, J. C., and Sheets, C. S. A comparative study of hexafluorodiethyl ether (Indoklon) and electroconvulsive therapy. *J. Nerv. Ment. Dis.,* 129:95–98, 1959.

Kurland, A. A., Krantz, J. C., and Truitt, E. B. Treatment of schizophrenia with sustained exposure to hexafluorodiethyl ether. *J. Nerv. Ment. Dis.,* 130:155–159, 1960.

Kurland, A. A., Turek, I. S., Brown, C. C., and Wagman, A. M. I. Electroconvulsive therapy and EEG correlates in depressive disorders. *Compr. Psychiatry,* 17:581–589, 1976.

Kusumo, K. S., and Vaughan, M. Effects of lithium salts on memory. *Br. J. Psychiatry,* 131:453–457, 1977.

Kwalwasser, S. Report on 441 cases treated with metrazol. *Psychiatr. Q.,* 14:527–546, 1940.

Laboucarie, J., and Barres, P. Aspects cliniques pathologiques et therapeutiques de l'anorexie mentale. *Evol. Psychiatr.,* 1:119–146, 1954.

Ladisch, W., Steinhauff, N., and Matussek, N. Chronic administration of electroconvulsive shock and norepinephrine metabolism in the rat brain. *Psychopharmacologia,* 15:296–304, 1969.

Lancaster, N. P., Steinert, R. R., and Frost, I. Unilateral electro-convulsive therapy. *J. Ment. Sci.,* 104:221–227, 1958.

Landis, C., Dillon, D., and Leopold, J. Changes in flicker-fusion threshold and in choice reaction time induced by electroconvulsive therapy. *J. Psychol.,* 41:61–80, 1956.

Langer, G., Heinze, G., Reim, B., and Matussek, N. Reduced growth hormone responses to amphetamine in "endogenous" depressive patients. *Arch. Gen. Psychiatry,* 33:1471–1475, 1976.

Langsley, D. G., Enterline, J. D., and Hickerson, G. X. Comparison of chlorpromazine and EST in treatment of acute schizophrenic and manic reactions. *Arch. Neurol. Psychiatry,* 81:384–391, 1959.

Lapin, I. B., and Oxenkrug, G. F. Intensification of the central serotoninergic processes as a possible determinant of the thymoleptic effect. *Lancet,* 1:132–136, 1969.

Larsen, E. F., and Vraa-Jensen, G. Changes in the brain following electroshock therapy. *Acta Psychiatr. Neurol. Scand.* 28:75–80, 1953.

Lassenius, B., Ottosson, J.-O., and Rapp, W. Prognosis in schizophrenia. The need for institutionalized care. *Acta Psychiatr. Scand.,* 49:295–305, 1973.

Laurell, B. (Ed.): Flurothyl convulsive therapy. *Acta Psychiatr. Scand. [Suppl.],* 213:1–79, 1970.

Laurell, B., and Perris, C. Seizure and postseizure electroencephalographic pattern. *Acta Psychiatr. Scand. [Suppl.],* 213:8–21, 1970.

Lebensohn, Z. M., and Jenkins, R. B. Improvement of parkinsonism in depressed patients treated with ECT. *Am. J. Psychiatry,* 132:283–285, 1975.

Lederis, K., and Cooper, K. E. *Recent Studies of Hypothalamic Function.* S. Karger, Basel, 434 pp., 1974.

Lee, J. C., and Olszewski, J. Increased cerebrovascular permeability after repeated electroshocks. *Neurology,* 11:515–519, 1961.

Leiter, L., and Grinker, R. R. Role of the hypothalamus in regulation of blood pressure; experimental studies, with observations on respiration. *Arch. Neurol. Psychiatry,* 31:54–86, 1934.

LeMay, M. Morphological cerebral asymmetries of modern man, fossil man, and nonhuman primate. *Annal. NY Acad. Sci.,* 280:349–366, 1976.

Lemere, F. The treatment of psychotic complications of porphyria with electroshock. *Am. J. Psychiatry,* 111:41–42, 1954.

Lennox, M. A., Ruch, T. C., and Guterman, B. The effects of benzedrine on the postelectroshock EEG. *Electroencephalogr. Clin. Neurophysiol.,* 3:63–69, 1951.

Levine, J., Schiele, B. C., and Bouthilet, L. *Principles and Problems in Establishing the Efficacy of Psychotropic Agents.* Super. Documents, Washington, D.C., PHS 2138, 392 pp., 1971.

Levy, N. A., and Grinker, R. R. Psychological observations in affective psychoses treated with combined convulsive shock and psychotherapy. *J. Nerv. Ment. Dis.,* 97:623–637, 1943.

Levy, N. A., Serota, H. M., and Grinker, R. R. Disturbances in brain function following convulsive shock therapy: Electroencephalographic and clinical studies. *Arch. Neurol. Psychiatry,* 47:1009–1029, 1942.

Levy, R. The clinical evaluation of unilateral electroconvulsive therapy. *Br. J. Psychiatry,* 114:459–463, 1968.

Lewis, J. K., and McKinney, W. T. The effect of electrically induced convulsions on the behavior of normal and abnormal rhesus monkeys. *Dis. Nerv. Syst.,* 37:687–693, 1976.

Lewis, N. D. C. Shock therapy of psychoses: Evidence for and against damage. *Bull. NY Acad. Med.,* 21:673–685, 1945.

Lewis, W. H., Jr., Richardson, D. J., and Gahagan, L. H. Cardiovascular disturbances and their management in modified electrotherapy for psychiatric illness. *N. Engl. J. Med.,* 252:1016–1020, 1955.

Lewis, W. H., Jr. Cardiovascular responses in psychiatric electrotherapy. *Dis. Nerv. Syst.* 17:81–83, 1956.
Liban, E., Halpern, L., and Rozonski, J. Vascular changes in the brain in a fatality following electroshock. *J. Neuropathol. Exp. Neurol.*, 10:309–318, 1951.
Liberson, W. T. Time factors in electric convulsive therapy. *Yale J. Biol. Med.*, 17:571–578, 1945.
Liberson, W. T. Brief stimulus therapy. Physiological and clinical observations. *Am. J. Psychiatry,* 105:28–29, 1948.
Liberson, W. T. Current evaluation of electric convulsive therapy—correlaion of the parameters of electric current with physiologic and psychologic changes. *Res. Publ. Assoc. Nerv. Ment. Dis.*, 31:199–231, 1953.
Liberson, W. T., Kaplan, J. A., Sherer, I. W., and Trehub, A. Correlations of EEG and psychological findings during intensive brief stimulus therapy. *Confin. Neurol.*, 16:116–125, 1956.
Lidbeck, W. L. Pathologic changes in the brain after electric shock: An experimental study on dogs. *J. Neuropathol. Exp. Neurol.*, 3:81–86, 1944.
Liljestrand, G. The prize in physiology and medicine. In: *Nobel—The Man and His Prizes.* Elsevier, Amsterdam, pp. 131–344, 1962.
Lindemann, E. Symptomatology and management of acute grief. *Am. J. Psychiatry,* 101:141–148, 1944.
Lindner, M., and Brouschek, R. Klinische Erfahrungen mit der Kurzreizmethode in der Elektrokrampftherapie. *Nervenarzt,* 24:163–164, 1953.
Linn, L., and Rosen, S. R. Brief shock therapy—an adjuvant to psychotherapy. *Psychiatr. Q.,* 24:506–514, 1950.
Lipsius, L. H. Electroconvulsive therapy and language. *Am. J. Psychiatry,* 132:459, 1975.
Lipton, M. A., and Goodwin, F. K. A controlled study of thyrotropin releasing hormone in hospitalized depressed patients. *Psychopharmacol. Bull.*, 11:28–29, 1975.
Lipton, M. A., Prange, A. J., Nemeroff, C. B., Breese, G. R., and Wilson, I. C. Thyrotropin-releasing hormone: Central effects in man and animals. In: E. Usdin, D. A. Hamburg, and J. D. Barchas (Eds.): *Neuro-regulators and Psychiatric Disorders.* Oxford University Press, New York, pp. 258–266, 1977.
Lipton, M. B., Tamarin, S., and Lotesta, P. Test evidence of personality change and prognosis by means of the Rorschach and Wechsler-Bellevue tests on 17 insulin-treated paranoid schizophrenics. *Psychiatr. Q.,* 25:434–444, 1951.
Little, A. F. M., and Reid, A. A. Recovery time from modified and unmodified ECT. *J. Ment. Sci.,* 103:270–274, 1957.
Loosen, P. T., Prange, A. J., and Wilson, I. C. Influence of cortisol on TSH response in depression. *Am. J. Psychiatry,* 135:244–246, 1978.
Loosen, P. T., Prange, A. J., Wilson, I. C., and Lara, P. P. Pituitary responses to thyrotropin releasing hormone in depressed patients: A review. *Pharmacol. Biochem. Behav. [Suppl.],* 5:95–101, 1976.
Loosen, P. T., Prange, A. J., Wilson, I. C., Lara, P. P., and Pettus, C. Thyroid stimulating hormone response after thyrotropin releasing hormone in depressed schizophrenic and normal women. *Psychoneuroendocrinology,* 2:137–148, 1977.
Lorimer, F. M., Segal, M. M., and Stein, S. N. The path of current distribution in the brain during electro-convulsive therapy. *Electroencephalogr. Clin. Neurophysiol.*, 1:343–348, 1949.
Loudon, J. B., and Waring, H. Toxic reactions to lithium and haloperidol. *Lancet,* 2:1088, 1976.
Lowinger, P., and Huston, P. E. Electric shock in psychosis with cerebral spastic paralysis. *Dis. Nerv. Syst.,* 14:2–4, 1953.
Lüttke, S., and Koch, R. D. Psychiatrische Schockbehandlung mit Bemegrid. *Dtsch. Gesundheitswesen,* 17:1027–1029, 1962.
Lynn, J. E., and Racy, J. The resolution of pathological grief after electroconvulsive therapy. *J. Nerv. Ment. Dis.,* 148:165–169, 1969.
Maclay, W. S. Death due to treatment. *Proc. R. Soc. Med.,* 46:13–20, 1953.
MacLean, P. D. The hypothalamus and emotional behavior. In: W. Haymaker, E. Anderson, and W. J. H. Nauta (Eds.): *The Hypothalamus.* Charles C Thomas, Springfield, Ill., pp. 659–678, 1969.
MacLean, P. D. Influence of limbic cortex on hypothalamus. In: K. Lederis, and K. E. Cooper (Eds.): *Recent Studies of Hypothalamic Functions.* S. Karger, Basel, pp. 216–231, 1974.
Madow, L. Brain changes in electroshock therapy. *Am. J. Psychiatry,* 113:337–347, 1956.
Magoun, H. W. *The Waking Brain.* Charles C Thomas, Springfield, Ill., 188 pp., 1958.

Mah, C. J., and Albert, D. J. Reversal of ECS-induced amnesia by post-ECS injections of amphetamine. *Pharmacol. Biochem. Behav.,* 3:1–5, 1975.
Malamud, N., and Sands, G. Neuropathological findings in disseminated lupus erythematosus. *Arch. Neurol. Psychiatry,* 71:723–731, 1954.
Maletzky, B. M. Seizure duration and clinical effect in electroconvulsive therapy. *Comp. Psychiatry,* 19:541–550, 1978.
Malik, M. O. A. Fatal heart block and cardiac arrest following ECT: A case report. *Br. J. Psychiatry,* 120:69–70, 1972.
Malzberg, B. The outcome of electric shock therapy in the New York civil state hospitals. *Psychiatr. Q.* 17:154–163, 1943.
Man, P. L., and Bolin, B. J. Further exploration of unilateral electroshock treatment. *Dis. Nerv. Syst.,* 30:547–551, 1969.
Mandel, M. R. Electroconvulsive therapy for chronic pain associated with depression. *Am. J. Psychiatry,* 132:632–636, 1975.
Mandell, A. J. *New Concepts in Neurotransmitter Regulation.* Plenum Press, New York, 316 pp., 1973.
Mann, S. H., De Pasquale, N., and Patterson, R. Cerebrospinal fluid-glutamic oxalacetic acid transaminase in patients receiving electroconvulsive therapy and in neurologic diseases. *Neurology,* 10:381–390, 1960,
Marhold, J., Zimanova, J., Lachman, M., Kral, J., and Vojtechovsky, M. To the incompatability of haloperidol with lithium salts. *Acta Nerv. Super.,* 16:199–200, 1974.
Marjerrison, G., James, J., and Reichert, H. Unilateral and bilateral ECT: EEG findings. *Can. Psychiatr. Assoc. J.,* 20(4):257–266, 1975.
Marjerrison. J. H., and Corsellis, J. A. N. Epilepsy and the temporal lobes. *Brain,* 89:499–530, 1966.
Marks, V., and Bannister, R. G. Pituitary and adrenal function in undernutrition with mental illness (including anorexia nervosa). *Br. J. Psychiatry,* 109:480–484, 1963.
Marti-Ibanez, F., Sackler, A. M., Sackler, M. D., and Sackler, R. R. (Eds.): *The Great Physiodynamic Therapies in Psychiatry.* Hoeber-Harper, New York, 190 pp., 1956.
Martin, P. A. Convulsive therapies: Review of 511 cases at Pontiac State Hospital. *J. Nerv. Ment. Dis.,* 109:142–157, 1949.
Martin, W., Ford, H. F., McDonald, E. C., and Towler, M. L. Clinical evaluation of unilateral EST. *Am. J. Psychiatry,* 121:1087–1090, 1965.
Masserman, J. H. Effects of sodium amytal and other drugs on the reactivity of the hypothalamus of the cat. *Arch. Neurol. Psychiatry,* 37:617–628, 1937.
Matakas, F., Cervos-Navarro, J., Roggendorf, W., Cristmann, U., and Sasaki, S. Spastic constriction of cerebral vessels after electric convulsive treatment. *Arch. Psychiatr. Nervenkr.* 224:1–9, 1977.
Matthew, J. R., and Constan, E. Complications following ECT over a three-year period in a state institution. *Am. J. Psychiatry,* 120:1119–1120, 1964.
Maxwell, R. D. H. Electrical factors in electroconvulsive therapy. *Acta Psychiatr. Scand.,* 44:436–448, 1968.
May, P. R. *Treatment of schizophrenia.* Science House, NewYork, 352 pp., 1968.
May, P. R., and Tuma, A. H. Follow up study of the results of treatment of schizophrenia. In: R. Spitzer and D. F. Klein (Eds.): *Evaluation of Psychological Therapies.* Johns Hopkins Press, Baltimore, pp. 256–284, 1976.
May, P. R. A., Tuma, A. H., and Dixon, W. J. Schizophrenia—a follow-up study of results of treatment: I. Design and other problems. *Arch. Gen. Psychiatry,* 33:474–478, 1976a.
May, P. R. A., Tuma, A. H., Yale, C., Potepan, P., and Dixon, W. J. Schizophrenia—a follow-up study of results of treatment: II. Hospital stay over two to five years. *Arch. Gen. Psychiatry,* 33:481–486, 1976b.
Mayer-Gross, W., and Walk, A. Cyclohexyl-ethyltriazol in convulsion treatment of schizophrenia. *Lancet,* 1:1324–1325, 1938.
McAndrew, J., Berkey, B., and Matthews, C. The effects of dominant and nondominant unilateral ECT as compared to bilateral ECT. *Am. J. Psychiatry,* 124:483–490, 1967.
McCabe, M. S. ECT in the treatment of mania: A controlled study. *Am. J. Psychiatry,* pp. 133, 1976.
McCabe, M. S., and Norris, B. ECT versus chlorpromazine in mania. *Biol. Psychiatry,* 12:245–254, 1977.
McDonald, I. M., Perkins, M., Marjerrison, G., and Podilsky, M. A controlled comparison of

amitriptyline and electroconvulsive therapy in the treatment of depression. *Am. J. Psychiatry,* 122:1427–1431, 1966.

McKenna, G., Engle, R. P., Brooks, H., and Dalen, J. Cardiac arrhythmias during electroshock therapy: Significance, prevention, and treatment. *Am. J. Psychiatry,* 127:530–533, 1970.

McKinnon, A. L. Electric shock therapy in a private psychiatric hospital. *Can. Med. Assoc. J.,* 58:478–483, 1948.

Meco, G., Casacchia, M., Carchedi, F., Falaschi, P., Rocco, A. and Frajese, G. Prolactin response to repeated electroconvulsive therapy in acute schizophrenia. *Lancet* 1:999, 1978.

Medlicott, R. W. Brief stimuli electroconvulsive therapy. *NZ Med. J.,* 47:29–37, 1948.

Meduna, L. J. Versuche uber die biologische Beeinflussung des Abaufes der Schizophrenia: Camphor und Cardiozolkrampfe. *Z. Ges. Neurol. Psychiatr.,* 152:235–262, 1935.

Meduna, L. J. *Die Konvulsionstherapie der schizophrenie.* Carl Marhold, Halle, 1937.

Meduna, L. J. General discussion of the cardiozol therapy. *Am. J. Psychiatry [Suppl.],* 94:40–50, 1938.

Meduna, L. J. Die Konvulsionstherapie der Schizophrenia. Rückblick und Ausblick. *Psychiatr. Neurol. Wochenschr.* 41:165–169, 1939.

Meduna, L. J. *Carbon Dioxide Therapy.* Charles C Thomas, Springfield, Ill., 236 pp., 1950.

Meduna, L. J. The convulsive treatment: A reappraisal. In: F. Marti-Ibanez, A. M. Sackler, M. D. Sackler, and R. R. Sackler (Eds.): *The Great Physiodynamic Therapies in Psychiatry.* Hoeber-Harper, New York, pp. 76–90, 1956.

Meduna, L. J., and Friedman, E. The convulsive-irritative therapy of the psychoses. *JAMA,* 112:501–509, 1939.

Meldrum, B. S., and Brierley, J. B. Prolonged epileptic seizures in primates. Ischemic cell change and its relation to ictal physiological events. *Arch. Neurol.,* 28:10–17, 1973.

Meldrum, B. S., Papy, J. J., Toure, M. F., and Brierley, J. B. Four models for studying cerebral lesions secondary to epileptic seizures. *Adv. Neurol.,* 10:147–161, 1975.

Mendels, J. Electroconvulsive therapy and depression: I. The prognostic significance of clinical factors. *Br. J. Psychiatry,* 111:675–681, 1965a.

Mendels, J. Electroconvulsive therapy and depression: II. Significance of endogenous and reactive syndromes. *Br. J. Psychiatry,* 111:682–686, 1965b.

Mendels, J. Electroconvulsive therapy and depression: III. A method for prognosis. *Br. J. Psychiatry,* 111:687–690, 1965c.

Mendels, J. The prediction of response to electroconvulsive therapy. *Am. J. Psychiatry,* 124:153–159, 1967.

Mendels, J. *The Psychobiology of Depression.* Spectrum Publications, New York, 175 pp., 1975.

Mendels, J., Van de Castle, R. L., and Hawkins, D. R. Electroconvulsive therapy and sleep. In: M. Fink, S. Kety, J. McGaugh, and T. A. Williams (Eds.): *Psychobiology of Convulsive Therapy.* V. H. Winston & Sons, Washington, D.C., pp. 41–46, 1974.

Merlis, S., and Hunter, V. Studies on mescaline: II. Electroencephalogram in schizophrenics. *Psychiatr. Q.,* 29:430–432, 1955.

Merritt, H. H., and Putnam, T. J. New series of anticonvulsant drugs tested by experiments on animals. *Arch. Neurol. Psychiatry,* 39:1003–1015, 1938.

Meyer, A., and Teare, D. Cerebral fat embolism after electrical convulsion therapy. *Br. Med. J.,* 2:42–44, 1945.

Meyer-Mickeleit, R. W. Das Elektroencephalogramm beim Elektrokrampf des Menschen. *Arch. Psychiatry,* 183:12–33, 1949.

Michael, R. P., and Gibbons, J. L. Interrelationships between the endocrine system and neuropsychiatry. *Int. Rev. Neurobiol.,* 5:243–292, 1963.

Michael, S. T., Menstrual disturbances during electric shock treatment. *Psychiatr. Q.,* 30:63–72, 1956.

Michael, S. T., and Brown, W. T. Blood lymphocytes and adrenal function in electric convulsive therapy of psychoses. *J. Nerv. Ment. Dis.,* 113:538–548, 1951.

Mikkelsen, W. P., and Hutchens, T. T. Lymphopenia following electrically induced convulsions in male psychotic patients. *Endocrinology,* 42:394–398, 1948.

Miller, D. H., Clancy, J., and Cummings, E. A comparison between unidirectional current nonconvulsive electrical stimulation given with Reiter's machine, standard alternating current electroshock and pentothal in chronic schizophrenia. *Am. J. Psychiatry,* 109:617–620, 1953.

Miller, E. Psychological theories of ECT: A review. *Br. J. Psychiatry,* 113:301–311, 1967.

Miller, E. Psychological theories of ECT: A review. *Int. J. Psychiatry,* 5:154–165, 1968.

Miller, E. The effect of ECT on memory and learning. *Br. J. Med. Psychol.,* 43:57–62, 1970.
Miller, L. H., Sandman, C. A., and Kastin, A. J. *Advances in Biochemical Psychopharmacology, Vol. 17, Neuropeptide Influences on the Brain and Behavior.* Raven Press, New York, 298 pp., 1977.
Millet, J. A. B., and Mosse, E. P. On certain psychological aspects of electroshock therapy. *Psychosom. Med.,* 6:226–236, 1945.
Milligan, W. L. Psychoneuroses treated with electrical convulsions. *Lancet,* 2:516–520, 1946.
Mindus, P., Cronholm, B., and Levander, S. E. Does piracetam counteract the ECT-induced memory dysfunctions in depressed patients? *Acta Psychiatr. Scand.,* 51:319–326, 1975.
Mitchell, P. H. Electric convulsion therapy in treatment of prolonged stupor. *Br. Med. J.,* 4783:535–538, 1952.
Modigh, K. Electroconvulsive shock and postsynaptic catecholamine effects: Increased psychomotor stimulant action of apomorphine and clonidine in reserpine pretreated mice by repeated ECS. *J. Neural Transm.,* 36:19–32, 1975.
Modigh, K. Long-term effects of electroconvulsive shock therapy on synthesis turnover and uptake of brain monoamines. *Psychopharmacology,* 49:179–185, 1976.
Moore, M. T. Electrocerebral shock therapy: A reconsideration of former contraindications. *Arch. Neurol. Psychiatry,* 57:693–711, 1947.
Moore, N. P. The maintenance treatment of chronic psychotics by electrically induced convulsions. *J. Ment. Sci.,* 89:257–269, 1943.
Moriarty, J. D., and Siemens, J. C. Electroencephalographic study of electric shock therapy. *Arch. Neurol. Psychiatry,* 57:712–718, 1947.
Moriarty, J. D., and Weil, A. A. Combined convulsive therapy and psychotherapy of the neuroses. *Arch. Neurol. Psychiatry,* 50:685–690, 1943.
Morison, R. S., and Dempsey, E. W. A study of thalamo-cortical relations. *Am. J. Physiol.,* 135:281–292, 1942.
Morrison, J. R. Catatonia: Retarded and excited types. *Arch. Gen. Psychiatry,* 28:39–41, 1973.
Morrison, J. R. Catatonia: Prediction of outcome. *Compr. Psychiatry,* 15:317–324, 1974.
Morrison, J., Clancy, J., Crowe, R. L., and Winokur, G. The Iowa 500: I. Diagnostic validity in mania, depression and schizophrenia. *Arch. Gen. Psychiatry,* 27:457–461, 1972.
Moruzzi, G., and Magoun, H. W. Brain stem reticular formation and activation of the E.E.G. *Electroencephalogr. Clin. Neurophysiol.,* 1:455–473, 1949.
Mosovich, A., and Katzenelbogen, S. Electroshock therapy, clinical and electroencephalographic studies. *J. Nerv. Ment. Dis.,* 107:517–530, 1948.
Moss, R. L. Effects of hypothalamic peptides on sex behavior in animal and man. In: M. A. Lipton, A. DiMascio, and K. F. Killam (Eds.): *Psychopharmacology: A Generation of Progress.* Raven Press, New York, pp. 431–440, 1978.
Moyes, I. C. A. ECT and cAMP excretion. *Br. Med. J.,* 3:829, 1972.
Muller, D. J. ECT in LSD psychosis: A report of three cases. *Am. J. Psychiatry,* 128:351–352, 1971.
Müller, M. Die Insulin- und Cardiazolbehandlung in der Psychiatrie. *Fortschr. Neurol. Psychiatr.,* 11:455–486, 1939.
Murillo, L. G., and Exner, J. E., Jr. The effects of regressive ECT with process schizophrenics. *Am. J. Psychiatry,* 130:269–273, 1973a.
Murillo, L. G., and Exner, J. E., Jr. Response to J. Spensley. *Am. J. Psychiatry,* 130:1163–1164, 1973b.
Murray, N. The use of succinylcholine in electro-shock therapy. *Confin. Neurol.,* 13:320–324, 1953.
Myers, R. D. Temperature regulation: Neurochemical systems in the hypothalamus In: W. Haymaker, E. Anderson, and W. J. H. Nauta (Eds.): *The Hypothalamus.* Charles C Thomas, Springfield, Ill., pp. 506–523, 1969.
Myerson, A. Experience with electric-shock therapy in mental disease. *N. Engl. J. Med.,* 224:1081–1085, 1941.
Myerson, A. Borderline cases treated by electric shock. *Am. J. Psychiatry.* 100:355–357, 1943.
Myerson, A. Prolonged cases of grief reaction treated by electric shock. *N. Engl. J. Med.,* 230:255–256, 1944.
Naidoo, D. The effects of reserpine (Serpasil) on the chronic disturbed schizophrenic: A comparative study of rauwolfia alkaloids and electroconvulsive therapy. *J. Nerv. Ment. Dis.,* 123:1–13, 1956.
Narang, R. L., Chaudhury, R. R. and Wig, N. N. Effect of electroconvulsive therapy on the antidiuretic hormone level in the plasma of schizophrenic patients. *Indian J. Med. Res.* 61:766–770, 1973.

REFERENCES

National Commission for the Protection of Human Subjects of Biomedical and Behavioral Research. *Psychosurgery—Report and Recommendations.* DHEW OS 77-0001, U.S. Govt. Printing Office, Washington, D.C., 76 pp., 1977.

Negrin, J. Intracranial electrotherapy: Observations with the Sedac unit. *Dis. Nerv. Syst.,* 18:152-153, 425-430, 1957.

Nelson, J. C. and Bowers, M. B. Delusional unipolar depression—Description and drug response. *Arch. gen. Psychiat.* 35:1321-1328, 1978.

Neubuerger, K. T., Whitehead, R. W., Rutledge, E. K., and Ebaugh, F. G. Pathologic changes in the brains of dogs given repeated electric shock. *Am. J. Med. Sci.,* 204:381-387, 1942.

Noble, P., and Lader, M. The symptomatic correlates of the skin conductance changes in depression. *J. Psychiatr. Res.,* 9:61-69, 1971.

Nordin, G., Ottosson, J.-O., and Roos, B.-E. Influence of convulsive therapy on 5-hydroxyindoleacetic acid and homovanillic acid in cerebrospinal fluid in endogenous depression. *Psychopharmacologia,* 20:315-320, 1971.

Norman, R. M. The neuropathology of status epilepticus. *Med. Sci. Law,* 4:46-51, 1964.

Norman, R. M., Sandry, S., and Corsellis, J.A.N. The nature and origin of pathoanatomical change in the epileptic brain. In: P. T. Vinken and G. W. Bruyn (Eds.): *Handbook of Clinical Neurology.* Holland, Amsterdam, pp. 611-620, 1974.

Norris, A. S., and Clancy, J. Hospitalized depressions: Drugs or electrotherapy? *Arch. Gen. Psychiatry,* 5:276-279, 1961.

Nowill, W. K., Wilson, W., and Borders, R. Succinylcholine chloride in electroshock therapy. II. Cardiovascular reactions. *Arch. Neurol. Psychiatry,* 71:189-197, 1954.

Nussbaum, K., and Kurland, A. A. Intravenous hexaflurodiethyl ether (Indoklon) modified by succinylcholine chloride. Clinical studies in convulsive psychiatric treatment. *Curr. Ther. Res.,* 4:44-56, 1962.

Nussbaum, K., and Kurland, A. A. Bis (2,2,2-triflurethyl) ether (Indoklon) modified with succinylcholine (Anectine) as a convulsant in psychiatric treatment. *J. Neuropsychiatry,* 4:143-149, 1963.

Nyirö, J., and Jablonsky, A. Einige Daten zur Prognose der Epilepsie, mit besonderer Rücksicht auf die Konstitution. *Psychiatr. Neurol. Wochenschr.,* 31:547-549, 1929.

Nymgaard, K. Studies on the sedation threshold. A. Reproducibility and effect of drugs. B. Sedation threshold in neurotic and psychotic depression. *Arch. Gen. Psychiatry,* 1:530-536, 1959.

Nyström, S. On relation between clinical factors and efficacy of E.C.T. in depression. *Acta Psychiatr. Scand. [Suppl.],* 181:115-118, 1964.

O'Dea, J. P. K., Gould, D., Hallberg, M., and Wieland, R. G. Prolactin changes during electroconvulsive therapy. *Am. J. Psychiatry,* 135:609-611, 1978.

Offner, F. Stimulation with minimal power. *J. Neurophysiol.,* 9:387-390, 1946.

O'Flanagan, P., Timothy, J., and Gibson, H. Further observations on use of combined photic and chemically induced cortical dysrhythmia in psychiatry. *J. Ment. Sci.,* 97:174-190, 1951.

Öhman, R., Balldin, J., Walinder, J., and Wallin, L. Prolactin response to electroconvulsive therapy. *Lancet,* 1:936-938, 1976.

Ollendorff, R. H. V. High dosage chlorpromazine therapy in acute and chronic schizophrenia. *Am. J. Psychiatry,* 116:729-736, 1960.

Oltman, J. E., and Friedman, S. Analysis of temporal factors in manic-depressive psychoses, with particular reference to the effect of shock therapy. *Am. J. Psychiatry,* 107:57-68, 1950.

O'Toole, J. K., and Dyck, G. Report of psychogenic fever in catatonia responding to electroconvulsive therapy. *Dis. Nerv. Syst.,* 38:852-853, 1977.

Ottosson, J.-O. Experimental studies of the mode of action of electroconvulsive therapy. *Acta Psychiatr. Neurol. Scand. [Suppl. 145],* 35:1-141, 1960.

Ottosson, J.-O. Electroconvulsive therapy of endogenous depression: An analysis of the influence of various factors on the efficacy of therapy. *J. Ment. Sci.,* 108:694-703, 1962a.

Ottosson, J.-O. Electroconvulsive therapy—Electrostimulatory or convulsive therapy? *J. Neuropsychiatry,* 3:216-220, 1962b.

Ottosson, J.-O. Seizure characteristics and therapeutic efficiency in electroconvulsive therapy: An analysis of the antidepressive efficiency of grand mal and lidocaine-modified seizures. *J. Nerv. Ment. Dis.,* 135:239-251, 1962c.

Ottosson, J.-O. Psychological or physiological theories of ECT. *Int. J. Psychiatry,* 5:170-174, 1968.

Ottosson, J.-O. Systemic biochemical effects of ECT. In: M. Fink, S. Kety, J. McGaugh, and T. Williams (Eds.): *Psychobiology of Convulsive Therapy.* V. H. Winston & Sons, Washington, D.C., pp. 209-220, 1974.

Pacella, B. L., and Barrera, E. S. Spontaneous convulsions following convulsive shock therapy. *Am. J. Psychiatry,* 101:783–788, 1945.

Pacella, B. L., Barrera, E. S., and Kalinowsky, L. Variations in the electroencephalogram associated with electric shock therapy in patients with mental disorders. *Arch. Neurol. Psychiatry,* 47:367–384, 1942.

Pacella, B. L., and Impastato, D. J. Focal stimulation therapy. *Am. J. Psychiatry,* 110:576–578, 1954.

Pacella, B. L., Piotrowski, Z., and Lewis, N. D. C. The effects of electric convulsive therapy on certain personality traits in psychiatric patients. *Am. J. Psychiatry,* 104:83–91, 1947.

Packman, P. M., Meyer, D. A., and Verdun, R. M. Hazards of succinylcholine administration during electrotherapy. *Arch. Gen. Psychiatr.,* 35:1137–1141, 1978.

Palmer, D. M., Sprang, H. E., and Hans, C. L. Electroshock therapy in schizophrenia: A statistical survey of 455 cases. *J. Nerv. Ment. Dis.,* 114:162–171, 1951.

Pancheri, P. Esperienze cliniche con elettroshock unilaterale. *Sist. Nerv.,* 21:223–233, 1969.

Papeschi, R., Randrup, A., and Lal, S. Effect of ECT on dopaminergic and noradrenergic mechanisms. *Psychopharmacologia,* 35:149–158, 1974.

Papez, J. W. A proposed mechanism of emotion. *Arch Neurol. Psychiatry,* 38:725–743, 1937.

Parliamentary Correspondent: Proposed inquiry into electroconvulsion therapy. *Lancet,* 1:220–221, 1978.

Parsons, E. H., Gildea, E. F., Ronzoni, E., and Hulbert, S. Z. Comparative lymphocytic and biochemical responses of patients with schizophrenia and affective disorders to electro-shock, insulin shock, and epinephrine. *Am. J. Psychiatry,* 105:573–580, 1949.

Paterson, A. S. Experiences with electrical stimulation of limited parts of the brain in the baboon and man. *Confin. Neurol.,* 12:311–314, 1952.

Paterson, A. S. *Electrical and Drug Treatments in Psychiatry.* Elsevier, Amsterdam, 248 pp., 1963.

Paterson, A. S., and Milligan, W. L. Electronarcosis: A new treatment of schizophrenia. *Lancet,* 2:198–201, 1947.

Pavan, L., Semerano, A., and Agius, S. Rilievi sulla applicazione dell'elettroshock monopolare. *Sist. Nerv.,* 21:234–236, 1969.

Peck, R. E. *The Miracle of Shock Treatment.* Exposition Press, New York, 78 pp., 1974.

Peet, M., and Turner, P. (Eds.): Proceedings of a Symposium on Mianserin, October, 1977. *Br. J. Clin. Pharmacol.,* 5:1–99S, 1978.

Penfield, W. *The Mystery of the Mind.* Princeton University Press, New Jersey, 123 pp., 1975.

Penn, H., Racy, J., Lapham, L., Mandel, M., and Sandt, J. Catatonic behavior, viral encephalopathy, and death. *Arch. Gen. Psychiatry,* 27:758–761, 1972.

Perrin, G. M. Cardiovascular aspects of electric shock therapy. *Acta Psychiatr. Neurol. Scand.,* 36:1–45, 1961.

Perris, C. The heuristic value of the distinction between bipolar and unipolar affective disorders. In: J. Angst (Ed.): *Classification and Prediction of Outcome in Depression.* F. K. Schattauer Verlag, Stuttgart, pp. 75–84, 1974.

Perris, C., and Brattemo, C.-E. The sedation threshold as a method of evaluating anti-depressive treatments. *Acta Psychiatr. Scand. [Suppl. 39],* 169:111–119, 1963.

Petito, C. K., Schaefer, J. A., and Plum, F. The blood brain barrier in experimental seizures. In: H. M. Pappius, and W. Feindel (Eds.): *Dynamics of Brain Edema.* Springer-Verlag, Berlin, pp. 38–42, 1976.

Phillips, O. C., and Capizzi, L. S. Anesthesia mortality. *Clin. Anesth.,* 10:220–244, 1974.

Piekenbrock, T. C., Taylor, R. C., and Becka, D. R. EEG during electroconvulsive therapy with succinylcholine. *Arch. Neurol. Psychiatry,* 76:653–659, 1956.

Piette, Y. Contribution a l'etude du mecanisme therapeutique de l'electrochoc. *Brux. Med.,* 35:2479–2491, 1955.

Piette, Y. L'electroencephalogramme de la crise convulsive de l'electrochoc. *Acta Neurol. Belg.,* 58:219–230, 1958.

Pilowsky, I., and Boulton, D. M. Development of a questionnaire-based decision rule for classifying depressed patients. *Br. J. Psychiatry,* 116:647–650, 1970.

Pilowsky, I., Levine, S., and Boulton, D. M. The classification of depression by numerical taxonomy. *Br. J. Psychiatry,* 115:937–945, 1969.

Pilowsky, I., and McGrath, M. D. Effect of ECT on responses to a depression questionnaire: Implications for taxonomy. *Br. J. Psychiatry,* 117:685–688, 1970.

Pinel, J. P. J., and Van Oot, P. H. Generality of the kindling phenomenon: Some clinical implications. *Can. J. Neurol. Sci.,* 2:467–475, 1975.

Pinel, J. P. J., and Van Oot, P. H. Intensification of the alcohol withdrawal syndrome following periodic electroconvulsive shocks. *Biol. Psychiatry,* 12:479–486, 1977.

Piotrowski, Z. Rorschach method as prognostic aid in insulin shock treatment of schizophrenics. *Psychiatr. Q.,* 15:807–822, 1941.

Pitts, F. N., Jr. Medical aspects of ECT. *Semin. Psychiatry,* 4:27–32, 1972.

Pitts, F. N., Jr., Desmarias, G. M., Stewart, W., and Schaberg, K. Induction of anesthesia with methohexital and thiopental in electroconvulsive therapy. *N. Engl. J. Med.,* 273:353–360, 1965.

Pitts, F. N., Jr. and Guze, S. Psychiatric disorders and myxedema. *Am. J. Psychiatry,* 118:142–147, 1961.

Pitts, F. N., Jr. and Patterson, C. W. Electroconvulsive therapy (ECT) of iatrogenic hypothalamic-hypopituitarism (CRF-ACTH Type). *Am. J. Psychiat. in press.*

Pitts, F. N., Jr., Woodruff, R. A., Jr., Craig, A. G., and Rich, C. L. The drug modification of ECT. II. Succinylcholine dosage. *Arch. Gen. Psychiatry,* 19:595–599, 1968.

Platman, S. R., Fieve, R. R., and Pierson, R. N. Effect of mood and lithium carbonate on total body potassium. *Arch. Gen. Psychiatry,* 22:297–300, 1970.

Plum, F., Howse, D. C., and Duffy, T. E. Metabolic effects of seizures. *Res. Publ. Assoc. Res. Nerv. Ment. Dis.,* 53:141–157, 1974.

Plum, F., Posner, J. B., and Troy, B. Cerebral metabolic and circulatory responses to induced convulsions in animals. *Arch. Neurol.,* 18:1–13, 1968.

Polatin, P., Strauss, H., and Altman, L. Transient organic mental reactions during shock therapy of the psychoses: A clinical study. *Psychiatr. Q.,* 14:457–465, 1940.

Pollack, M., and Fink, M. Sociopsychological characteristics of patients who refuse convulsive therapy. *J. Nerv. Ment. Dis.,* 132:153–157, 1961.

Pollack, M., and Fink, M. Disordered perception of simultaneous stimulation of face and hand: A review and theory. In: J. Wortis (Ed.): *Biological Psychiatry,* Vol. 4, Plenum Press, New York, pp. 362–369, 1962.

Pollack, M., Kahn, R. L., Karp, E., and Fink, M. Tachistoscopic perception after induced altered brain functions: Influence of mental set. *J. Nerv. Ment. Dis.,* 134:422–430, 1962.

Pollack, M., Klein, D. F., Willner, A., Blumberg, A. G., and Fink, M. Imipramine-induced behavioral disorganization in schizophrenic patients: Physiological and psychological correlates. In: J. Wortis (Ed.): *Biological Psychiatry,* Vol. 7, Plenum Press, New York, pp. 53–61, 1965.

Pollack, M., Rosenthal, F., and Macey, R. Changes in electroshock convulsive response with repeated seizures. *Exp. Neurol.,* 7:98–106, 1963.

Pollack, M., Siegel, N., Kahn, R. L., and Fink, M. Social aspects of psychiatric treatment in three hospitals: Methodological problems. *VA Coop. Chemother. Studies Psychiatry,* 6:202–206, 1961.

Pollitt, J. D. Suggestions for a physiological classification of depression *Br. J. Psychiatry,* 111:489–495, 1965a.

Pollitt, J. *Depression and its Treatment.* William Heinemann Medical Books, London, 114 pp., 1965b.

Popper, K. R. Science: problems, aims, responsibilities. *Fed. Proc.,* 22:961–972, 1963.

Porot, M., Moulinoux, C., de Mori, V., Coudert, A.-J., and Plenat, M. Electrochocs, antidépresseurs et anesthésie. *L'Encephale* 1:367–373, 1975.

Posner, J. B., Plum, F., and Van Poznak, A. Cerebral metabolism during electrically induced seizures in man. *Arch. Neurol.,* 20:388–395, 1969.

Post, R. M., Cramer, H., and Goodwin, F. K. Cyclic AMP in cerebrospinal fluid of manic and depressive patients. *Psychol. Med.,* 7:599–605, 1977.

A Practicing Psychiatrist. The experience of electroconvulsive therapy. *Br. J. Psychiatry,* 111:365–367, 1965.

Prange, A. J., Nemeroff, C. B., and Lipton, M. A. Behavioral effects of peptides: Basic and clinical studies. In: M. A. Lipton, A. DiMascio, and K. F. Killam (Eds.): *Psychopharmacology: A Generation of Progress.* Raven Press, New York, pp. 441–463, 1978a.

Prange, A. J., Nemeroff, C. B., Lipton, M. J., Breese, G. R., and Wilson, I. C. Peptides and the central nervous system. In: L. L. Iversen, S. D. Iversen, and S. H. Snyder (Eds.): *Handbook of Psychopharmacology, Vol. 13,* Plenum Press, New York, pp. 1–107, 1978b.

Prange, A. J., Wilson, I. C., Lara, P. P., Alltop, L. B., and Breese, G. R. Effects of thyrotropin-releasing hormone in depression. *Lancet,* 2:999–1002, 1972.

Price, T. R. P. and Levin, R. The effects of electroconvulsive therapy on tardive dyskinesia. *Am. J. Psychiatr.* 135:991–993, 1978.

Pritchard, M. Prognosis of schizophrenia before and after pharmacotherapy: I. Short term outcome. *Br. J. Psychiatry,* 113:1345–1352, 1967a.
Pritchard, M. Prognosis of schizophrenia before and after pharmacotherapy: II. Three-year follow up. *Br. J. Psychiatry,* 113:1353–1359, 1967b.
Proctor, L. D., and Goodwin, J. E. Comparative electroencephalographic observations following electroshock therapy using raw 60 cycle alternating and unidirectional fluctuating current. *Am. J. Psychiatry,* 99:525–530, 1943.
Proctor, L. D., and Goodwin, J. E. Clinical and electro-physiological observations following electroshock. *Am. J. Psychiatry,* 101:707–800, 1945.
Pryor, G. T. Effects of repeated ECS on brain weight and brain enzymes. In: M. Fink, S. Kety, J. McGaugh, and T. Williams (Eds.): *Psychobiology of Convulsive Therapy.* V. H. Winston & Sons, Washington, D.C., pp. 171–184, 1974.
Pryor, G. T., and Otis, L. S. Brain biochemical and behavioral effects of 1, 2, 4 or 8 weeks' electroshock treatment. *Life Sci.,* 8:387–399, 1969.
Pryor, G. T., Peache, S., and Scott, M. K. The effect of repeated electroconvulsive shock on avoidance conditioning and brain monoamine oxidase activity. *Physiol. Behav.,* 9:623–628, 1972a.
Pryor, G. T., Scott, M. K., and Peache, S. Increased monoamine oxidase activity following repeated electroshock seizures. *J. Neurochem.,* 19:891–893, 1972b.
Quitkin, F., Rifkin, A. and Klein D. F.: Imipramine response in deluded depressed patients. *Am. J. Psychiatr.* 135:806–811, 1978.
Rachlin, H. L., Goldman, G. S., Gurvitz, M., Lurie, A., and Rachlin, L. Follow-up study of 317 patients discharged from Hillside Hospital in 1950. *J. Hillside Hosp.,* 5:17–40, 1956.
Read, C. F., Steinberg, L., Liebert, E., and Finkelman, I. Use of Metrazol in the functional psychoses. *Am. J. Psychiatry,* 95:781–786, 1939.
Redlich, F. C., and Freedman, D. X. *The Theory and Practice of Psychiatry.* Basic Books, New York, 880 pp., 1966.
Redlich, F. C., Hollingshead, A. B., Roberts, B. H., Robinson, H. A., Freedman, L. Z., and Meyers, J. K. Social structure and psychiatric disorders. *Am. J. Psychiatry,* 109:729–734, 1953.
Rees, L. Electronarcosis in the treatment of schizophrenia. *J. Ment. Sci.,* 95:625–637, 1949.
Regestein, Q. R., Alpert, J. S., and Reich, P. Sudden catatonic stupor with disastrous outcome. *JAMA,* 238:618–620, 1977.
Regestein, Q. R., Murawski, B. J., and Engle, R. P. A case of prolonged, reversible dementia associated with abuse of electroconvulsive therapy. *J. Nerv. Ment. Dis.,* 161:200–203, 1975.
Regestein, Q. R., and Roper, P. The treatment of psychiatric patients by simultaneous use of electroconvulsive and pharmacoconvulsive therapy. *Can. Med. Assoc. J.,* 95:875–877, 1966.
Reichert, H., Benjamin, J., Keegan, D., and Marjerrison, G. Bilateral and non-dominant unilateral ECT. I. Therapeutic efficacy. *Can. Psychiatr. Assoc. J.,* 21:69–78, 1976a.
Reichert, H., Benjamin, J., Neufeldt, A. H., and Marjerrison, G. Bilateral and non-dominant unilateral ECT. II. Development of prograde effects. *Can. Psychiatr. Assoc. J.* 21:79–86, 1976b.
Reichlin, S., Baldessarini, R. J., and Martin, J. B. *The Hypothalamus.* Res. Publ. Assoc. Nerv. Ment. Dis., Vol. 56. Raven Press, New York, 490 pp., 1978.
Reichlin, S., and O'Neal, L. W. Thyroid hormone levels after electroshock-induced convulsions in man. *J. Clin. Endocrinol.,* 22:385–388, 1962.
Reiss, M. Unusual pituitary activity in a case of anorexia nervosa. *J. Ment. Sci.,* 89:270–273, 1943.
Remick, R. A., and Maurice, W. L. ECT in pregnancy. *Am. J. Psychiatry,* 135:761–762, 1978.
Renaud, L. P. Peptides as neurotransmitters or neuromodulators. In: M. A. Lipton, A. DiMascio, and K. F. Killam (Eds.): *Psychopharmacology: A Generation of Progress.* Raven Press, New York, pp. 423–430, 1978.
Rennie, T. A. C. Prognosis in manic-depressive and schizophrenic conditions following shock treatment. *Psychiatr. Q.,* 17:642–654, 1943.
Revitch, E. Observations on organic brain damage and clinical improvement following protracted insulin coma. *Psychiatr. Q.,* 28:79–92, 1954.
Rich, C. L., Woodruff, R. A., Jr., Cadoret, R., Craig, A. G., and Pitts, F. N., Jr. Electrotherapy: the effects of atropine on EKG. *Dis. Nerv. Syst.,* 30:622–626, 1969.
Richardson, D. J., Lewis, W. H., Jr., Gahagan, L. H., and Sheehan, D. Etiology and treatment of cardiac arrhythmias under anesthesia for electroconvulsive therapy. *NY State J. Med.,* 57:881–885, 1957.
Riddell, S. A. The therapeutic efficacy of ECT. *Arch. Gen. Psychiatry,* 8:546–556, 1963.
Rinaldi, F., Manacorda, A., and Mazzarella, B. L'elettroshock unilaterale: Osservazioni elettroence-

falografiche in una serie di pazienti sottoposti a trattamento elettroconvulsivante sull'emisfero non dominante. *Folia Neuropsychiatr.,* 10:481–494, 1967.
Robbins, E. S., Weinstein, S., Berg, S., Rifkin, A., Wechsler, D., and Oxley, B. The effect of electroconvulsive treatment upon the perception of the spiral aftereffect, a presumed measure of cerebral dysfunction. *J. Nerv. Ment. Dis.,* 128:239–242, 1959.
Roberts, A. H. The value of E.C.T. in delirium. *Br. J. Psychiatry,* 109:653–655, 1963.
Roberts, J. M. Prognostic factors in the electroshock treatment of depressive states: I. Clinical features from history and examination. *J. Ment. Sci.,* 105:693–702, 1959 a.
Roberts, J. M. Prognostic factors in the electroshock treatment of depressive states: II. The application of specific tests. *J. Ment. Sci.,* 105:703–713, 1959 b.
Robin, A. The College memorandum on ECT. *Br. J. Psychiatry,* 132:316–317, 1978.
Robin, A. A., and Harris, J. A. A controlled comparison of imipramine and electroplexy. *J. Ment. Sci.,* 108:217–219, 1962.
Robinson, G. W., Jr., and De Mott, J. D. How important is liver damage in the use of anectine controlled electroshock? *Confin. Neurol.,* 14:275–281, 1954.
Robinson, H. A., Redlich, F. C., and Myers, J. K. Social structure and psychiatric treatment. *Am. J. Orthopsychiatry,* 24:307–316, 1954.
Rohde, P., and Sargant, W. Treatment of schizophrenia in general hospitals. *Br. Med. J.,* 2:67–70, 1961.
Rose, J. T. The Funkenstein test—A review of literature. *Acta Psychiatr. Scand.,* 38:124–153, 1962.
Rose, J. T. Reactive and endogenous depressions—Response to E.C.T. *Br. J. Psychiatry,* 109:213–217, 1963.
Rose, L., and Watson, A. Flurothyl (Indoklon). *Anaesthesia,* 22:425–434, 1967.
Rosenblatt, S., Chanley, J. D., Sobotka, H., and Kaufman, M. R. Interrelationships between electroshock, the blood-brain barrier and catecholamines. *J. Neurochem.,* 5:172–176, 1970.
Ross, D. Psychotic casualties in New Guinea with special reference to use of convulsive therapy in forward areas. *Med. J. Aust.,* 1:830–833, 1946.
Ross, J. R., and Malzberg, B. A review of the results of the pharmacological shock therapy and the metrazol convulsive therapy in New York State. *Am. J. Psychiatry,* 96:297–316, 1939.
Rosvold, H. E., Kaplan, S. J., and Stevenson, J. A. F. Effects of electroconvulsive shock on the adrenal cortex of the rat. *Proc. Soc. Exp. Biol. Med.,* 80:60–62, 1952.
Roth, L. H. Involuntary civil commitment. The right to treatment and the right to refuse treatment. *Psychiatr. Ann.,* 7:50–76, 1977.
Roth, M. Changes in the EEG under barbiturate anesthesia produced by electro-convulsive treatment and their significance for the theory of ECT action. *Electroencephalogr. Clin. Neurophysiol.,* 3:261–280, 1951.
Roth, M. A theory of E.C.T. action and its bearing on the biological significance of epilepsy. *J. Ment. Sci.,* 98:44–59, 1952.
Roth, M., Garside, R., and Gurney, C. Classification of depressive disorders. In: J. Angst (Ed.): *Classification and Prediction of Outcome in Depression.* F. K. Schattauer Verlag, Stuttgart, pp. 3–26, 1974.
Roth, M., Kay, D. W. K., and Kiloh, L. G. The results of biological (physical) treatment in psychiatry and their bearing on the classification of mental disease. In: M. Rinkel (Ed.): *Biological Treatment of Mental Illness.* L. C. Page, New York, pp. 71–112, 1966.
Roth, M., Kay, D. W. K., Shaw, J., and Green, J. Prognosis and pentothal induced electroencephalographic changes in electro-convulsive treatment. *Electroencephalogr. Clin. Neurophysiol.,* 9:225–237, 1957.
Roth, M., and Rosie, J. M. The use of electroplexy in mental disease with clouding of consciousness. *J. Ment. Sci.,* 99:103–111, 1953.
Rothschild, D., van Gordon, D. J., and Varjabedian, A. Regressive shock therapy in schizophrenia. *Dis. Nerv. Syst.,* 12:147–151, 1951.
Roubicek, J. *Šokové Léčení duševních chorob.* Prometheus Press, Prague, 132 pp., 1946.
Roubicek, J. Mutism and electric shock treatment. *Zvlastni Otisk Neurol. Psychiatr. Cesk.,* 10:1–9, 1948.
Roubicek, J. Studie o pruchodu elektrickeho proudu mozkem. Etude sur le passage du courant electrique dans l'encephale. *Sb. Lek.* 49:21–44, 1949.
Roubicek, J. Electrošok a electroencefalogram. *Cesk. Psychiatr.,* 2:90 95, 1959.
Roudeau, Y., Nadeau, G., and Delage, J.: An appraisal of histamine therapy in schizophrenia. *J. Clin. Exp. Psychopathol.* 16:1–9, 1955.

Rovere, D. Clinical-statistical analysis for forms of recidivism in schizophrenia. *Riv. Psychiatr.,* 2:409–413, 1967.
Rowntree, D. W., and Kay, W. W. Clinical, biochemical and physiological studies in cases of recurrent schizophrenia. *J. Ment. Sci.,* 98:100–121, 1952.
Royal College of Psychiatrists. Memorandum on the use of electroconvulsive therapy. *Br. J. Psychiatry,* 131:261–272, 1977.
Royce, J. R., and Rosvold, H. E. Electroshock and the rat adrenal cortex. *Arch. Neurol. Psychiatry,* 70:516–527, 1953.
Rozman, R. S., and Kurland, A. A. The effect of flurothyl and electroshock on pulmonary diffusion. *Behav. Neuropsychiatry,* 2:20–22, 1970.
Rubin, R. T., and Mandell, A. J. Adrenal cortical activity in pathological emotional states: A review. *Am. J. Psychiatry,* 123:387–400, 1966.
Russell, G. F. M. Body weight and balance of water, sodium and potassium in depressed patients given electro-convulsive therapy. *Clin. Sci.,* 19:327–336, 1960.
Russell, G. F. M., Loraine, J. A., Bell, E. T., and Harkness, R. A. Gonadotrophin and oestrogen excretion in patients with anorexia nervosa. *J. Psychosom. Res.,* 9:79–85, 1965.
Ryan, R. J., Swanson, D. W., Faiman, C., Mayberry, W. E., and Spadoni, A. J. Effects of convulsive electroshock on serum concentrations of follicle-stimulating hormone, leutenizing hormone, thyroid stimulating hormone and growth hormone in man. *J. Clin. Endocrinol. Metab.,* 30:51–58, 1970.
Sachar, E. J. (Ed.) *Hormones, Behavior, and Psychopathology.* Raven Press, New York, 307 pp., 1976.
Sachar, E. J., Finkelstein, J., and Hellman, L. Growth hormone responses in depressive illness. *Arch. Gen. Psychiatry,* 25:263–269, 1971a.
Sachar, E. J., Frantz, A. G., Altman, N., and Sassin, J. Growth hormone and prolactin in unipolar and bipolar depressed patients: Responses to hypoglycemia and L-dopa. *Am. J. Psychiatry,* 130:1362–1367, 1973a.
Sachar, E. J., Hellman, L., Fukushima, D. K., and Gallagher, T. F. Cortisol production in depressive illness: A clinical and biochemical clarification. *Arch. Gen. Psychiatry,* 23:289–298, 1971b.
Sachar, E. J., Hellman, L., Roffwarg, H., Halpern, F., Fukushima, D., and Gallagher, T. F. Disrupted 24-hour patterns of cortisol excretion in psychotic depression. *Arch. Gen. Psychiatry,* 28:19–24, 1973b.
Sachs, E., Jr. Acetylcholine and serotonin in the spinal fluid. *J. Neurosurg.,* 14:22–27, 1957.
Sainz, A. Clarification of the action of successful treatment in the depressions. *Dis. Nerv. Syst. [Suppl.],* 20:53–57, 1959.
Sakel, M. *Pharmacological Treatment of Schizophrenia.* Nervous and Mental Disease, Publ. Co. New York, 136 pp., 1938.
Sakel, M. The classical Sakel shock treatment: A reappraisal. In: F. Marti-Ibanez, A. M. Sackler, M. D. Sackler, and R. R. Sackler (Eds.): *The Great Physiodynamic Therapies in Psychiatry.* Hoeber-Harper, New York, pp. 13–75, 1956.
Salgado, A. L. D., Fernandez-Durango, R., and Lopez del Campo, J. G. *Applications and Clinical Uses of Hypothalamic Hormones.* American Elsevier, New York, 351 pp., 1976.
Salomon, K., and Gabrio, B. W. Plasma calcium fractions after electric convulsion treatment. *Arch. Neurol. Psychiatry,* 62:99–104, 1949.
Salzman, C. Electroconvulsive therapy. In: R. Shader (Ed.): *Manual of Psychiatric Therapies.* Little, Brown & Co., Boston, pp. 115–124, 1975.
Salzman, C. ECT and ethical psychiatry. *Am. J. Psychiatry,* 134:1006–1009, 1977.
Salzman, L. An evaluation of shock therapy. *Am. J. Psychiatry,* 103:669–679, 1947.
Sandifer, M. G., Albert, R. F., and Wilson, I. C. Patient preference: Indoklon vs. electroshock therapy. *J. Nerv. Ment. Dis.,* 134:184–186, 1962.
Sandison, R. A. The psychology of electric convulsion therapy. *J. Ment. Sci.,* 96:734–744, 1950.
Sand-Strömgren, L. S. Unilateral vs. bilateral electroconvulsive therapy. *Acta Psychiatr. Scand. [suppl.],* 240:1–65, 1973.
Sand-Strömgren, L. S. Therapeutic results in brief-interval unilateral ECT. *Acta Psychiatr. Scand.,* 52:246–255, 1975.
Sand-Strömgren, L. S. The influence of depression on memory. *Acta Psychiatr. Scand.,* 56:109–128, 1977.
Sand-Strömgren, L., Christensen, A.-L., and Fromholt, P. The effects of unilateral brief-interval ECT on memory. *Acta Psychiatr. Scand.,* 54:336–346, 1976.

Sand-Strömgren, L. S., and Juul-Jensen, P. EEG in unilateral and bilateral electro-convulsive therapy. *Acta Psychiatr. Scand.*, 51:340–360, 1975.
Sargant, W., and Slater, E. *An Introduction to Somatic Methods of Treatment in Psychiatry.* Williams & Wilkins, Baltimore, 171 pp., 1944.
Sargant, W., and Slater, E. *An Introduction to Physical Methods of Treatment in Psychiatry.* Williams & Wilkins, Baltimore, 351 pp., Ed. III, 1954.
Sargent, W., and Slater, E. *An Introduction to Physical Methods of Treatment in Psychiatry.* Williams & Wilkins, Baltimore, Ed. V., 346 pp., 1963.
Savitsky, N., and Karliner, W. Further studies on short courses of electric shock treatments. *Am. J. Psychiatry,* 104:197–199, 1947.
Savitsky, N., and Karliner, W. Reflex studies in electroshock treatments. *Arch. Neurol. Psychiatry,* 59:481–484, 1948.
Savitsky, N., and Karliner, W. Electroshock therapy and multiple sclerosis. *NY J. Med.,* 51:788, 1951.
Savitsky, N., and Karliner, W. Electroshock in the presence of organic disease of the nervous system. *J. Hillside Hosp.,* 2:3–22, 1953.
Savitsky, N., and Tarachow, S. The question of shorter courses of electroshock therapy in the depressions. *J. Nerv. Ment. Dis.,* 101:115–120, 1945.
Sawyer, C. H. Regulatory mechanisms of secretion of gonadotrophic hormones. In: W. Haymaker, E. Anderson, and W. J. H. Nauta (Eds.): *The Hypothalamus.* Charles C Thomas, Springfield, Ill., pp. 389–430, 1969.
Scanlon, W. G., and Mathas, J. Electroencephalographic and psychometric studies of Indoklon convulsive treatment and electroconvulsive treatment (a preliminary report). *Int. J. Neuropsychiatry,* 3:276–281, 1967.
Schally, A. V. Hypothalamic regulatory hormones: Experimental and clinical studies. In: A. L. C. Salgado, R. Fernandez-Durango, and J. G. Lopez del Campo (Eds.): *Applications and Clinical Uses of Hypothalamic Hormones.* American Elsevier, New York, pp. 3–18, 1976.
Scharrer, E., and Scharrer, B. Secretory cells within the hypothalamus. *Res. Publ. Assoc. Nerv. Ment. Dis.,* 20:170–174, 1940.
Schiele, B. C., and Schneider, R. A. The selective use of electroconvulsive therapy in manic patients. *Dis. Nerv. Syst.,* 10:291–297, 1949.
Schilder, P. Localization of the body image (postural model of the body). *Res. Publ. Assoc. Nerv. Ment. Dis.,* 15:466–484, 1932.
Schilder, P. Notes on the psychology of metrazol treatment of schizophrenia. *J. Nerv. Ment. Dis.,* 89:133–144, 1939.
Schildkraut, J. J. The catecholamine hypothesis of affective disorders: A review of supporting evidence. *Am. J. Psychiatry,* 122:509–522, 1965.
Schildkraut, J. J., and Draskoczy, P. R. Effects of electroconvulsive shock on norepinephrine turnover and metabolism: basic and clinical studies. In: M. Fink, S. Kety, J. McGaugh, and T. A. Williams (Eds.): *Psychobiology of Convulsive Therapy.* V. H. Winston & Sons, Washington, D.C., pp. 143–170, 1974.
Schmidt, W. R., and Jarcho, L. W. Persistent dyskinesias following phenothiazine therapy. *Arch. Neurol.,* 14:369–377, 1966.
Scholz, W. *Die Krampfschädigungen des Gehirns.* Springer-Verlag, Berlin, 144 pp., 1951.
Schou, M. Lithium in psychiatric therapy and prophylaxis. *J. Psychiatr. Res.,* 6:67–95, 1968.
Schou, M. Prophylactic lithium maintenance treatment in recurrent endogenous affective disorder. In: S. Gershon and B. Shopsin (Eds.): *Lithium. Its Role in Psychiatric Research and Treatment.* Plenum Press, New York, pp. 269–294, 1973.
Schyve, P. M., Smithline, F., and Meltzer, H. Neuroleptic-induced prolactin elevation and breast cancer: An emerging clinical issue. *Arch. Gen. Psychiatry,* 35:1291–1303, 1978.
Seager, C. P. A comparison between the results of unmodified and modified electroplexy (E.C.T.) *J. Ment. Sci.,* 104:206–220, 1958.
Seager, C. P. Controlled trial of straight and modified electroplexy. *J. Ment. Sci.,* 105:1022–1028, 1959.
Seager, C. P., and Bird, R. L. Imipramine with electrical treatment in depression—a controlled trial. *J. Ment. Sci.,* 108, 456:704–707, 1962.
Sebag-Montefiore, S. E. Flurothyl (Indoklon) in depression. *Br. J. Psychiatry,* 124:616–617, 1974.
Seidman, J., Schreiber, M., Cohen, S., and Richards, R. *Procedure for Electro-Convulsive Treatment.* V.A. Hospital, Los Angeles, Preprint, March, 1956.

Shader, R. I., and DiMascio, A. *Psychotropic Drug Side-Effects: Clinical and Theoretical Perspectives.* Williams & Wilkins, Baltimore, 290 pp., 1970.
Shagass, C. The sedation threshold. A method for estimating tension in psychiatric patients. *Electroencephalogr. Clin. Neurophysiol.,* 8:221–233, 1954.
Shagass, C. A measurable neurophysiological factor of psychiatric significance. *Electroencephalogr. Clin. Neurophysiol.,* 9:101–108, 1957.
Shagass, C. *Evoked Brain Potentials in Psychiatry.* Plenum Press, New York, 274 pp., 1972.
Shagass, C., and Jones, A. L. A neurophysiological test for psychiatric diagnosis: Results in 750 patients. *Am. J. Psychiatry,* 114:1002–1010, 1958.
Shagass, C., Muller, K., and Acosta, H. B. The pentothal "sleep" threshold as an indicator of affective change. *J. Psychosom. Res.,* 3:253–270, 1959.
Shagass, C., and Naiman, J. The sedation threshold as an objective index of manifest anxiety in psychoneurosis. *J. Psychosom. Res.,* 1:49–57, 1956.
Shah, D. K., Wig, N. N. and Chaudhury, R. R. Antidiuretic hormone levels in patients with weight gain after chlorpromazine therapy. *Indian J. Med. Res.* 61:771–776, 1973.
Shattock, F. M., and Micklem, L. P. An investigation of the adrenocortical response of mental patients to ECT and insulin hypoglycemia. *J. Ment. Sci.,* 98:287–293, 1952.
Shaw, D. M. The practical management of affective disorders. *Br. J. Psychiatry,* 130:432–451, 1977.
Sheldon, J. H. Anorexia nervosa. *Proc. R. Soc. Med.,* 32:738–740, 1939.
Shepherd, M. Clinical trial of the treatment of depressive illness. *Br. Med. J.,* 1:881–886, 1965.
Shoor, M., and Adams, I. H. The intensive electroshock therapy of chronic disturbed psychotic patients. *Am. J. Psychiatry,* 107:279–282, 1950.
Siegel, N., Kahn, R. L., Pollack, M., and Fink, M. Social class, diagnosis, and treatment in three psychiatric hospitals. *Soc. Probl.,* 10:191–196, 1962.
Siegel, S. *Nonparametric Statistics for the Behavioral Sciences.* McGraw-Hill, New York, 312 pp., 1956.
Siekert, R. G., Williams, S. C., and Windle, W. F. Histologic study of the brains of monkeys after experimental electric shock. *Arch. Neurol. Psychiatry,* 63:79–86, 1950.
Silbermann, I. The psychical experiences during the shocks in shock therapy. *Int. J. Psychoanal.,* 21:179–200, 1940.
Silverman, M. Organic stupor subsequent to a severe head injury treated with ECT. *Br. J. Psychiatry,* 110:648–650, 1964.
Silverman, M. Catatonic stupor responsive to ECT. *Br. Med. J.,* 1:582, 1977.
Simpson, G. M., Lee, J. H., Cuculic, Z., and Kellner, R.: Two dosages of imipramine in hospitalized endogenous and neurotic depressives. *Arch. Gen. Psychiatr.* 33:1093–1102, 1976.
Skoda, C., Nestlingerova, E., and Nestarcova, K. Retention rates of schizophrenia during period of shock and pharmacotherapy and in relation to the open door system. *Acta Nerv. Super.,* 10:343–344, 1968.
Small, I. F. Inhalant convulsive therapy. In: M. Fink, S. Kety, J. McGaugh, and T. A. Williams (Eds.): *Psychobiology of Convulsive Therapy.* V. H. Winston & Sons, Washington, D.C., pp. 65–77, 1974.
Small, I. F., Sharpley, P., and Small, J. G. Influence of Cylert upon memory changes with ECT. *Am. J. Psychiatry,* 125:837–840, 1968*a*.
Small, I. F., and Small, J. G. Ictus and amnesia. *Recent Adv. Biol. Psychiatry,* 10:144–159, 1968.
Small, I. F., and Small, J. G. Electroencephalographic (EEG), evoked potential, and direct current (DC) responses with unilateral electroconvulsive treatment (ECT). *J. Nerv. Ment. Dis.,* 152:396–404, 1971*a*.
Small, I. F., and Small, J. G. The clinical use of flurothyl. In: W. B. Essman, and L. Valzelli (Eds.): *Curr. Dev. Psychopharmacol,* 2:64–78, 1975.
Small, I. F., Small, J. G., Milstein, V., and Sharpley, P. Interhemispheric relationships with somatic therapy. *Dis. Nerv. Syst.,* 34:170–177, 1973.
Small, J. G. EEG and neurophysiological studies of convulsive therapies. In: M. Fink, S. Kety, J. McGaugh, and T. A. Williams (Eds.): *Psychobiology of Convulsive Therapy.* V. H. Winston & Sons, Washington, D.C., pp. 47–63, 1974.
Small, J. G., Kellams, J. J., Milstein, V., and Small, I. F. Lithium in combination with ECT—Possible negative interactions. *Personal communication,* 1978*a*.
Small, J. G., and Small, I. F. CNV correlations with psychiatric diagnosis. *Arch. Gen. Psychiatry,* 25:550–554, 1971*b*.
Small, J. G., and Small, I. F. Clinical results; Indoklon vs. ECT. *Semin. Psychiatry,* 4:13–26, 1972.

Small, J. G., and Small, I. F. Pharmacology-neurophysiology of lithium. In: S. Gershon and B. Shopsin (Eds.): *Lithium. Its Role in Psychiatric Research and Treatment*. Plenum Press, New York, pp. 83–106, 1973.

Small, J. G., Small, I. F., and Milstein, V. Electrophysiology of EST. In: M. A. Lipton, A. DiMascio, and K. F. Killam (Eds.): *Psychopharmacology: A Generation of Progress*. Raven Press, New York, pp. 759–769, 1978b.

Small, J. G., Small, I. F., Milstein, V., and Dian, D. A. Effects of ACTH 4–10 on ECT-induced memory dysfunctions. *Acta Psychiatr. Scand.*, 55:241–250, 1977.

Small, J. G., Small, I. F., Perez, H. C., and Sharpley, P. EEG and neurophysiological studies of electrically induced seizures. *J. Nerv. Ment. Dis.*, 150:479–489, 1970.

Small, J. G., Small, I. F., Sharpley, P., and Moore, D. F. A double-blind comparative evaluation of fluorothyl and ECT. *Arch. Gen. Psychiatry*, 19:79–86, 1968b.

Smith, J. J. Treatment of acute alcoholic states with ACTH and adrenocortical hormones. *Q. J. Studies Alcohol.*, 11:190–198, 1950.

Smith, K., Surphlis, W. R. P., Gynther, M. D., and Shimkunas, A. M. ECT—chlorpromazine and chlorpromazine compared in the treatment of schizophrenia. *J. Nerv. Ment. Dis.*, 144:284–292, 1967.

Smith, R. J. Electroshock experiments at Albany violate ethics guidelines. *Science*, 198:383–386, 1977.

Smith, S. The use of electroplexy (ECT) in psychiatric syndromes complicating pregnancy. *J. Ment. Sci.*, 102:796–800, 1956.

Smitt, J. W., and Wegener, C. F. On electric convulsive therapy with particular regard to a parietal application of electrodes, controlled by intracerebral voltage. *Acta Psychiatr. Neurol.*, 19:529–549, 1944.

Sobel, D. E. Fetal damage due to ECT, insulin coma, chlorpromazine or reserpine. *Arch. Gen. Psychiatry*, 2:606–611, 1960.

Solomon, H. C., Rose, A. S., and Arnot, R. E. Electric shock treatment in general paresis. *J. Nerv. Ment. Dis.*, 107:377–381, 1948.

Solomon, H. C., and Yakovlev, P. I. *Shock Therapy in the Military Services. A Manual of Military Neuropsychiatry*. W. B. Saunders, Philadelphia, 764 pp., 1944.

Spencer, J. Psychiatry and convulsant therapy. *Med. J. Aust.*, 1:844–847, 1977.

Spensley, J. Ataractic drugs versus ECT in schizophrenia. *Am. J. Psychiatry*, 130:1162–1163, 1973.

Spiegel, E. A. Quantitative determination of convulsive reactivity by electric stimulation of brain with skull intact. *J. Lab. Clin. Med.*, 22:1274–1276, 1937.

Spiegel, E., and Spiegel-Adolf, M. Permeability changes in the brain induced by metrazol and insulin convulsions. *J. Nerv. Ment. Dis.*, 93:750–755, 1941.

Spiegel, E. A., and Spiegel-Adolf, M. Physiological and physicochemical mechanisms in electroshock treatment. *Confin. Neurol.*, 13:38–63, 1953.

Spreche, D. A quantitative comparison of electroconvulsive therapy with hexafluorodiethyl ether. *J. Neuropsychiatry*, 5:132–137, 1964.

Squire, L. R. Amnesia for remote events following electroconvulsive therapy. *Behav. Biol.*, 12:119–125, 1974.

Squire, L. R. A stable impairment in remote memory following electroconvulsive therapy. *Neuropsychologia*, 13:51–58, 1975.

Squire, L. R. ECT and memory loss. *Am. J. Psychiatry*, 134:997–1001, 1977.

Squire, L. R., and Chace, P. M. Memory functions six to nine months after electroconvulsive therapy. *Arch. Gen. Psychiatry*, 32:1557–1564, 1975.

Squire, L. R., Chace, P. M., and Slater, P. C. Retrograde amnesia following electroconvulsive therapy. *Nature*, 260:775–777, 1976a.

Squire, L. R., and Miller, P. L. Diminution of anterograde amnesia following electroconvulsive therapy. *Br. J. Psychiatry*, 125:490–495, 1974.

Squire, L. R., and Slater, P. C. Forgetting in very long-term memory as assessed by an improved questionnaire technique. *J. Exp. Psychol.*, 104:50–54, 1975.

Squire, L. R. and Slater, P. C. Bilateral and unilateral ECT: Effects on verbal and nonverbal memory. *Am. J. Psychiatry* 135:1316–1320, 1978.

Squire, L. R., Slater, P. C., and Chace, P. M. Retrograde amnesia: Temporal gradient in very long-term memory following electroconvulsive therapy. *Science*, 187:77–79, 1975.

Squire, L. R., Slater, P. C., and Chace, P. M. Anterograde amnesia following electroconvulsive therapy: No evidence for state-dependent learning. *Behav. Biol.*, 17:31–41, 1976b.

Squire, L. R., Slater, P. C., and Chace, P. M. Reactivation of recent or remote memory before electroconvulsive therapy does not produce retrograde amnesia. *Behav. Biol.,* 18:335–343, 1976c.

Stainbrook, E. Shock therapy: Psychologic theory and research. *Psychol. Bull.,* 43:21–60, 1946.

Stanley, W. J., and Fleming, H. A clinical comparison of phenelzine and electro-convulsive therapy in the treatment of depressive illness. *J. Ment. Sci.,* 108:708–710, 1962.

Stein, J., Roth, B., Schultz, H., and Müller, J. Die bioelektrisch kontrollierte Krampfbehandlung der endogene Psychosen in Narkose und Relaxation. III: Das Hirnstrombild des Electrokrampfes. *Arch. Psychiatr. Nervenkr.,* 211:448–459, 1968.

Stern, J. A., and Sila, B. Autonomic responsivity and electric convulsive therapy. *J. Neuropsychiatry,* 1:100–103, 1959.

Stern, J. A., Sila, B., and Word, T. J. Observations on the effect of electroconvulsive therapy and pharmacotherapy on the psychogalvanic response. *J. Neuropsychiatry,* 2:149–152, 1961.

Stern, J. A., and Word, T. J. Changes in cardiac response of the albino rat as a function of electroconvulsive seizures. *J. Comp. Physiol. Psychol.,* 54:389–394, 1961.

Stern, K., Askonas, B. A., and Cullen, A. M. The influence of electroconvulsive treatment on blood sugar, total number of leucocytes and lymphocytes. *Am. J. Psychiatry,* 105:585–588, 1949.

Sternberg, D. E., and Jarvik, M. E. Memory functions in depression. *Arch. Gen. Psychiatry,* 33:219–224, 1976.

Stevenson, G. H., and Geoghegan, J. J. Prophylactic electroshock. *Am. J. Psychiatry,* 107:743–748, 1951.

Stevenson, J. A. F. Neural control of food and water intake. In: W. Haymaker, E. Anderson, and W. J. H. Nauta (Eds.): *The Hypothalamus.* Charles C Thomas, Springfield, Ill., pp. 524–621, 1969.

Stief, A., and Tokay L. Beiträge zur Histopathologie der experimentellen Insulinvergiftung. *Z. Gesamte Neurol. Psychiatr.,* 139:434–461, 1932.

Stinson, B., Kempf, N., Lilly, V., and Schmidt, G. Prediction of response to electro-shock therapy in chronic mental patients. *Dis. Nerv. Syst.,* 33:123–125, 1972.

Stokes, P. E. Studies on the control of adrenocortical function in depression. In: T. A. Williams, M. Katz, and J. A. Shield (Eds.): *Recent Advances in the Psychobiology of the Depressive Illnesses.* U.S. Govt. Printing Office, Washington, D.C., #HSM 70-9053, pp. 199–220, 1972.

Stones, M. J. Electroconvulsive treatment and short-term memory. *Br. J. Psychiatry,* 122:591–594, 1973.

Strain, J. J., and Bidder, T. G. Transient cerebral complication associated with multiple monitored electroconvulsive therapy. *Dis. Nerv. syst.,* 32:95–100, 1971.

Strain, J. J., Brunschwig, L., Duffy, J. P., Agle, D. P., Rosenbaum, A. L., and Bidder, T. G. Comparison of therapeutic effects and memory changes with bilateral and unilateral ECT. *Am. J. Psychiatry,* 125:294–304, 1968.

Strauss, E. B., and MacPhail, A. Steep-wave electroplexy. *Lancet,* 2:896–899, 1946.

Strauss, H., Ostow, M., and Greenstein, L. *Diagnostic Electroencephalography.* Grune & Stratton, New York, 282 pp., 1952.

Sullivan, P. R. Treatment of schizophrenia: The place of ECT. *Dis. Nerv. Syst.,* 35:467–469, 1974.

Sutherland, E. M., Oliver, J. E., and Knight, D. R. EEG, memory and confusion in dominant, non-dominant and bi-temporal ECT. *Br. J. Psychiatry,* 115:1059–1064, 1969.

Suzuki, O., Takanohashi, M., and Yagi, K. Protective effect of dexamethasone on enhancement of blood-brain barrier permeability caused by electroconvulsive shock. *Arzneim. Forsch.,* 26:533–534, 1976.

Sweeney, D., Nelson, C., Bowers, M., Maas, J., and Heninger, G.: Delusional versus non-delusional depression: Neurochemical differences. *Lancet* 1:100–101, 1978.

Swift, M. R., and LaDu, B. N. A rapid screening test for atypical cholinesterase. *Lancet,* 1:513–574, 1966.

Szirmai, I., Boldizsar, F., and Fischer, J. Correlation between blood gases, glycolytic enzymes and EEG during electroconvulsive treatment in relaxation. *Acta Psychiatr. Scand.,* 51:171–181, 1975.

Takahashi, S., Kondo, H., Yoshimura, M., and Ochi, Y. Antidepressant effect of thyrotropin releasing hormone (TRH) and the plasma thyrotropin levels in depression. *Folia Psychiatr. Neurol. Jpn.,* 27:305–314, 1973.

Taschev, T. The course and prognosis of depression on the basis of 652 patients deceased. In: J. Angst (Ed.): *Classification and Prediction of Outcome in Depression.* F. K. Schattauer Verlag, Stuttgart, pp. 157–172, 1974.

Taylor, J. H. Control of grand-mal epilepsy with electroshock. *Dis. Nerv. Syst.,* 7:284–285, 1946.
Taylor, M. A., and Abrams, R. A. Catatonia. *Arch. Gen. Psychiatry.,* 34:1223–1228, 1977.
Taylor, M. A. and Abrams, R. A.: The prevalence of schizophrenia. *Am. J. Psychiatr.* 135:945–948, 1978.
Taylor, R. H., Gross, M., and Ruby, I. J. Nonconvulsive electrostimulation and the pituitary-adrenocortical system. *J. Nerv. Ment. Dis.,* 114:337–383, 1951.
Tedeschi, D. H., Swinyard, E. A., and Goodman, L. S. Effects of variations in stimulus intensity on maximal electroshock seizure pattern, recovery time and anticonvulsant potency of phenobarbital in mice. *J. Pharmacol. Exp. Therap.,* 116:107–113, 1956.
Terry, G. C. *Fever and Psychoses.* Hoeber, New York, 167 pp., 1939.
Tetlow, A. G., Newman, G., Anton, A. H., and Gravenstein, J. S. The cardiovascular and catecholamine response to flurothyl convulsion therapy and a comparison with the response to ECT. *Int. J. Clin. Pharmacol.,* 3:203–208, 1968.
Tewfik, G. I., and Wells, B. G. The use of Arfonad for the alleviation of cardio-vascular stress following electro-convulsive therapy. *J. Ment. Sci.,* 103:636–644, 1957.
Thenon, J. Electrochoque monolateral. *Acta Neuropsiquiatr. Argentina,* 2:292–296, 1956.
Thompson, G. N. Electroshock and other therapeutic considerations in sexual psychopathy. *J. Nerv. Ment. Dis.,* 109:531–539, 1949.
Thorell, J. I., and Adielsson, G. Antidepressive effects of electroconvulsive therapy and thyrotrophin-releasing hormone. *Lancet,* 1:43, 1973.
Thorpe, F. T. Prefrontal leucotomy in treatment of post-encephalitic conduct disorder. *Br. Med. J.,* 1:312–314, 1946.
Thorpe, J. G. The current status of prognostic test indicators for electroconvulsive therapy. *Psychosom. Med.,* 24:554–568, 1962.
Tietz, E. B. Further experiences with electronarcosis. *J. Nerv. Ment. Dis.,* 106:150–158, 1947.
Tillotson, K. J., and Sulzbach, W. A comparative study and evaluation of electric shock therapy in depressive states. *Am. J. Psychiatry,* 101:455–459, 1945.
Tomlinson, P. J. Insulin and electric therapy in general paresis. *Psychiatr. Q.,* 18:413–421, 1943.
Townsend, J. C., Russell, R. W., and Patton, R. A. Durations of convulsions in rats as functions of the intensity, duration and cumulative effects of electroshock stimulation. *J. Nerv. Ment. Dis.,* 115:49–56, 1952.
Turek, I. S. EEG correlates of electroconvulsive treatment. *Dis. Nerv. Syst.,* 33:584–589, 1972.
Turek, I. S. Combined use of ECT and psychotropic drugs: Antidepressants and antipsychotics. *Compr. Psychiatry,* 14:495–502, 1973.
Turek, I. S., and Block, B. Memory changes with ECT in depression. *Br. J. Clin. Pract.,* 28:94–95, 1974.
Turek, I. S., and Hanlon, T. E. The effectiveness and safety of electroconvulsive therapy (ECT). *J. Nerv. Ment. Dis.,* 164:419–431, 1977.
Turner, W. J., Lowinger, L., and Huddleson, J. H. The correlation of pre-electroshock electroencephalogram and therapeutic results in schizophrenia. *Am. J. Psychiatry,* 102:299–300, 1945.
Tyler, E. A., and Lowenbach, H. Polydiurnal electric shock treatment in mental disorder. *NC Med. J.,* 8:577–582, 1947.
Ueno, Y, Aoki, N., Yabucki, T., and Kuraishi, F. Electrolyte metabolism in blood and cerebrospinal fluid in psychoses. *Folia Psychiatr. Neurol. Jpn.,* 15:304–326, 1961.
Uhrbrand, L., and Faurbye, A. Reversible and irreversible dyskinesia after treatment with perphenazine, chlorpromazine, reserpine and electroconvulsive therapy. *Psychopharmacologia,* 1:408–418, 1960.
Ulett, G. A. Preliminary observations on convulsive and subconvulsive treatments induced by intermittent photic stimulation. *Am. J. Psychiatry,* 109:741–748, 1953.
Ulett, G. A. Experience with photic stimulation in psychiatric research. *Am. J. Psychiatry,* 114:127–133, 1957.
Ulett, G. A., Das, K., Hornung, F., Davis, D., and Johnson, M. Changes in the photically-driven EEG following electroconvulsive therapy. *J. Neuropsychiatry,* 3:186–189, 1962.
Ulett, G. A., Gleser, G. C., Caldwell, B. W., and Smith, K. The use of matched groups in the evaluation of convulsive and subconvulsive photoshock. *Bull. Menninger Clin.,* 18:138–146, 1954.
Ulett, G. A., and Johnson, M. W. Effect of atropine and scopolamine upon electroencephalographic changes induced by electroconvulsive therapy. *Electroencephalogr. Clin. Neurophysiol.,* 9:217–224, 1957.

Ulett, G. A., Smith, K., and Gleser, G. C. Evaluation of convulsive and subconvulsive shock therapies utilizing a control group. *Am. J. Psychiatry,* 112:795–802, 1956.
Vale, W., Rivier, C., Rivier, J., and Brown, M. Adenohypophyseal and other extracentral nervous system roles of hypothalamic regulatory peptides. In: M. A. Lipton, A. DiMascio, and K. F. Killam (Eds.): *Psychopharmacology: A Generation of Progress.* Raven Press, New York, pp. 403–421, 1978.
Valentine, M. Intensive electroplexy. *J. Nerv. Ment. Dis.,* 109:95–112, 1949.
Valentine, M., Keddie, K. M. G., and Dunne, D. A comparison of techniques in electroconvulsive therapy. *Br. J. Psychiatry,* 114:989–996, 1968.
Valzelli, L., and Garattini, S. Effect of electroshock on indoleamine metabolism and aggressive behavior. In: M. Fink, S. Kety, J. McGaugh, and T. A. Williams (Eds.): *Psychobiology of Convulsive Therapy.* V. H. Winston & Sons, Washington, D.C., pp. 221–230, 1974.
van Praag, H. M. *Depression and Schizophrenia—A Contribution on their Chemical Pathologies.* Spectrum Publications, New York, 260 pp., 1977.
van Riezen, H., Rigter, H., and Greven, H. M. Critical appraisal of peptide pharmacology. In: L. Miller, C. Sandman, and A. J. Kastin (Eds.): *Neuropeptide Influences on the Brain and Behavior.* Raven Press, New York, pp. 11–28, 1977.
Verhoeven, W. M., van Praag, H. A., Botter, P. A., Sunier, A., van Ree, J. M., and de Wied, D. (Des-Tyr[1])-γ-Endorphin in schizophrenia. *Lancet,* 1:1046–1047, 1978.
Verstraeten, P. La thérapeutique convulsante de la psychose maniaco-dépressive. *Ann. Med. Psychol.,* 95:654–659, 1937.
Vigas, M., Stowasserova, N., Nemeth, S., and Jurcovicova, J. Effect of electroconvulsive therapy without anticonvulsive premedication on serum growth hormone in man. *Horm. Res.,* 6:65–70, 1975.
Vigas, M., Wiederman, V., Nemeth, S., Jurcovicova, J., and Zigo, L. Alpha-adrenergic regulation of growth hormone release after electroconvulsive therapy in man. *Neuroendocrinology,* 21:42–48, 1976.
Vigersky, R. A., and Loriaux, D. L. Anorexia nervosa as a model of hypothalamic dysfunction. In: R. A. Vigersky (Ed.): *Anorexia Nervosa.* Raven Press, New York, pp. 109–122, 1977.
Volavka, J. Neurophysiology of ECT. *Semin. Psychiatry,* 4:55–65, 1972.
Volavka, J. Is EEG slowing related to therapeutic effect of convulsive therapy? In: M. Fink, S. Kety, J. McGaugh, and T. A. Williams (Eds.): *Psychobiology of Convulsive Therapy.* V. H. Winston & Sons, Washington, D.C., pp. 35–40, 1974.
Volavka, J., Feldstein, S., Abrams, R. A., Dornbush, R., and Fink, M. EEG and clinical change after bilateral and unilateral electroconvulsive therapy. *Electroencephalogr. Clin Neurophysiol.,* 32:631–639, 1972.
von Angyal, L., and Gyrafas, K. Über die Cardiozol-Krampfbehandlung der Schizophrenie. *Arch. Psychiatry,* 106:1–12, 1936.
von Baeyer, W. R. *Die Moderne Psychiatrische Schockbehandlung.* Georg Thieme Verlag, Stuttgart, 160 pp., 1951.
von Braunmühl, A. Fünf Jahre Schock- und Krampf-behandlung in Eglfing-Haar. Ein Rechenschaftsbericht. *Arch. Psychiatry,* 114:410–440, 1942.
von Graffenried, B., del Pozo, E., Roubicek, J., Krebs, E., Pöldinger, W., Burmeister, P., and Kerp, L. Effects of the synthetic enkephalin analogue FK 33–824 in man. *Nature,* 272:729–730, 1978.
von Hagen, K. O. Chronic intractable pain—discussion of its mechanism and report of eight cases treated with electroshock. *JAMA,* 65:773–777, 1957.
Walter, W. G. Electroencephalography in cases of mental disorder. *J. Ment. Sci.,* 88:110–121, 1942.
Walter, W. G. *The Curve of the Snowflake.* Norton & Co., New York, 282 pp., 1956.
Ward, P. J. ECT and cardiac arrhythmia. *Br. Med. J.,* 4:229, 1974.
Wasterlain, C. S. Mortality and morbidity from serial seizures. *Epilepsia,* 15:155–176, 1974.
Weaver, L. A., Ives, J. O., Williams, R., and Nies, A. A comparison of standard alternating current and low-energy brief pulse electrotherapy. *Biol. Psychiatr,* 12:525–544, 1977.
Weaver, L., Ives, J. and Williams, R.: The threshold number of pulses in bilateral and unilateral ECT. *Biol. Psychiatr.* 13:227–241, 1978.
Weaver, L., Ravaris, C., Rush, S., and Paananen, R. Stimulus parameters in electroconvulsive shock. *J. Psychiatr. Res.,* 10:271–281, 1974.
Weaver, L., Williams, R., and Rush, S. Current density in bilateral and unilateral ECT. *Biol. Psychiatry,* 11:303–312, 1976.

REFERENCES

Weckowicz, T. E., Yonge, K. A., Cropley, A. J., and Muir, W. Objective therapy predictors in depression: A multivariate approach. *J. Clin. Psychol. [Suppl.],* 27:3–29, 1971.
Weeks, A. W., and Alexander, L. The distribution of electric current in the animal body. *J. Ind. Hyg. Toxicol.,* 21:517–525, 1939.
Weigert, E. Psychoanalytic notes on sleep and convulsion treatment in functional psychoses. *Psychiatry,* 3:189–209, 1940.
Weil, A. A., and Brinegar, W. C. Electroencephalographic studies following electric shock therapy. *Arch. Neurol. Psychiatry,* 57:719–729, 1947.
Weil, P. Regressive electroplexy in schizophrenics. *J. Ment. Sci.,* 96:514–520, 1950.
Weil-Malherbe, H. The effect of convulsive therapy on plasma adrenaline and noradrenaline. *J. Ment. Sci.,* 101:156–162, 1955.
Weil-Malherbe, H., and Szara, S. I. *The Biochemistry of Functional and Experimental Psychoses.* Charles C Thomas, Springfield, Ill., 406 pp., 1971.
Weinberger, D. R., and Kelly, M. J. Catatonia and malignant syndrome: A possible complication of neuroleptic administration. *J. Nerv. Ment. Dis.,* 165:263–268, 1977.
Weinberger, D. R., and Wyatt, J. R. Catatonic stupor and neuroleptic drugs. *JAMA,* 239:1846, 1978.
Weinstein, E. A., and Kahn, R. L. Personality factors in denial of illness. *Arch. Neurol. Psychiatry,* 69:355–367, 1953.
Weinstein, E. A., and Kahn, R. L. *Denial of Illness.* Charles C Thomas, Springfield, Ill., 166 pp. 1955.
Weinstein, E. A., Kahn, R. L., and Bergman, P. S. The effect of electroconvulsive therapy on intractable pain. *Arch. Neurol. Psychiatry,* 81:37–42, 1959.
Weinstein, E. A., Kahn, R. L., and Sugerman, L. A. Ludic behavior in patients with brain disease. *J. Hillside Hosp.,* 3:98–106, 1954a.
Weinstein, E. A., Kahn, R. L., Sugerman, L. A., and Linn, L. Diagnostic use of amobarbital sodium ("amytal sodium") in brain disease. *Am. J. Psychiatry,* 109:889–894, 1953.
Weinstein, E. A., Kahn, R. L., Sugerman, L. A., and Malitz, S. Serial administration of the "amytal test" for brain disease: Its diagnostic and prognostic value. *Arch. Neurol. Psychiatry,* 71:217–226, 1954b.
Weinstein, E. A., Linn, L., and Kahn, R. L. Psychosis during electroshock therapy: Its relation to the theory of shock therapy. *Am. J. Psychiatry,* 109:22–26, 1952.
Weinstein, E. A., and Malitz, S. Changes in symbolic expression with amobarbital sodium ("amytal sodium"). *Am. J. Psychiatry,* 110:198–206, 1954.
Weinstein, M. R., and Fischer, A. Combined treatment with ECT and antipsychotic drugs in schizophrenia. *Dis. Nerv. Syst.,* 32:801–808, 1971.
Weiss, D. M. Changes in blood pressure with electroshock therapy in a patient receiving chlorpromazine hydrochloride (Thorazine). *Am. J. Psychiatry,* 111:617–619, 1955.
Weitzel, W. D. Changing law and clinical dilemmas. *Am. J. Psychiatry,* 134:293–295, 1977.
Weitzman, E. Temporal organization of neuroendocrine function in relation to sleep-walking cycle in man. In: K. Lederis, and K. E. Cooper (Eds.): *Recent Studies of Hypothalamic Function.* S. Karger, Basel, pp. 26–38, 1974.
Wells, D. A. Electroconvulsive treatment for schizophrenia. A ten-year survey in a university hospital psychiatric department. *Compr. Psychiatry,* 14:291–298, 1973.
Wessels, W. H. A comparative study of the efficacy of bilateral and unilateral electroconvulsive therapy with thioridazine in acute schizophrenia. *S. Afr. Med. J.,* 46:890–892, 1972.
White, R. K., Shea, J. J., and Jonas, M. A. Multiple monitored electroconvulsive treatment. *Am. J. Psychiatry,* 125:622–626, 1968.
de Wied, D. Vasopressin in affective illness. *Lancet* 1:273, 1978 (Letter).
Wilcox, K. W. The pattern of cognitive reorientation following loss of consciousness. *Mich. Acad. Sci. Arts Lett.,* 41:357–366, 1956.
Wilcox, P. H. Electroshock therapy. A review of over 23,000 treatments using unidirectional currents. *Am. J. Psychiatry,* 104:100–112, 1947.
Will, O. A., Jr., Rehfeldt, F. C., and Neumann, M. A. A fatality in electroshock therapy: Report of a case and review of certain previously described cases. *J. Nerv. Ment. Dis.,* 107:105–126, 1948.
Williams, M. Memory studies in electric convulsion therapy. *J. Neurol. Neurosurg. Psychiatry,* 13:30–35, 1950a.
Williams, M. Memory studies in electric convulsion therapy: II. The persistence of verbal response patterns. *J. Neurol. Neurosurg. Psychiatry,* 13:314–319, 1950b.

Williams, M. Memory disorders associated with electroconvulsive therapy. In: C. W. M. Whitty, and O. L. Zangwill (Eds.): *Amnesia.* Butterworths, London, pp. 139–149, 1966.

Wilson, I. C., and Gottlieb, G. Unilateral convulsive shock therapy. *Dis. Nerv. Syst.,* 28:541–545, 1967.

Wilson, I. C., Vernon, J. T., Guin, T., and Sandifer, M. G. A controlled study of treatments of depression. *J. Neuropsychiatry,* 4:331–337, 1963.

Wilson, W. P., Hickam, J. B., Nowill, W. K., and Frayser, R. Succinylcholine chloride in electroshock therapy. *Arch. Neurol. Psychiatry,* 72:550–554, 1954.

Wilson, W. P., and Wilson, N. J. Observations on the duration of photically elicited arousal responses in depressive psychoses. *J. Nerv. Ment. Dis.,* 133:438–440, 1961.

Winokur, A., and Utiger, R. D. Thyrotropin-releasing hormone: Regional distribution in rat brain. *Science,* 185:267–268, 1974.

Winokur, G., Clayton, P. J., and Reich, T. *Manic Depressive Illness.* C. V. Mosby, St. Louis, 186 pp., 1969.

Wittenborn, J. E., Plante, M., Burgess, F., and Livermore, N. The efficacy of electroconvulsive therapy, iproniazid and placebo in the treatment of young depressed women. *J. Nerv. Ment. Dis.,* 133:316–332, 1961.

Wittenborn, J. E., Plante, M., Burgess, F., and Maurer, H. A comparison of imipramine, electroconvulsive therapy and placebo in the treatment of depressions. *J. Nerv. Ment. Dis.,* 135:131–137, 1962.

Witton, K. Efficacy of ECT following prolonged use of psychotropic drugs. *Am. J. Psychiatry,* 119:79–80, 1962.

Wolff, G. E. Electric shock treatment. *Am. J. Psychiatry,* 111:748–750, 1955.

Wolff, G. E. Electro-convulsive treatment: A help for epileptics. *Am. Practitioner,* 7:1791–1793, 1956.

Woodruff, R. A., Jr., Pitts, F. N., Jr., and Craig, A. Electrotherapy: The effects of barbiturate anesthesia, succinylcholine and pre-oxygenation in EKG. *Dis. Nerv. Syst.,* 30:180–185, 1969.

Woodruff, R. A., Jr., Pitts, F. N., Jr., and McClure, J. N., Jr. The drug modification of ECT. I: Methohexital, thiopental and pre-oxygenation. *Arch. Gen. Psychiatry,* 18:605–611, 1968.

Wortis, J. The history of insulin shock treatment. In: M. Rinkel, and H. Himwich (Eds.): *Insulin Shock Treatment in Psychiatry.* Philosophical Library, New York, pp. 19–44, 1959.

Yalow, R., Varsano-Aharon, N., Echemendia, E., and Berson, S. HGH and ACTH secretory responses to stress. *Horm. Metab. Res.,* 1:3–8, 1969.

Ylikorkala, O., Kauppila, A., Haapalahti, J., and Karppanen, H. The effect of electric convulsion therapy on the circulating concentrations of pituitary hormones, cortisol and cyclic adenosine monophosphate. *Clin. Endocrinol.,* 5:571–574, 1976.

Zamora, E. W., and Kaelbling, R. Memory and electroconvulsive therapy. *Am. J. Psychiatry,* 122:546–554, 1965.

Zarcone, V., Gulevich, G., and Dement, W. Sleep and electroconvulsive therapy. *Arch. Gen. Psychiatry,* 16:567–573, 1967.

Zeidenberg, P., Smith, R., Greene, L., and Malitz, S. Psychotic depression in a patient with progressive muscular dystrophy: Treatment with multiple monitored electroconvulsive therapy. *Dis. Nerv. Syst.,* 37:21–23, 1976.

Zeifert, M. Metrazol therapy in manic-depressive and involutional psychoses. *Psychiatr. Q.,* 13:498–502, 1939.

Zeifert, M. Results obtained from the administration of 12,000 doses of Metrazol to mental patients. *Psychiatr. Q.,* 15:772–778, 1941.

Zinkin, S., and Birtchnell, J. Unilateral electroconvulsive therapy: Its effects on memory and its therapeutic efficacy. *Br. J. Psychiatry,* 114:973–988, 1968.

Ziskind, E., Somerfeld-Ziskind, E., and Ziskind, L. Convulsive therapy (metrazol) in affective psychoses: Controlled series covering 3 year period. *Bull. Los Angeles Neurol. Soc.,* 8:43–52, 1943.

Ziskind, E., Somerfeld-Ziskind, E., and Ziskind, L. Metrazol and electric convulsive therapy of the affective psychoses: Controlled series of observations covering period of 5 years. *Arch. Neurol. Psychiatry,* 53:212–217, 1945.

Zubin, J. Memory functioning in patients treated with electric shock therapy. *J. Pers.,* 17:33–41, 1948.

Zung, W. W. K. Photic arousal response in depressed patients during ECT. *Acta Psychiatr. Scand.,* 45:295–302, 1969.

Author Index

Numbers in parentheses represent the pages on which the reference information appears.

Abely, P., 163,(239)
Abiuso, P. 239
Abrams, R., 22,28,32,34,35, 37,47,60,62,84,86,87,93, 100,112,116,117,131,150, 163,174,175,184,199,200, 201,206,207,209,214,215, (239),(253),(281)
Abse, W., 164,(239)
Achte, K.A., 36,(239),(241)
Ackner, B., 15,64,(239)
Adams, I.H., 35,44,(278)
Adams, R.D., (244)
Addersley, D.J., 227,(239)
Aden, G.C., 31, (240)
Adielsson, 148,(281)
Adler, M.W., 203,205,(240)
Adorno, T.W., 68, (240)
Aird, R.B., 145,157,163, 168,202,(240)
Alanen, Y.O., (241)
Albert, D.I., 124, (268)
Alexander, F.G., 13,22,43, 48,49,86,(240)
Alexander, L., 118, 191, 192,193,194,(240)
Alexander, S.P., 202,234, (240)
Allen, J.P., 38,48,(240)
Alpern, H.P., 118,(240)
Alpers, B.J., 42,44,157, 180,(240)
Altman, L.I., 64, (240)
Altschule, M.D., 49,147, 148,155,156,168,213, (240)
Anchel, D., 13,32,37,47, 112,131,166,206,(264)
Anderson, E., 161,(240)
Androp, S., 12,22,36,193, (241)
Angel, C., 145,(241)
Anton, A.H., 156,(241)
Appel, K.E., (241)
Apo, M., 36, (239),(241)
Arajarvi, T., 40,(241)
Arfwiddson, L., 24, (241)
Arn, L., (241)
Arneson, G.A., 38,48,49, 145,157,(241)
Arnold, O.H., 162,212,(241)

Ashby, W.R., 95,143,161,163, 168, (241),(242)
Ashton, R., 125,(241)
Asnis, G., 38,48,74,75,77,79, 176,(241)
Assael, M.I., 45,96,(241)
Avery, D., 27,53,55,(241)
Ayd, F., 17,53,(239),(241)
Ayres, C.M., 33,36,(241)

Babington, R.G., 46,(241)
Baker, A.A., 32,33,37,48,49, (241),(242)
Baldessarini, R.J., 149,151, 176,(241),(242)
Balduzzi, E., 38,237,(242)
Ballin, H.M., 169,(255)
Bankhead, A.J., 49,(242)
Bannister, R.G., 212,237, (254),(268)
Banta, H.D., 51,(242)
Banting, 7
Barker, J.C., 48,49,(242)
Barnacle,C.H., 39,(242)
Barrera, S.E., 45,157,(242), (272)
Barres, P., 38,237,(266)
Barron, S.P., 49, (242)
Bartlett, J.R., 15,(244)
Barton, J.L., 22,24,40,208, (242)
Bassett, M., 95, (242)
Battie, W., 5, (242)
Bayles, S., 118,192,(242)
Bazzi, T., 206, (243)
Beck, P.J., 54,67,(242)
Bellet, S., 213,(242)
Belton, 200
Bender, L., 39,134,(242)
Bennett,A.E., 23,30,190, 212,(242)
Bennie,E.H., 24,(242)
Bente, D., 104,(242)
Berent, S., 112,(242)
Beresford, H.R., 43,44,48, 144,(242),(243)
Berg, S., 33,34,(243)
Berger, H., (243)
Bergman, P.S., 197,(243)
Berkwitz, N.J., 193,(243)

Bernstein, I.C., 34,35,38, 183,237,(243)
Berson, S., 148,(243)
Beskow, J., (241)
Beuret, L., 148,161,(243)
Bianchi, J.A., 30, 190,(243)
Bidder, T.G., 22,47,112, 115,117,131,200,206,214, (243),(245),(280)
Biggs, J.T., 53,(243)
Bilikiewicz, A., 200,(243)
Bini, L., 11,190,191,196,206, (243),(246)
Bird,G., 24,207,(241)
Birtchnell, J., 116,117,200, 228,(284)
Bjerner, B., 144,145,(243)
Björum, N., 145,(243)
Blachly, P.H., 22,41,47,87,93, 105,195,206,213,231,(240), (243)
Black, F.W., 39, (243)
Blackman, L., 215,(243)
Blackwell, B., 17, (241)
Blaurock, M.F., 86,97,197,(243)
Bliss, E.L., 147,237,(243)
Block, B., 112, (281)
Blomquist, C., 108,(247)
Blumberg,64, (243)
Blumenthal, J., 45,(243)
Boardman, R.H., 15,(243), (246)
Böck-Greissau, W., 212,(241)
Bodlander, F.M.S., 52,(244)
Bodley, 200
Bohus, 177, (249), (250)
Bolin, B.J., 116,(268)
Bolwig, T.G., 17,145,163,(244)
Bond, E.D., 33,(244)
Bondy, S.C., 168,169,(250)
Bonner, C.A., 184, (244)
Borowitz, A.H., 33,(244)
Borkowski, W., 212,(260)
Boucher, F., 94,(245)
Boulton, D.M., 62,(272)
Bourne, H., 39,207,(244)
Bowditch, S.C., (240)
Bowen, C.D., (243)
Bowman, K.N., 8,(244)
Bowman-Barany, M., 31,(244)
Boyd, 38,50,(244)

AUTHOR INDEX

Bradley, P., 151,(244)
Brambilla, F., (244)
Branch, C.H.H., (243)
Bratfos, O., 23,(244)
Brattemo, C.-E., 64,104,(272)
Brazier, M.A.B., (244)
Breakey, W.R., 34,35,38,183, (244)
Breitner, C., 197,(244)
Brengelmann, J.C., 112,124, (244)
Brewer, C., 53,(244)
Bridenbaugh, R.H., 112,207, (244)
Bridges, P.K., 15,(244)
Brierly, J.B.,43, (269)
Brill, N.Q., 15,24,25,32,36, 37,(244)
Brinegar, W.C., 97,(283)
Brockman, R.J., 29,46,(244)
Brody, M.B., 112,(244)
Brooks, B.R., 44,(245)
Broman, T., (243)
Bross, R., 34,(245)
Brouschek, R., 193,(267)
Brown, D., 38,49,50,145, 148,155,156,163,175,176, 213,236,(244)
Brown, M., (245)
Brown, G., (251)
Brown, W., (269)
Bruce, E.M., 23,25,(245)
Brune, G.G., 185,(245)
Brunschwig, L., 107,200, (243),(245)
Brussel, J.A., 35,(245)
Bucher, 96
Buckingham, J.C., 180,(245)
Buckman, C., 226,(245)
Bunce, L., 228,(254)
Bunney, W.E., 185,236, (245),(252)
Burkett, (241)
Busse, E.W., (242)
Butler, T., 48, 49,(241)

Cade, J., 145,(245)
Callaway, E., 94,96,(245)
Cameron, D.E., 37,50,140, 141,165,166,206,(245)
Cammer, L., 215,(245)
Campbell, J.E., 40,52,177, (245)
Cannicott, S.M., 116,117, 165,166,197,200,(245)
Capizzi, L.S., 52,53,(272)
Caplan, G., 38,(245)
Carman, J.S., 145,176,(245)

Carney, M.W.P., 39,59,60,61, 145,163,194,(245)
Carpenter, W., 236,(245)
Carroll, B., 175,177,236,(246)
Carse, J., 156,(246)
Cash, P.T., 212,(246)
Catalano, C., 17,(246)
Cerletti, U., 10,11,162,169, 190,191,196,(246)
Cerquetelli, G., 17,(246)
Cervos-Navarro, J., 43,157, (255)
Chace, P.M., 112,116,122, 123,(279)
Chafetz, M.E., 35,(246)
Chase, L.S., 190,(246)
Chatrian, G.E., 85,86,87, (246)
Checkley, S.A., 175,(246)
Cheney, L.O., 35,(246)
Cherkin, A., 118,(246)
Chessen, D.H., 49,213,(246)
Chiarello, C.J., 30,59,190, (243),(256)
Childers, R.T., 33,34,(246)
Choi, S.J., 144,(246)
Churchill-Davidson, H.C., 49, (246)
Chusid, J.G., 85,87,88,89, 96,97,(246)
Cicardo, V.H., 146,(246)
Clancy, J., 23,(271)
Clare, A., 161,220,(246)
Clark, G., 157,(246)
Cleghorn, R.A., 148,(247), (257)
Clemedson, C.J., 146,(247)
Cline, J.E., (240)
Clower, C.G., 147,(247)
Clyman, E.A., 228,(247)
Coble, P., 95,(247)
Cohen, B.D., 54,95,112, 116,166,168,(242),(247)
Cohen, L., 54,95,112,116, 166,168,(243)
Cole, J.O., 24,(247)
Collins, R.C., 44,52,(247)
Colon, E.J., 157,(247)
Colville, K.I., 156,(247)
Constan, C., 49,(268)
Cooper, K.E., 177,(266)
Coppen, A.J., 24,144,145, (247)
Corsellis, J.A.N., 23,43,49, (247),(268)
Cossa, P., 202,(255)
Costain, D.W., 17,149,(247)
Costello, C.G., 117,200, (247)

Cotter, L.H., 23,39,(247)
Cotton, J.M., (240)
Craddock, W.L., 213,(247)
Cram, J.E., (240)
Crammer, J.L., 175,(246)
Cremerius, J., 85,87,94,97, (247)
Crome, N., 53,(245)
Crome, P., (247)
Cronholm, B., 24,26,107,108, 109,111,117,118,121,122, 124,193,196,204,234,(247), (248)
Cronick, C.H., 30,(248)
Cronin, D., 117,200,(248)
Cropper, C.F., 155,157,194, (248)
Crumpton, E., (244)
Cumming, J., 147,(247)
Currier, G.E., 33,(248)

D'Agostino, A.M., 55,(248)
Dally, P., 224,(256)
Danziger, L., 32,33,37,162, (248)
Darling, H.F., 39,(248)
Dattner, B., 6, (248)
Davidson, J.R.T., 23,27,(248)
Davies, R.K., 196,(248)
Davis, J., 24,26,53,54,157,175, 191,(247),(248),(264)
Davison, 200
Dawson, M.E., 95,(248)
Delay, J., 13,156,163,(248)
Delgado, H., (248)
Delgado, J.M.R., 190,202,(248)
d'Elia, G., 22,24,28,29,85,86, 93,94,105,108,109,113,115, 116,117,125,150,166,198,199, 200,201,206,228,(241),(248), (249)
Delitala, G., 148,(249)
Deliyiannis, S., 155, (249)
Delmas-Marsalet, P., 163,191, 193,(249)
Demars, J.P.C., 50,(249)
Dement, W.C., 95,(247)
de Mott, J.D., 213,(275)
Dempsey, E.W., 174,(270)
Denber, H.C.B., 104,(249)
Denney, D., (240)
Dennis, M., 204,(262)
De Robertis, E., 157,(249)
Desclin, L., 180,(249)
Deshaies, G., 48,144,155,(249)
Detre, T., 32,38,(249)
de Vito R.A., 200,(239)
De Wet, J.S., 37,(249)

AUTHOR INDEX

Dewhurst, K., 38,(249)
de Wied, D., 177,178,236, (250)
Diaz-Guerrero, R., 104,(250)
Dietz, P.E., 75,76,(250)
Di Mascio, A., 50,(246),(278)
Dimsdale, J.E., 49,(250)
Di Perri, R., 200,(250)
Doan, D.I., 50,(250)
Dolenz, B.J., 197,204,(250)
Doongaji, D.R., 34,201,(250)
Dornbush, R.L., 107,109, 113,114,115,116,117, (239),(250)
Doust, J.W.L., 157,(250)
Drake, F.R., (244)
Draskoczy, P.R., 149,(277)
Dressler, D.M., 38,(250)
Drewry, P.H., 35,(246)
Driver, M.V., 202,(250)
Drooby, A.S., 37,(250)
Dudley, W.H., Jr., 38,(250)
Dunkelman, R., (239)
Dunn, A.J., 168,169,(250)
Dyck, G., 35,(271)
Dysken, M., 38,149,169, (250)

Eastwood, M.R., 16,17,75, 76,77,(250)
Ebaugh, F.G., (251)
Edenberg, M.F., 202,(250)
Edwalds, R.M., 202,(251)
Ehrensing, R.H., 177,236, (251)
Eiduson, S., 145,(244), (251)
El-Islam, M.F., 34,99,(251)
Elithorn, A., 147,(251)
Ellison, E.A., 33,132,(251)
Elmore, J.I., 47,131,(251)
Emrich, H.M., 178,(251)
Ende, M., 38,(251)
Engel, G.L., 49,(251)
Epstein, J., 30,192,197, (251)
Esecover, H., 140,(251)
Esquibel, A., 203,(251)
Essig, C.F., 87,(251)
Essman, W.B., 144,146,161, 168,169,170,176,(251)
Ettigim, P.G., 148,175,176, 236,(251)
Evans, J.P.M., 149,169,(251)
Ewald, K., 23,156,162,(252)
Exner, J.E., Jr., 16,33,37,47, 96,112,123,131,166,(252), (270)

Fahy, P., 23,26,(252)
Faragalla, F.F., 145,176,(252)
Faurbye, A., 50,(281)
Fawcett, J.A., 185,236,(252)
Feinberg, I., 64,(252)
Feldman, H., 37,38,(265)
Feldman, P., (259)
Ferguson, H.C., (252)
Ferraro, A., (252)
Feuillet, C., (252)
Fieschi, C., (252)
Fink., M., 2,3,15,16,17,22, 24,25,26,29,30,41,42, 46,47,50,52,59,64,65,66, 67,68,71,72,85,88,89,91, 93,94,96,97,99,100,101, 104,112,117,118,119, 120,121,124,125,126, 128,131,132,133,134, 135,136,137,139,140, 143,150,151,165,167. 168,174,176,181,185, 186,193,194,200,203, 204,206,207,209,214, 215,(239),(241),(244), (252),(253),(257),(261), (262),(264),(265),(273)
Finner, R.W., 29,46,87, 209,210,(253)
Fischer, A., 33,(283)
Fish, B., 40,(254)
Fishbein, I.L., 12,23,(254)
Fisher, H., 125,212,(254)
Fitzpatrick, G., (245)
Flach, F.F., 145,176,(254)
Fleming, T., 23,143,161, 168, (254),(279)
Fleminger, J.J., 116,117, 200,228,(254)
Folger, R., 139,(259)
Folk, J., 38,(250)
Folstein, M., 33,63,(254)
Ford, H., 33,200,(254)
Forssman, H., 50,(254)
Foster, F.G., 33,95,(265)
Foulon, L., 107,(254)
Fox, B., 107,(254)
Frankel, F., 16,40,48,56, 73,75,76,77,78,205, 208,214,215,219,220, 237,(254)
Frantz, A.M., (240)
Freedman, D.X., 32,161,(274) (274)
Freeman, C., 11,24,50,140, 141,186,(254)
French, O., 49,(254)
Frenkel-Brunswick, E., (240)
Freund, J.D., 203,(254)

Frewin, S.J., (245)
Friedberg, J., 16,73,(254)
Friedman, E., 23,190,191,196, 202,(254),(269)
Frizel, D., 145,(254)
Fromholt, P., 109,117,(254)
Frosch, F., 164,165,(254)
Frost, I., 116,200,(254)
Frostig, J.P., 13,194,(255)
Fukuda, T., 64,163,(255)
Fulton, J.F., 11,177,(240), (255)
Funk, I.C., 35,(255)
Funkenstein, D.H., 59,64,149, 169,185,(255)
Funkhouser, J.B., 39,(255)
Furst, W., (242)

Gabriel, A.R., (243)
Gabrio, B.W., 156,(276)
Gahagan, L.H., (240)
Gaitz, C.M., 34,(255)
Galaburda, A.M., 93,(255)
Gallagher, E.B., 68,69,(255)
Gallinek, A., 38,131,237,(255)
Gambill, J.M., 37,(255)
Game, J.A., (241)
Gander, D.R., 119,203,204,205, (255)
Group for the Advancement of Psychiatry (GAP), 73,(255)
Garattini, S., 149,(255),(282)
Garcia, J.H., 43,157,(255)
Garrett, E.S., 37,47,(255)
Gastaut, H., 202,(255)
Gayle, R.F., III, 33,34,193, (254),(255)
Gelenberg, A.J., 35,183,(255)
Geller, M.R., 38,(255)
Gellhorn, E., 64,148,149,163, 166,185,(255),(264)
Geoghegan, J.J., 31,40,207,(280)
George, R., 180,(258)
Gerbino, L., 24,(256)
Gershon, S., 54,(256)
Gerstmann, J., 134,(256)
Gibbons, J.L., 144,236,(256), (269)
Gibbs, F.A., (243)
Giberti, F., 200,(256)
Gibson, A.C., 146,(256)
Gilbert, H.P., 213,(247)
Gillin, J.C., 95,(256)
Gillis, A., 40,(245),(256)
Glassman, A.H., 28,53,(256), (256)
Gleser, G.C., (244)
Globus, J.H., 45,157,(256)

AUTHOR INDEX

Glueck, B.C., 32,33,37,47, 112,131,(256)
Goddard, G., (256)
Gold, L., 59,64,175,178, 182,(256)
Goldfarb, W., 33,(256)
Goldman, D., 17,112,192, (256)
Goldstein, K., 134,(256)
Golla, E., 167,(256)
Goller, E.S., 24,25,33,(256)
Gomez, J., 48,220,224,(256)
Gonzalez, J.R., 34,(256)
Goodwin, F.K., 86,167,193, 208,213,(267)
Goodwin, J.E., (274)
Gorden, A.E., 177,(256)
Gordh, T., 213,(256)
Gordon, H.L., 13,133,162, 163,(257)
Gottlieb, G., 33,35,115,117, 197,(257),(284)
Gowing, D., 22,41,47,85,87, 93, 105, 206,231,(243)
Graber, H.K., 37,(257)
Graham, B.F., 148,(257)
Grahame-Smith, D.G., 17, 149,170,(257)
Gralnick, A., 42,50,(257)
Grant, Q.A., 63,(239)
Granville-Grossman, K., 48, 49,(257)
Gravenstein, J.S., 205,(257)
Grayson, H.M., (244)
Green, J., 17,29,149,150, 178,179,208,209,(257)
Green, M., (253)
Green, W., (257)
Greenblatt, M., 16,22,25,26, 134,(239),(257)
Gregoire, F., 175,(257)
Griffiths, W.J., 49,(246)
Grinker, R.R., 39,140,148, (257),(266)
Grinspoon, L., 34,(258)
Grosser, G.H., 40,73,74,76, 79, (258)
Grunebaum, H., (240)
Gunn, D.R., 205,(258)
Guttman, E., 33,(258)
Guze, S.B., 38,147,(258)
Gyarfos, K., 34,(282)

Haard, G., 213,219,(258)
Haase, H.J., 50,(258)
Haddenbrock, S., 23,156, 162,(252)

Halliday, A.M., 115,116,117, 200,228,(258)
Halpern, B., 67,(241)
Hamadah, K., 144,(258)
Hamilton, M., 12,23,33,34,60, 64,71,227,(239),(251),(258)
Hanlon, T.E., 162,(281)
Harakal, C., (239)
Harper, R.G., 107,111,113,117, (258)
Harris, A., 23,25,26,178,179, 180,(239)
Harris, T., (242)
Hartelius, H., 44,(258)
Hartman, A.M., (241)
Hartshorn, E.A., 53,(258)
Hastings, D.W., 40,207,(258)
Haug, J.O., 23,(244)
Havens, L., 41,42,45,47,49, 211,212,(258)
Hayes, K.J., 174,202,(258)
Haymaker, W., 177,178,179, (240),(258)
Head, H., 134,(258)
Heath, E., 24,36,197,(259)
Heggtveit, H.A., 49,(259)
Heilbrunn, G., 38, 44, 157, (259)
Hellman, L.I., (244)
Hemphill, R., 11, 163, 212, (259)
Henry, G.M., 54,(259)
Herrington, R.N., 24,(259)
Hertz, M.M., (244)
Heshe, A.J., 48,49,68,76,77, (259)
Hess, N., 125,178,(241)
Heuyer, G., 40, 47,(259)
Hift, E., 40,(259)
Hill, D., 64,96,140,(259)
Hillard, J.R., 139,(259)
Himwich, 185,(245)
Hines, H.M., (245)
Hinterhuber, H., 200,(259)
Hippius, H., 17,22,32,38,39, 48,49,161,186,208,210, 215,(262)
Hirano, A., 157,(259)
Hoagland, H., 87,94,97,147, 167,168,(259)
Hobson, R.F., 59,60,61,(259)
Hoch, P., 7,17,22,41,53,210, 214,(262),(263)
Hodges, J.R., 180,(245)
Hoekstra, C.S., 212,(246)
Hoenig, J., 35,(259)
Hohman, L.B., 38,(259)
Hökfeldt, T., 180,(259)

Hollender, M.H., 38,(260)
Hollingshead, A.B., 79,(260)
Hollister, L.E., 177,(260)
Höllt, V., 178,(251)
Holmberg, G., 87,108,143, 155,161,168,169,206, 209,210,212,213,226, 234,(260)
Holm-Jensen, J., (244)
Holovachka, A., 226,(260)
Holt, W.L., 40,(260)
Hordern, A., 27,(260)
Horsley, 11
Hoyt, R., 148,(260)
Hrenoff, M.K., (240)
Huddleson, 29,46,(260)
Huggins, P.K., 211,213,(260)
Hughes, J., 42,44,49,85,155, 157,(240),(260)
Hullin, R.P., (245)
Hunt, H.F., 111,(260)
Hunter, J., 104,174,(260)
Hurwitz, T.D., 161,(260)
Hussar, A.E., 48,49,155,157, (260)
Huston, P.E., 12,23,27,33,35, 38,50,54,(250),(257),(260), (267)
Hutchens, J.T., (260),(269)
Hutchinson, 23

Ilaria, R., 17,22,143,149,161, 168,169,176,205,208,(260)
Imahara, J.K., 34,(256)
Imlah, N.W., 24,207,(261)
Impastato, D.I., 48,49,50,164 165,192,197,200,228,(243), (245),(254),(261),(272)
Inglis, J., 107,201,261
Itil, T., 151,174,(261)
Ives, J.O., 227,(261)
Jablonsky, A., 9, (271)
Jackson, H.H., 134,(261)
Jacobsen, 11
Jacobsohn, N., (244)
Jacoby, M.G., 33,37,(261)
Jaffe, J., 26,140,141,(261)
Jameson, G.K,33,(254)
Janis, I.L., 109,124,164, 165,(261)
Janowsky, D.S., 179,(261)
Janssen, P.A.J., 50,(258)
Jarcho, L.W., 50,(277)
Jarecki, H.C., 32,38,(249)
Jarvik, M.E., 54,122,(280)
Jasper, H.H., 94,174,260, (261)

AUTHOR INDEX

Jenkins, R.B., 38,176,(266)
Jensen, E., 148,200,(261)
Johnson, L., 97,102,103,153, (261)
Johnson, M., (281)
Jones, A.L., 104,(278)
Jori, A., 150,(261)
Josephs, D., 193,(255)
Juba, A., (261)
Jung, R., 85,87,94,97,(247)
Juul-Jensen, P., 85,86,89, 105,(277)

Kaelbling, R., 95,109,116,117, 168,(261),(284)
Kafi, A., 118,203,204,(262)
Kahlbaum, K.L., 184,(262)
Kahn, R.L., 48,59,65,66,67, 68,69,70,71,80,88,89,94, 96,97,99,100,101,104,125, 126,127,132,133,134,135, 136,138,139,165,167,181, (253),(262),(283)
Kala, A.K., 34,35,38,183, (244)
Kalinowsky, L., 6,7,11,12,13, 31,32,38,39,41,47,48,49, 53,186,194,205,208,210, 214,215,(242),(262),(263)
Kallio, I.V.I., 147,(263)
Kantor, S.J., 28,53,(263)
Kaplan, A.I., 80,(263)
Karagulla, S., 23,27,(263)
Karliner, W., 12,38,40,45, 96,119,131,165,200,203, 204,205,207,228,(261), (263), (277)
Kastin, A.J., 177,236,(251), (263)
Katz, J.L., 237,(263)
Katzenelbogen, S., 97,145, (263),(270)
Kay, W., 24,183,207,(263), (275)
Keddie, 200
Kelly, D., 35,37,183,(263)
Kendall, B., 71,193,(263)
Kendell, R.E., 16,(263)
Kendler, K.S., 175,(263)
Kennard, M.A., 97,(264)
Kennedy, C.J.C., 13,32,37, 47,112,131,166,206,(264)
Kendwall, J.W., (240)
Kent, G.H., 184,(244)
Kerman, E.G., 40,(264)
Kershbaum, A., (242)
Kessler, M., 148,166,(264)

Kety, S., 143,149,168,169,171, (264)
Kiersey, D.K., 64,(264)
Kieve, H., 33,(256)
Killam, K.F., (246)
Kiloh, L.G., 22,23,25,26,65, (264)
Kimble, D.P., 118,(240)
Kindwall, J., 32,33,37,162, 215,(264)
King, P.D., 23,33,37,(264)
Kino, F.F., 31,33,131,(264)
Kinross-Wright, V., 33,(264)
Kirby, G.H., 184,(264)
Kirkegaard, C., 72,175,(264)
Kizer, J.S., 180,(264)
Klaesi, 7
Klein, D.F., 71,134,185, (264),(265)
Klerman, G.L., 71,(265)
Kline, N.S., 178,236,(265)
Klotz, M., 94,(265)
Knott, J.R., 87,(265)
Koch, R.D., 203,(267)
Koella, W.P., 180,(265)
Koenig, J.H., 37,(265)
Kolb, L.C., 48,(265)
Kooi, K.A., 96,(265)
Kopin, I.J., 149,(265)
Korin, H., 109,110,111,112, 125,135,140,(265)
Kort, K., 147,(248)
Kraeplin, E., 29
Kraicer, J., 176,(265)
Kramer, J.C., 185,(265)
Krantz, J.C., 15,86,203, 265)
Krell, A., (245)
Kriss, A., 86,(265)
Kristiansen, E.S.A., 23,(265)
Kronfol, Z., 113,(265)
Krzyzowski, J., 200,(243)
Kukopulos, A., 63,(265)
Kupfer, D.J., 95,(265)
Küppers, E., 30,190,(265)
Kurland, A., 15,101,118,128, 203,204,205,(265),(266), (271),(276)
Kusumo, K.S., 54,(266)
Kwalwasser, S., 190,(266)

Laboucarie, J., 38,237,(266)
Lader, M., 95,(271)
Ladisch, W., 149,(266)
LaDu, B.N., 223,(280)
Lancaster, N.P., 116,197, 200,228,(266)

Landis, C., 125,(266)
Langer, G., 175,236,(266)
Langsley, D.G., 31,33,(266)
Lapin, I.B., 169,(266)
Larsen, E.F., 49,(266)
Lascelles, C.F., (245)
Lassenius, B., 36,(266)
Laurell, B., 22,29,85,86,87, 118,119,203,209,(241), (266)
Lavin, N.J., (241)
Lebensohn, Z.M., 38,176,(266)
Lederis, K., 177,(266)
Lee, J.C., 145,(266)
Lefkowits, H.J., 80,(263)
Leiter, L., 148,(266)
LeMay, M., 93,(266)
Lemere, F., 38,(266)
Lennox, M.A., 104,(266)
Levin, R., 38,(273)
Levine, J., 22,(245), (266)
Levinson, D.J., (240)
Levy, N., 94,96,112,116,117, 140,200,(266)
Lewis, N., 28,48,49,97,156, (242),(266)
Liban, E., 43,(267)
Liberson, W.T., 13,86,89,118, 193,195,206,208,(267)
Lidbeck, W.L., 45,(267)
Liebert, E., 44,(259)
Liljestrand, G., 7, (267)
Lindemann, E., 39,(267)
Lindner, M., 193,(267)
Linn, L., 140,(267)
Lipsius, L.H., 131,(267)
Lipton, M.A., 67,177,(246), (267)
Little, A.F.M., 211,(267)
Locher, L.M., 12,23,27,55,(260)
Lomas, J., (244)
Loosen, P.T., 175,(267)
Loriaux, F.M., 237,(267),(282)
Lorimer, F.M., 147,174,202, (243)
Loudon, J.B., 54,(267)
Lowenbach, H., 37,43,157,166, 202,206, (240), (281)
Lowinger, L., 29,38,46,(260)
Luttke, S., 203,(267)
Lynn, J.E., 39,(267)

Maclay, W.S., 48,49,(267)
MacLean, H.V., 140,180,(257)
MacPhail, A., (280)
Madow, L., 43,49,(267)
Magoun, H., 174,178,(267),(270)

AUTHOR INDEX

Mah, C.J., 124,(268)
Malamud, N., 38,(268)
Maletzky, B.M., 29,210,230, (268)
Malik, M.O.A., 49,155,157, (268)
Malitz, S., 65,(283)
Malzberg, B., 32,37,190,(275)
Man, P.L., 116,(268)
Mandell, A., 35,38,149,236, (268),(276),
Mann, S.H., 146,(268)
Marhold, J., 54,(268)
Marjerrison, G., 201,(268)
Markowe, M., (244)
Marks, V., 237,(268)
Marti-Ibanez, F., 6,17,(268)
Martin, P., 42,48,86,93,197, 200,(268)
Masserman, 148,(268)
Matakas, F., 157,(268)
Mathas, J., 118,128,(277)
Matsuda, Y., 64,163,(254)
Matthew, J.R., 49,200,(268)
Maurice, W.L., 217,(274)
Maxwell, R.D.H., 194,195,196, (268)
May, P.R., 22,36,37,(268)
Mayer-Gross, W., 202,(268)
Mazzarello, 200
McAndrew, J., 125,128,200, 228,(268)
McCabe, M.S., 31,51,55,(268)
McDonald, I.M., 23,24,26,(269)
McGaugh, J.,(239)
McGrath, M.D., 62,(272)
McHugh, R.B., 37,(257)
McKenna, G., 49,156,(269)
McKinney, W.T., 132,(266)
McKinnon, A.L., 33,(269)
McLeod, 7
Meco, G., (269)
Medlicott, R.W., 192,(269)
Meduna, L.J., 8,9,10,15,162, 189,190,202,(269)
Meldrum, B.S., 43,44,(269)
Mendels, J., 59,61,62,95,149, 175,236,(246),(269)
Merlis, S., 104,(269)
Merritt, H.H., 190,(269)
Mersky, H., (245)
Messina, 200
Meyer, A., 42,49, (247),(269)
Meyer-Mickeleit, R.W., 85,87, (269)
Meyerson, 39
Michael, R., 149,156,236,(269)
Micklem, L., 156,(278)
Migeon, C.J., 147,237,(243),

Mikkelsen, W.P., 147,(269)
Miller, E., 32,36,37,107,109,112, 123,124, 161,164,177,194, 236,(269),(270)
Millet, J.A.B., 164,(270)
Milligan, W.L., 35,206,(270), (272)
Mindus, P., 124,(270)
Mitchell, P.H., 38,(270)
Mockbee, C.W., 47,(255)
Modigh, K., 17,149,169,(270)
Molander, L., 108,124,(247), (248)
Moniz, 11
Moore, M., 38,40,53,207,(270)
Moriarty, J.D., 97,140,193, (270)
Morrison, R., 174,184,(270)
Moruzzi, G., 174,(270)
Mosovich, A., 97,(270)
Moss, R.L., 178,180,(270)
Mosse, E.P., 164,(270)
Moyes, I.C., 144,(270)
Muller, D.J., 228, (270)
Murillo, L.G., 47,96,112, 131,166,(252),(270)
Murray, N., 212,(270)
Myers, J.M., 180,(241)
Myerson, A., 12,165,(270)

Naidos, D., 24,25,32,37, (270)
Naiman, J., 64,(278)
Narang, R.L., (270)
National Commission for the Protection of Human Subjects of Biomedical and Behavioral Research, 15,17,(271)
Nauta, W.J., (241)
Negrin, J., 197,(271)
Nelson, J.C., (271)
Nelson, D.H., (243)
Neuberger, K.T., 157,(271)
Noble, P., 95,(271)
Nordin, G., 150,(271)
Norman, E., 197,(259)
Norris, A., 23,55,(268)
Notermans, J.L., 157,(247)
Nowak, H., 200,(259)
Nowill, W.K., 49,156,(271)
Nussbaum, K., 204,205,(271)
Nyirö, J., 9, 271
Nymgaard, K., 64,(271)
Nyström, S., 61,(271)

O'Dea, J.P.K., 148,185,(271)

Offner, F., 191,(271)
O'Flanagan, 202, (271)
Öhman, R., 148,185,(271)
Oldham, A.J., (239)
Oliver, 200
Ollendorf, R.H.V., 33,(271)
Olszewski, J., 145,(266)
Oltman, J.E., 23,(271)
O'Neal, L.W., 156,(274)
O'Regan, T.J., (244)
Otis, L.S., 146,(274)
O'Toole, J.K., 35, (271)
Ottosson, J.-O., 24,26,29,60, 85,88,104,107,108,111,117, 118,121,122,124, 143,145, 146,150,161,166,167,168, 169,171,172,174,193,194, 196,204,206,209,210,234, (241),(248),(271)
Ourso, R., 38.145,(241)
Oxenkrug, G.F., 169,(266)

Pace, J., (240)
Pacella, B.L., 45,67,85,87, 88,89,197,(242),(246), (261),(272)
Pachter, M., 48,49,157,(260)
Packman, P.M., 213,(272)
Padula, L., 119,203,204,205, (263)
Palmer, D.M., 33,45,(272)
Pampiglione, G., 64,(239)
Pancheri, P., 200,(272)
Papacostas, C.A., (240)
Papeschi, R., 149,(272)
Papez, J.W., 178,(272)
Parkhurst, B.H., (240)
Parr, G., 96, (259)
Parsons, E.H., 156,(272)
Paterson, A.S., 32,35,194, 197,215,(272)
Patton, J.D., 140,(259)
Paulson, O.B., (244)
Pavan, L., 200,(272)
Peacocke, J.E., 16,17,76, (250)
Peck, R.E., 215,(272)
Peet, M., 53,(272)
Pellier, S., 48,(249)
Penfield, W., 179,(272)
Penn, H., 34,35,(272)
Perrin, G.M., 48,49,155, 157,(272)
Perris, C., 64,85,86,87,93, 104,(241),(249),(266), (272)
Persson, G., (241)
Petersen, M.C., 85,86,87 (246)

AUTHOR INDEX

Petito, C.K., 157,(272)
Phillips, O.C., 52,53,(272)
Piekenbrock, T.C., 56,85, 87,(272)
Piette, Y., 85,163,(272)
Pilowsky, I., 62,(272)
Pincus, G., 147,(259)
Pinel, J.P.J., 3,45,46,(272), (273)
Pinsley, I., (245)
Piotrowski, Z., 67,(273)
Pitts, F.N., 38,50,211,215, 240,(273)
Platman, S.R., 144,(273)
Plenge, P., (243)
Plum, F., 44,144,156,(243)
Poetzl, 8
Polatin, P., 47,167,(273)
Pollack, M., 50,65,80,86,87, 127,128,133,135,140,185, 209,(262),(273)
Pollitt, J.D., 181,(273)
Porot, M., 223,(273)
Posner, J.B., 44,(243),(273)
Post, R.M., 144,(273)
Prange, A.J., 17,22,143,149, 161,168,169,176,177,205, 208,(260),(273)
Pratt, D., (240)
Price, T.R.P., (273)
Pritchard, M., 36,(274)
Proctor, L.D., 86,167,193,208, (274)
Promisel, E., (240)
Proper, M., (239)
Pryor, G.T., 146,149,176,(274)
Putnam, T.J., 190,(269)

Quitkin, F., 28,(274)

Racy, J., 39,(267)
Rachlin, H.L., 35,(274)
Rafaelson, O.J., (243),(244)
Ranson, S.W., (240)
Raotma, 29,105,109,200, 206,212,228,(249)
Raschka, L.B., 156,(250)
Redderson, C.L., (241)
Redlich, F.C., 32,79,161,260, (274)
Rees, L., (274)
Regestein, Q.R., 47,183,203, (274)
Reichert, H., 111,116,199,201, (274)
Reichlin, S., 156,177,(274)
Reid, A.A., 211,(267)

Reidenberg, M.M., (240)
Reis, M., (274)
Reiss, M., 54,148,237, (259),(274)
Remick, R.A., 217,(274)
Renard, E., 144,155,(249)
Renaud, L.P., 178,180,(274)
Rennie, T.A., 30,(274)
Revitch, E., 168,186,(274)
Rhode, 34
Rich, C.L., 214,(274)
Richardson, D.J., 156,(274)
Riddell, S.A., 21,22,24,36, 107,161, (274)
Rinaldi, F., 200,(275)
Rinkel, M., (244)
Robbins, E.S., 125, (275)
Roberts, A., 38,59,60,64, 145,(275)
Robins, A., 23,24,25,26, (258),(275)
Robinson, G.W., 79,213,(275)
Roeder, E., 48,49,76,77,78, (259)
Rohde, 37,(275)
Roizin, L., 44,(252)
Roper, 203, (274)
Rose, J.T., 29,64,203,205, (275)
Rosen, S.R., 140,(267)
Rosenblatt, S., 145,(275)
Rosie, J.M., 34,38,183,(275)
Ross, D., 32,37,39,(275)
Rosvold, H.E., 148,(260), (276)
Roth, M., 34,35,37,38,59, 65,71,85,88,94,96,97,98, 101,135,163,167,181,183, 220,(275)
Rothschild, D., 13,37,(275)
Roubicek, J., 13,34,87,202, (239),(275)
Roudeau, Y., 35,(275)
Rovere, D., (276)
Rowntree, D.W., 183,(276)
Royal College of Psychiatrists, 16,220,(276)
Royce, J.R., 147,(276)
Rozman, R.S., 205,(276)
Rubin, R.T., 185,(276)
Russell, G.F.M., 144,237,(276)
Rusy, B.F., (239)
Ryan, R.J., 148,(276)

Sachar, E.J., 148,175,177, 236,(276)
Sachs, E., 150,(276)
Saferstein, S., (241)

Safford, H., 148,(255)
Sainz, A., 24,25,194,(276)
Sakel, M., 7,8,15,162,(276)
Salgado, A.L.D., 177,(276)
Salomon, K., 156,(276)
Salzman, C., 16,35,39,215, (276)
Samuels, L.T., (243)
Sandifer, M.G., 204,(276)
Sandison, R.A., 164,(276)
Sands, G., 37,(268)
Sand-Strömgren, L.S., 54,78, 85,86,89,105,108,112,116, 117,166,198,200, 209,(276), (277)
Sanford, R.N., (240)
Sargant, W., 13, 22,32,34,37, 38,39,83,161,205,208,215, (263),(275),(277)
Sarkaria, D.S., 157,(246)
Savitsky, N., 12,38,131,(277)
Sawyer, C.H., 179,(277)
Scanlon, W.G., 118,128,(277)
Schally, W.G., 177,(277)
Scharrer, E., 178,(277)
Scheflen, A.E., (241)
Schiele, B.C., 31,(277)
Schilder, P., 134,140,164,165, (277)
Schildkraut, J.J., 149,(277)
Schmidt, W.R., 50,(277)
Schneider, J., 31,35,(245)
Schneider, R.A., (277)
Scholz, W., 29,43,(277)
Schou, M., 24,54,(277)
Schyve, P.M., 54,(277)
Seager, C.P., 24,207,211,(277)
Sebag-Montefiore, S.E., 204,(277)
Segal, M.M., (243)
Seidman, J., 215,(277)
Selesnick, S.T., 5,(240)
Semerano, 200
Shader, R.I., 50,(278)
Shagass, C., 59,64,65,95,104, (278)
Shanahan, W.M., 30,(251)
Shattock, F.M., 156,(278)
Shaw, D.N., 53,56,144,215, (247),(278)
Sheffield, B.F., 39,163,194,(245)
Sheldon, J.H.. 237,(278)
Shepherd, M., 23,25,26,(278)
Shoor, M., 35,37,(278)
Shopsin, B., 54,(256)
Siegel, N., 59,80,(278)
Siekert, R.G., 157,(278)
Siemens, J.C., 97,193,(270)
Sila, B., 95,(280)
Silberman, I., 164,(278)

AUTHOR INDEX

Silfverskiöld, B.P., 213,(256)
Silverman, M., 38,39,190,(278)
Silverman, A., (242)
Silverman, S., (246)
Simpson, G.M., 28,(278)
Skoda, C., 36,(278)
Slater, P., 13,22,32,38,39,112, 123,156,161,183,205,208, 215,(279)
Small, I.F., 29,31,85,86,87,90, 93,95,122,200,203,204,205, 209,(278),(279)
Small, J., 29,31,85,86,87,89, 93,96,105,118,119,124, 128,183,200,203,204,205, 209,(278),(279)
Smedberg, D., 23,(260)
Smith, K., 3,33,34,37,50,72, 148,(279)
Smitt, J.W., 202,(279)
Snaith, R.P., (242)
Sobel, D.E., 50,(279)
Solomon, H.C., 38,39,(279)
Spencer, J., 139,220,(279)
Spiegel, J., 39,144,145,146, 161,163,185,190,(257)
Spiegel-Adolph, M., 144,145, 146,161,163,168,169,185, (279)
Spotoft, H., (244)
Spreche, D.A., 118,128,203, 204,205,(279)
Squire, L.R., 16,107,111,112, 113,116,117,122,123,124, 198,(279)
Stainbrook, E., 148,165,(261)
Stajduhar, P.P., 95,(257)
Stanley, W.J., 23,(280)
Steckler, P.P., 38,(260)
Stein, J., 87, (280)
Stern, J.A., 95,156,(280)
Sternberg, D.E., 122,(280)
Stevenson, G.H., 40,180,207, (255)
Stiasny, S., 75,77,250
Stief, A., 162,(280)
Stinson, B., 35,(280)
Stokes, P.E., 148,175,(280)
Stones, M.J., 115,116,(280)
Strain, J.J., 22,47,112,115, 117,124,125,131,200,206, 214,(243),(245),(280)
Strait, L.A., 145,163,(240)
Strauss, E.B., 96,(280)
Sugerman, A., 47,131,(251)
Sullivan, P.R., 33,49,(280)
Sulzbach, W.A., 23,(281)

Sutherland, E.M., 93,94,115, 200,240,(280)
Suzuki, O., 146,157,(280)
Swanson, D.W., 148,161,(243)
Sweeney, D., 28,(280)
Swensson, A., (243)
Swift, M.R., 223,(280)
Szara, S., 149,(283)
Szirmai, I., 44,144,(280)

Takahashi, S., 177,(280)
Tala, E.O.J., 147,(263)
Tarachow, S., 12,(277)
Taschev, T., 55,(280)
Taylor, M.A., 32,35,38,117, 168,174,175,184,201, (239),(280),(281)
Teare, D., 42,(269)
Tedeschi, 86
Tetlow, A.G., 204,205,(281) (281)
Tewfik, G.I., 48,156,(281)
Thenon, J., 197,(281)
Thesleff, S., 212,(260)
Thompson, G.N., 39,(281)
Thorell, J.I., 148,(281)
Thorpe, J.G., 31,33,64,65, (264),(281)
Tillotson, K.J., (240),(281)
Tietz, E.B., 35,194,(281)
Tillotson, K.J., 23,(281)
Tokay, L., 162,(280)
Tomlinson, P.J., 38,(281)
Torrens, J.K., (242)
Townsend, J.C., 86,(281)
Truitt, 203
Tuma, 22,33,36,(268)
Turek, I.S., 17,22,37,48, 96,97,162,(281)
Turner, P., 53,97,(272)
Tyler, E.A., 37,166,206, (281)

Ueno, Y., 145,(281)
Uhrbrand, L., 50,(281)
Ulett, G.A., 16,22,24,25, 94,102,153,194,202, (244),(281),(282)
Utiger, R.D., 177,(284)
Uy, D.S., (241)

Vale, W., 178,180,(282)
Valentine, M., 37,86, 117,194,200,(282)

Valzelli, L., 149,(282)
van Houten, Z., 33,37,(261)
Van Oot, P.H., 3,46,(272),(273)
van Praag, H.M., 148,149, 169,176,(282)
Van Riezen, H., 236,(282)
Vaughan, M., 54,(266)
Verhoeven, W.M., 178,(282)
Verstraeten, P., 10,(282)
Vigas, M., 148,(282)
Vigersky, R.A., 237,(282)
Viitamaki, O., (241)
Vogel, V.H., 48,(265)
Volavka, J., 85,90,93,101, 209,(239),(282)
Von Angyal, L., 34,(282)
Von Baeyer, W.R., 13,163,(282)

Waggoner, R.W., 116,117,166, (245)
Wagner-Jauregg, J., 6,7
Walk, A., 202,(268)
Wall, J.H., (258)
Walsh, B.T., 237,(263)
Walter, W.G., 11,163,183, 212,(259),(282)
Ward, P.J., 12,23,156,(258)
Waring, H., 54,(267)
Warren, F.Z., 203,(254)
Wasterlain, C.S., 44,(282)
Watson, A., 203,205,275
Watts, J.W., 11,(254)
Weaver, L.A., 77,118,174, 191,196,(282)
Weckowicz, T.E., 62,63,(283)
Wedeking, P.W., 146,(241)
Weeks, A.W., 43,(283)
Wegener, C.F., 202,(279)
Wehrheim, H.K., 40,207, (263)
Weickhardt, 10
Weigert, E., 12,140,164,185, 189,(283)
Weil, A.A., 37,44,97,157, (259), (270)
Weil-Malherbe, H., 149,169,(283)
Weinberger, D.R., 34,35,183,(283)
Weinstein, E.A., 33,38,47,65,66, 99,104,131,134,135,136,164, 165,(283)
Weiss, D.M., 34,(283)
Weitzel, W.D., 220,(283)
Weitzman, E., 177,(283)
Wells, B., 33,48,156,(281)
Wender, L., 192,193,(251)

Wender, L., 192,193,(251)
Wessels, W.H., 34,(283)
White, J.M., 22,64,112,206, (258)
Widepalm, K., 117,209,(249)
Wiens, A.N., 109,11,113,117
Wilbur, C.B., 23,(242)
Wilcox, P., 116,119,193,208, (254)
Wilkinson, W.E., 38,(259)
Will, D.A., Jr., 43,49,(283)
Williams, M., 107,109,(239),(283)
Willner, M.D., 97,(264)
Wilson, I.C., (257),(283)
Wilson, W.P., (283)
Winokur, G., 27,53,55,177, 184,(283)
Wistedt, B., (241)

Wittenborn, J.E., 25,(284)
Witton, 34,(284)
Wolff, G.E., 33,38,(284)
Woodruff, R.A., 155,211, (284)
Word, T.J., 95,(280)
Worthing, H.J., 32,37,131, (263)
Wortis, J., 7,(284)
Wyatt, R.J., 35,145,183, (245)

Yakovlev, P., 39
Yalow, R., 148,(243),(284)
Ylikorkala, O., 149,(284)
Youngblood, W.W., 180,(264)

Zamora, E.W., 109,115,116, 117,
Zarcone, V., 95,(284)
Zeidenberg, P., 38,(284)
Zeifert, M., 12,32,33,(284)
Zinkin, S., 116,117,200,(284)
Ziskind, E., 12,27,30,194,(284)
Zubin, J., 109,(284)
Zung, W.W.K., 93,94,(284)

Subject Index

Acetylcholine
  biochemical role, 151-153
  in ECT, 151-153, 169, 235
ACTH, see Adrenocorticotropin
Acute schizophrenia, 32-34; see also Schizophrenia
Addison's disease and ECT, 147
Adolescents and ECT, 57
Adrenal glands and ECT, 147
Adrenergic system, in ECT response, 145, 149, 169
Adrenocorticotropin(ACTH)
  antidepressant activity, 180, 236
  biochemical stimulation, 236
  in ECT efficacy hypothesis, 168
  ECT stimulation of, 148
Age and ECT prognosis, 59, 60, 68, 216, 218
Agonines, 162
Alternating current stimulation; see also Electrical currents
  brief-pulse stimulation compared with, 192-193
  in ECT induction, 190-193
  equipment producing, 191, 229
  modified current stimulation compared with, 192-196
  unidirectional pulse stimulation compared with, 193-196
Amitriptyline, 23, 24, 27, 53, 144
Amnesia
  age and, 109
  anesthetics and, 108
  anoxia and, in ECT, 108, 118
  antidepressant drugs and, 53-54, 107-111, 117, 166
  antidepressant effect, separation, 194-195, 201
  brain damage and, 45
  as contraindication for ECT, 218, 230
  in depressive psychosis, 108, 122, 128
  duration of, after seizures, 108-112
  ECT efficacy and, 107-110, 128, 163, 155-166, 215
  electric current modification in, 108, 117-118, 194
  electrode placement and, 52, 113-117, 194, 197, 198, 201

flurothyl and ECT compared in, 118-121
frequency of ECT and, 112
literature on, 107
long-term (retrograde), 108-109, 122-124
in multiple ECTs, 112-113
in organic mental syndrome, 113
oxygen inhalation in reduction of, 108, 213-214, 226
patient self-reporting on, 121-122
in pentylenetetrazol seizures, 189
persistent, and treatment termination, 230, 232
as post-ECT risk, 41
reduction of, by ECT operational techniques, 108, 227-228
regressive ECT and, 166
repression in, 165-166
retrograde, 108-109, 122-124
as risk, in ECT, 41, 42, 45, 52
role of, in convulsive therapy, 107-108, 128-129, 165-166
schizophrenia and, 109, 122
seizure duration and severity in, 108-109
shock-countershock and, 234
in temporal sequence recall, 123
tricyclic drug therapy in, 53-54
Amobarbital
  in denial of illness, 127, 135, 165
  denial test protocol and, 136
  effect on EEG, 102
  in ECT modification, 210
  in ECT prognosis, 65-66
  language change effects, 134, 135, 137
Amphetamine, 104, 124
Anectine, see Succinylcholine
Anemia, pernicious, 38
Anesthetics; see also Barbiturates; Drug modified ECT; and specific anesthetic drugs by name
  administrative procedures, 225-226, 229-230
  in amnesia reduction, 108
  in cardiac arrhythmia reduction, 156
  in chronic schizophrenia therapy, 36
  in depression therapy, 24, 25, 98
  in ECT modification, 204, 210-212
  fatalities, 52-53
  operational complications, 223
  in panic reduction, 50, 164, 210

295

SUBJECT INDEX

Anesthetics (contd.)
  in risk reduction pretreatment, 41, 43
    49, 53, 211
  succinylcholine and, 211
Animal studies
  of ACTH production, in rats, 180
  of adrenal corticosteroid response, in
    rats, 147
  of atropine, in EEG changes, 102
  of behavioral effects of ECS, in monkeys, 131-132; in rats, 132
  of brain damage due to seizures, 44-45
  of brain weight changes, in rats, 146-147
  of cardiac arrhythmias, in modified ECS, 156
  of cardiovascular response to ECS, 145, 146, 156
  of cerebral effects of ECS, 157
  of conditioned response and ECS, in rats, 166
  of ECT effects on catecholamine levels, in rats, 149-150
  of flurothyl and ECT compared, 205
  of memory reinforcement and ECS, 111
  of peptide hormone effects, 177-178
  of protein metabolism, 146-147
  of REM deprivation, in cats, 95
  of spontaneous seizure kindling, 46
Anorexia nervosa, 38, 237
Anosognosia, 65-67, 165; see also Denial of illness
Anoxia, cerebral
  in amnesia, 108, 118
  in brain damage, 44
Anticholinergic drugs
  EEG response to, 103-104, 167, 169, 174
  memory performance effects of, 124
Anticonvulsant drugs, in ECT modification, 212
Antidepressant therapy
  in affective disorders, 215
  amnesia and, 53-54, 107-111, 117, 168
  biochemical data, 175-178
  in convulsive therapy, 171-172, 175-178
  in depressive psychosis, 23-24, 27, 172-177; see also specific agents by name
  drugs in, see Chemical induction
    seizure therapy; Drug modified ECT;
    Pharmacotherapy; and specific agents
    by name
  ECT as, see ECT efficacy
  ECT compared with drugs in, 53-54; see also specific agents by name
  electrode placement in, 198-200
  peptide hormones in, 177-180

  in post-ECT treatment, 231
  research on, 236
  in schizophrenia, 54
  suicide rate reduction, 27
  tricyclic drugs as, see Tricyclic antidepressant drugs
  TSH in, 236
Antipsychotic drugs; see also specific antipsychotic agents by name
  combined with TCAD, delusional depression, 28
  ECT similarities, 185
  efficacy compared with ECT, 51
  maintenance ECT replaced by, 207
  regressive ECT replaced by, 37, 206
  in schizophrenia, 35-37, 54, 185; see also Schizophrenia
Anxiety, 218
Aphasia, 131
Apnea, 49, 52
Atropine, in ECT modification, 49, 102-103, 155-157, 214
Attitude change and ECT, 138-140
Auditory memory and electrode placement, 114-116
Autonomic functions in ECT, 149, 163, 216-217
Azozol, in seizure induction, 46

Barbiturate(s)
  amine levels in ECT, 149
  anesthesia, contraindications, 233
  in ECT prognosis, 104
  in ECT premedication, 12, 41, 50, 102, 210-212
  EEG slow wave activity and, 94, 102
  insulin coma, compared with, 15
  memory performance effects, 124
  seizure threshold elevation, 211-212
Behavior
  brain function changes and, 134
  denial type, see Denial behavior
  hypothalamus' role, 178-179
  modification, 3-4
  peptide hormones and, 177-178
Bilateral electrode placement; see also Electrode placement
  EEG slow wave response, 174
  efficacy, 174-175
  frequency, 229
  location of, 78, 196, 197
  memory disruption, 113-116, 122
  seizure duration, 209
  unilateral compared with, 28, 91, 113-117, 198-202
Biochemical changes, seizure induced
  in brain tissue, 143-144, 146-147

SUBJECT INDEX

Biochemical changes, seizure induced (contd.)
   catecholamine turnover, 149-150
   cerebrovascular permeability, 145-146
   ECT efficacy and, 168-170, 175-178, 235
   mineral metabolism, 144-145
   neuroendocrine effects, 147-149
   neurohormonal effects, 149-153
   oxygen consumption, cerebral, 143-144
   timing and efficacy of, 143
Bite-block, 229-230
Blood-brain barrier, see Cerebrovascular system
Blood composition and ECT, 156
Blood pressure, ECT effects on, 64, 155, 169
Brain; see also specific organs and tissues by name
   damage to, see Brain damage
   electrical current pathways in, 202
   enzymes, ECT effects on, 146-147
   functional disruptions in, see Cerebral dysfunctions
   hemispheres, see Cerebral hemisphere asymmetry
   monoamine activity of, 173-176
   oxygen consumption in seizures, 143-144, 156
   seizure as basic to ECT efficacy, 29, 105-106, 143, 199
   toxicity as psychosis hypothesis, 162
Brain damage
   amnesia and ECT, 45
   blood supply impairment, 43-44
   as convulsive therapy risk, 42-43
   EEG indications of, 45, 96
   psychological test indicators of, 45
   types of, in repeated seizures, 43-44
Brainstem
   autonomic functions, 178
   in ECT efficacy, 163, 172, 173, 235
   modulators of, in ECT efficacy, 235
   monoamine regulation, 176
Brain tumor, ECT use in, 38, 219
Brevital, see Methohexital
Brief-pulse stimulation therapy (BST)
   alternating current stimulation compared with, 192-193
   in depressive psychosis, 194
   efficacy, 192-194, 229
   equipment, 229
   low-energy type, 195-196
   unidirectional stimulation compared with, 193

Calcium metabolism, 144-145, 176
California F-scale, 68-70, 133, 138-139
Camphor
   intravenous, 41

   mental illness treatment, 9-10
   seizure induction, 189, 202
Canada, ECT usage, 75-76
Carbon dioxide therapy, 10
Cardiac arrest, as ECT risk, 157, 214
Cardiac arrhythmia
   in drug modified ECT, 211-214, 222
   reduction, 155-156
Cardiazol, see Pentylenetetrazol
Cardiovascular system
   in pretreatment examination, 222-223
   risks, 222-223
   seizure effects, 145-146, 155, 213-214, 222-223
Catatonia
   characterization of, 34-35, 183-184
   ECT efficacy, 35, 38, 51, 56, 183-184, 237
   ECT use indicated, 77, 216, 218, 237
   maintenance drug therapy, 231
   mania and, 184
   numbers of seizures, 208
   schizophrenia diagnosis and, 34, 35, 183, 184, 185, 237
   types, 51
Catecholamines and ECT, 149-151, 175-176
Cerebral dysfunction
   behavioral changes and, 134
   ECT efficacy and, 235
   EEG slow-wave activity, 139
   language changes, 134
   psychological test changes, 139
Cerebral hemisphere asymmetry
   bilateral stimulation and, 173-174
   ECT differential responses in, 113-117
   ECT electrode placement, 113-114
   hidden figure perception, 128
   in memory testing, 113-117
   in verbal/nonverbal recall, 113-114
Cerebral oxygen consumption, 143-144, 156
Cerebral spastic paralysis, 38
Cerebrovascular system; see also Brain
   blood flow and ECT, 156
   permeability and ECT, 145-146, 155-157, 168, 169
Chemical induction seizure therapy, 202-214; see also Drug modified ECT; Pharmacotherapy; and specific chemical agents by name
   antidepressant effects of, 204
   duration, 86-87
   EEG patterns, 86-89
   electroconvulsive induction compared with, 203-204
   flurothyl in, see Flurothyl
   hazards, 41-42, 202-203
Chemotherapy, see Pharmacotherapy
Children, ECT efficacy and, 39-40, 57
Chlorpromazine
   in acute schizophrenia, 34

Chlorpromazine *(contd.)*
  combined with ECT in depression, 24, 34
  compared with ECT in mania, 31
  compared with insulin coma, 8, 15
Choline, in ECT response, 151, 169
Cholinergic system, 167, 169
Cholinesterase, in ECT response, 151-152, 169
Chronic schizophrenia, *see* Schizophrenia
Cocaine brain permeability and ECT, 145
Confabulation, 131, 140
Confusional state
  acute and ECT efficacy, 38
  in multiple ECT, 231
  treatment termination and, 230
Consent, *see* Patient consent
Convulsions, *see* Seizures
Convulsive photoshock, 25-26
Convulsive therapy; *see also* Chemical induction seizure therapy; Electroconvulsive therapy; Seizures
  brainstem, role, 163, 172, 173, 178-180, 235
  characteristics, 2-4, 8-9, 171-172
  chemically induced, *see* Chemical induction seizure therapy
  dementia praecox and, *see* Schizophrenia
  in depressive psychosis, *see* Depressive psychosis
  diagnostic indications, 215-217; *see also* ECT efficacy
  drugs in, *see* Drug modified ECT
  EEG monitoring of, *see* Electroencephalograms
  electrophysiological equivalence, various types, 174
  explanatory hypotheses, 171-186, 235; *see also* Electroconvulsive therapy efficacy
  by insulin, *see* Insulin coma therapy
  in manic-depressive psychosis, 22-29, 182-183
  memory impairment, 107-125, 165-166; *see also* Amnesia
  military applications, 12, 39
  partial (incomplete), 12-13, 22, 49, 50, 233
  psychological aspects, 181-182
  risks, 12-13, 41-57, 229-231
  research, 5-17, 22, 161-170, 189
  schizophrenia and, 12, 16, 21, 32-34, 57, 185-186
  specificity in diagnosis, 171-172, 185-186
  therapeutic efficacy, 161-169; *see also* Electroconvulsive therapy efficacy
  types, 2-19
Cortisol and ECT, 148, 175
Corticosteroids, elevation and ECT, 147
Critical-flicker fusion frequency, 125

Curare in ECT, 12, 41, 49, 102, 211, 212
Current, *see* Electrical current
Cyclic AMP and ECT, 144
Cyclohexylethyltriazol, 202

Delirium
  ECT usage, 77
  mania distinguished from, 29
  in organic mental syndrome, 131
  as post-ECT risk, 42
Delusions, 27-28; *see also* Depressive psychosis and delusions
Dementia praecox, *see* Schizophrenia
Denial of illness (anosognosia)
  amobarbital, 135, 136
  characteristics, 134, 165
  ECT efficacy, 165, 167
  ECT prognosis, 65-66, 70, 104
  hidden figure perception, 127
  in neurophysiologic-adaptive hypothesis, 167
  personality evaluation, 66, 70
  psychotherapy, 140, 141
  in speech analysis, 134
Denmark, ECT usage, 76-78
Depression, *see* Depressive psychosis
Depressive psychosis
  amnesia, 108, 122, 128
  antidepressant drugs, 23-24, 27, 172-177; *see also specific agents by name*
  bipolar, *see* Manic-depressive psychosis
  brief-pulse stimulus therapy, 194
  cyclic AMP, 144
  death rate, 55
  with delusions, 27-28, 181
  diagnosis, 61, 181
  ECT efficacy, 21-29, 51-52, 172-184
  ECT prognosis, 59-60, 70-72, 181
  ECT safety, 53
  ECT specificity, 56, 181, 216-217, 236
  endogenous, characterized, 181
  endorphin in, 178
  flurothyl treatment, 203
  hormonal changes, 182, 236
  hypothalamic dysfunction and, 173, 175
  indication for ECT, 77-78, 215-217
  learning impairment in, 108, 109
  low energy-brief pulse stimulation in, 195
  maintenance ECT treatment, 231
  memory recall in, 109
  mineral metabolism and, 144-145
  monoamine hypothesis of, 23, 151
  mortality rate reduction with ECT, 27
  patient adaptations, 134
  plasma magnesium levels, 145
  post-seizure response, 101
  psychological, *see* Neurotic depression

SUBJECT INDEX

Depressive psychosis (*contd.*)
  punishment concept of ECT in, 164
  reactive, 77
  regressive ECT and, 166
  response of, to convulsive therapies, 22-29, 172-184
  seizure frequency, 205, 207
  seizure number, 208, 230
  sleep patterns and ECT, 95
  suicide rate, 55
  thiopental modified ECT, 98
  thyroid-releasing hormone (TRH) in, 175
  types of, characterized, 181
Diazepam, 24
Diencephalon
  cerebrovascular permeability and, 145-146
  chlorpromazine, 24, 34
  curare in, *see* Curare
  in delusions, 27-28, 181
  in depressive psychosis, 23-25
  diphenylhydantoin, 212
  disadvantages, 211
  in ECT efficacy, 162-163, 167, 186
  estrogens, 23
  in fracture reduction, 211-213
  gallamine triethiodide, 12, 212
  in hidden figure perception, 125-128
  imipramine, 24
  insulin, 210
  lidocaine, 26, 100, 210
  lithium with, 24, 31-32
  in maintenance ECT, 231
  memory performance and, 124-125
  mephenesin, 212
  methohexital, 12, 49, 203, 211
  muscle relaxation, 212-213
  oxygen in, *see* Oxygen inhalation
  pentylenetetrazol, 41, 156
  phenelzine in, 23, 24
  in pretreatment procedures, 12, 223-224
  prognosis, 211
  in risk reduction, 12, 41-42, 50, 57, 210-213
  electrode stimulation of, 197-198
  monoamine regulation of, 176
  role of, in CNS, 178
Diethazine, 103
Diphenhydramine, 104
Diphenylhydantoin, 212
L-DOPA, 175
Dopamine, 149, 169
Double-simultaneous stimulation, 125-126
Drugs, effect on EEG, 102-105
Drug dependence, ECT and, 57, 218
Drug modified ECT; *see also* Chemical induction seizure therapy; Pharmacotherapy; *and specific ECT modifying agents by name*
  amitriptyline, 24

amobarbital, 210
anesthetics, 204, 210-213
anticonvulsant drugs, 212
antidepressant drugs, 24, 27, 172-177
atropine, 49, 102-103, 155-157, 203, 214
barbiturates, *see* Barbiturate(s)
  cardiac arrhythmias, 156-157, 211-214, 222
  cardiovascular effects, 213, 222-223
  scopolamine, 102-103, 152, 210
  sedatives, 210
  in seizure modification, 210-211
  succinylcholine, *see* Succinylcholine
  thiopental *see* Thiopental
  l-tryptophan, 24
  unmodified ECT compared with, 211
  vascular effects, 155
Dyadic-type token ratio, 137
Dyskinesia, tardive, 38, 50

ECS (Electroconvulsive shock), *see* Animal studies
ECT, *see* Electroconvulsive therapy
EEG, *see* Electroencephalogram
Electrical current
  alternating, *see* Alternating current
  amnesia reduction, 52, 108, 194-195, 201
  brain damage, 43
  brain paths, 201-202
  brief pulse, *see* Brief-pulse stimulation therapy (BST)
  EEG and, 86, 89
  equipment, 191-196, 229
  hypothalamic functions, 173, 180
  instrument settings, 229
  low-energy brief pulse type, 191-196
  memory changes and, 117-118
  modifications of, 191
  monitoring of, in ECT, 226
  rectangular pulse, 191
  subconvulsive, *see* Subconvulsive current stimulation
  types of, in seizures, 78, 191-196, 220
  unidirectional, *see* Unidirectional current stimulation
Electrical current generators, 191-196
Electroconvulsive therapy (ECT); *see also* Chemical induction seizure therapy; Convulsive therapy; Seizures
  alternating current, *see* Alternating current stimulation
  amnesia and, *see* Amnesia
  anesthesia administration in, *see* Anesthetics
  anesthesiologist in, 225
  antidepressant effects of, *see* Antidepressant therapy
  anxiety and, 28, 218
  attitude changes, 138-139

Electroconvulsive therapy (*contd.*)
  autonomic effects, 95
  barbiturates and, *see* Barbiturate(s)
  behavioral approaches, 161-162
  benefit-risk ratio, 56-57
  bilateral, *see* Bilateral electrode placement
  biochemical effects of, *see* Biochemical changes
  blood component changes, 156
  brain damage, 42-46, 96
  brain pathways, 202
  brief-stimulus type, 192-196, 229
  cardiac arrests, 157, 214
  cardiovascular effects, 155-157
  in catatonia, *see* Catatonia
  cerebral hemisphere differential responses to, 113-117, 173-174
  cerebrovascular permeability and, 145-146, 157
  chemical induction seizure therapy compared with, 202-203; *see also* Chemical induction seizure therapy
  in children, 39-40, 57
  in chronic schizophrenia, 35-37; *see also* Schizophrenia
  clinical efficacy of, 20-40
  conditioning techniques, 39
  coronary insufficiency and, 157
  cost estimates, 75
  cost limitations, 79
  deaths, *see* Fatalities
  in depressive disorders, *see* Depressive psychosis
  diagnosis for, 21, 131, 134, 216, 218
  disorder specificity, 171-172, 185-186
  drug modification of, *see* Drug modified ECT
  drug therapy compared with, 36-37
  dyadic-type token ratio and, 137
  education and training for, 225, 237
  effects of, *see* Electroconvulsive therapy efficacy
  EEG and, *see* Electroencephalogran
  electrode placement, *see* Electrode placement
  endocrine hormone stimulation, 148
  explanatory hypotheses, 161-186
  exclusionary criteria, 218-219
  flurothyl therapy compared with, 29, 118-121, 203-205
  follow-up after, 231-232
  glissando type, 233
  historical development, 10-11, 12-17, 73-76, 190-191
  hospitalization reduction in, 54-55
  indications, 56-57, 77-78, 215-219
  induction methods, 190-214
  insulin coma therapy compared with, 33, 35, 163, 169
  kindling, 46
  language changes, 134-139
  learning recovery after, 110-111
  litigation rate, 56
  as maintenance treatment, *see* Maintenance ECT
  in mania treatment, *see* Mania
  in manic-depressive psychosis, *see* Manic-depressive psychosis
  medical facilities for, 224-225
  medical insurance and, 56, 237
  in medically ill, 53
  memory impairment and, *see* Amnesia
  military use, 12, 39
  mineral metabolism, 144-145
  missed seizures in unmodified, 49
  modified treatment, *see* Drug modified ECT
  monitoring, 226-227
  in mutism, 34
  neurohormonal effects, 149-153
  number of treatments, 208-209, 230-231
  oxygen consumption, 143-144; *see also* Oxygen inhalation
  with pacemaker, 219
  in Parkinsonism, 38, 50, 176
  patient's consent, 16, 73, 78-79, 219-221, 238
  patient preparation, 223-224
  patient resistance, 220
  perception modification, 125-128
  pharmacotherapy compared with, *see* Pharmacotherapy
  practitioners, 56
  precautions in, 229-230
  in pregnancy, 217
  pretreatment considerations, 222-224
  psychotherapy and, *see* Psychotherapy
  regressive, *see* Regressive ECT
  risks, 41-42, 50, 52-53, 57, 222-224, 229-230
  safety, 13-16
  schizophrenia, *see* Schizophrenia
  as secondary treatment, 216
  seizures in, *see* Seizures
  shock-countershock, 234
  socioeconomic factors, 55-56, 73, 79-80
  speech changes, 134-135; *see also* Language changes
  spontaneous seizures, 96
  subconvulsive treatment, *see* Subconvulsive current stimulation
  symmetrical, 174
  symptomatic indications for, 216-219
  tardive seizures, 96
  therapeutic efficacy of, *see* Electroconvulsive therapy efficacy
  "therapeutic window," 29, 230
  treatment survey, by localities, 77-78

SUBJECT INDEX

Electroconvulsive therapy (contd.)
  treatment termination criteria, 208, 230
  two-stage induction, 233
  unilateral, see Unilateral electrode placement
Electroconvulsive therapy efficacy; see also Electroconvulsive therapy, prognosis
  adrenal glands in, 147
  adrenocorticotropin (ACTH) and, 168
  in anorexia nervosa, 28, 237
  antidepressant activity, 26, 53-54, 107-110, 117, 144, 166, 172-173
  biochemical factors, 168-170, 175-178, 235
  in brain seizures, 29, 105-106, 143, 199
  brainstem in, 162-163, 172, 173, 235
  in catatonia, 183-184
  denial of illness syndrome and, 165
  in depressive psychosis, 172-175
  disorders modified by, 51-52, 216-217
  electrical current and, 175-176
  EEG slow-wave activity and, 167-168, 174
  electrophysical aspects of, 166-168, 173-175
  explanatory hypotheses for, 29, 105-106, 144, 171-186, 199, 235-236
  enzyme activity and, 168-169
  in manic-depressive psychosis, 182-183
  mental illness classification and, 182
  neurohormones and, 149, 180
  neurohumoral hypothesis of, 169, 235
  neurophysiological-adaptive hypothesis of, 167-168, 173
  norepinephrine turnover and, 149
  personality factors in, 181-182
  physical considerations in, 219
  postsynaptic responses in, 169-170
  predictive circumstances for, 217
  psychogenic explanations of, 163-166
  in schizophrenia, 184-186
  seizure duration and, 29, 199, 210
  sleep and, 168
Electroconvulsive therapy prognosis
  age, 59, 60, 68, 216, 218
  amobarbital test, 65-66
  barbiturate reactivity and, 104
  behavioral factors in, 59, 62, 104; see also Denial of illness; Language change
  blood pressure change and, 64
  Carney scoring of, 60-61
  clinical factors in, 59-60, 70-71
  depersonalization in, 63
  in depressive psychosis, 172, 181
  diagnostic factors in, 59-60, 70-71
  EEG, 64-65, 96-101, 173, 181
  Hobson scoring of, 59-60
  in hypothalamic related symptoms, 181
  illness length in, 63-64
  insomnia in, 95
  Mendels scoring of, 61, 62
  in neurotic depression, 181
  Nyström coefficients, 61
  personality factors, 59-61, 70-72, 181-182
  physiological factors in, 59, 64-65, 70
  postseizure EEG patterns and, 94
  problems of, 70-72
  psychological testing, 65-70
  Rohrschach test criteria, 67-68
  sedation threshold, 64, 104
Electrode placement, 16, 196-201
  in amnesia risk reduction, 52, 108, 113-117, 197, 198, 201
  anterior bifrontal, 201
  antidepressant efficacy in, 198-200
  auditory memory and, 114-116
  behavioral responses to, 100-101
  bilateral, see Bilateral electrode placement
  bilateral and unilateral compared, 198-201
  cerebral hemisphere dominance in, 228
  in cortical sites, 197
  in diencephalon stimulation, 197-198
  in ECT efficacy, 28-29, 174-175, 196-201
  in ECT risk reduction, 41
  in EEG monitoring, 105
  EEG seizure patterns and, 86, 89, 90-93
  electrical current pathways and, 202
  evoked response and, 95
  in focal seizures, 197-198
  frontoparietal, 196, 197
  in learning and recall, 114, 117
  in low-energy brief-pulse stimulation, 195
  number of seizures and, 209
  monopolar, 197
  moveable, hand held, 197
  in multiple monitored ECT, 93
  posterior, 197
  in schizophrenia, 199-201
  seizure duration and, 209
  skin contact in, 227-229
  spacing in, 228-229
  temporal, 196-197
  temporal-vertex, 196-197
  unilateral, see Unilateral electrode placement
Electroencephalogram (EEG)
  amnesia and slowing of, 109
  anticholinergic drugs and, 103-104, 151-152, 167
  atropine and, after ECT, 102-103
  barbiturates and slowing of, 94, 102
  behavior and slowing of, 174
  bilateral slow, and ECT responses, 173-175
  brain damage indication in, 45, 96
  California F-scale changes and, 139
  in catatonia, 183
  cerebral dysfunctions, induced and, 139
  drug modifications of, 102-103
  dyadic-type token ratio and, 137
  ECT effect on, 45, 85-95, 166-167, 227

Electroencephalogram (EEG)(contd.)
  in ECT follow-up procedures, 105, 231
  in ECT prognosis, 65, 96-101, 173, 181
  electrode placement and, 197-201
  of grand mal convulsion, in ECT, 86
  interseizure, 90-93
  lidocaine and, 100
  lithium therapy and, in mania, 183
  monitoring of, 105, 233
  multiple ECT and, 207, 233
  normalization of, after seizures, 96
  pre- and post-ECT relationships, 97
  prognosis indications of, 64-65, 167-168
  after regressive ECT, 123
  of seizures, 93, 105-106, 155, 227, 233
  in sleep, 95
  slow (delta) type, 94, 99-102, 109, 135, 151-152, 167, 173-174, 181
  speech changes and, 135
  studies of, 85, 95
  thiopental, and ECT, in, 97-98
Electromyogram (EMG), seizure monitoring by, 227
Electronarcosis, see Subconvulsive current stimulation
Electroshock; see also Electroconvulsive therapy
  innovation of, 10-11, 190-191
  term and usage, 3
Electroseizure therapy (EST); see also Electroconvulsive therapy
  characteristics of, 50
  use of term, 2-3
Endorphins, 177-178
Energy metabolism, convulsive seizures and, 143-144
Enkephalins, 177-178
Enzymes, brain, ECT effects on, 146-147
Epilepsy
  cerebral pathologies in, 43
  clinical, centrencephalic, 173-174
  convulsive drug induction of, 9-10
  ECT in, 38, 190
  EEG wave patterns in, 85, 86, 106
  schizophrenia and, 162, 189
  in schizophrenia therapy, 8-9
Epileptic focus, kindling, 45-46
Epinephrine, 149
EST, see Electroseizure therapy; Electroconvulsive therapy
Estrogens, 23
Ether, halogenated, 15
Euphoric-hypomanic adaptation, in patient improvement, 132, 134
Evoked responses, with ECT, 95

Fatalities
  with anesthesia, 52-53
  atropine in reduction of, 49
  in depression, 55
  incidence of, in ECT, 42, 48-49, 52
  by suicide, see Suicide
  reduction of, with ECT, 27, 49
Fever therapy, 6-7
Finland, ECT usage in, 78
Flaxedil, see Gallamine triethiodide
Flurothyl (hexafluorodiethylether, Indoklon)
  catecholamine levels and, 150
  clinical efficacy, 201-205
  ECT compared with, 15, 29, 118-128, 203-205
  EEG effects, 86-89
  memory impairment effects of, 118-121
  seizure complications with, 203-205
  seizure induction procedures with, 15, 86, 89, 118-120, 203, 209, 232
Fluphenazine, and ECT, in acute schizophrenia therapy, 34
Focus kindling, epileptic, 45-46, 197-198
Follicle-stimulating hormones (FSH), 148
Food withholding, in ECT conditioning, 39
Forgetting, ECT effects on, 108, 128; see also Amnesia; Memory
Fractures
  anesthetics in reduction of, 41, 53, 211, 212
  drugs in reduction of, 211-213
  as ECT risk, 41-42, 49

Gallamine triethiodide, 12, 212
Generators, electric current, 191-196, 229
Glaucoma, as ECT risk, 219, 222, 223
Glissando ECT, 233
Gonadotropins and ECT, 148
Gottschaldt embedded figures test, 126
Grand mal, see Epilepsy; Seizures
Growth hormone (GH), ECT effects on, 148, 175

Heart rate, ECT effects on, 155
Hexobarbital, 25, 210; see also Barbiturates
Hexafluorodiethylether, see Flurothyl
Hidden figures test, 126-128
Hobson ECT prognosis score, 59
Homovanillic acid (HVA), ECT effects on, 150
Hospitals, ECT usage in, by type, 73-79
5-Hydroxyindole acetic acid (5-HIAA), ECT effects on levels of, 149, 150
5-Hydroxytryptamine (5-HT), see Serotonin
Hypercapnia, 146
Hyperoxygenation, see Oxygen inhalation
Hypertension, ECT and, 64, 155, 169, 222
Hyperventilation, 94; see also Oxygen inhalation

Hypothalamic hormone regulation; see also
   Hypothalamus
   aminergic system effects and, 180
   behavioral and mood effects and, 176-177
   ECT effects and, 172-176, 180, 235
Hypothalamus; see also Hypothalamic
      hormone regulation
   biochemical stimulation of, 180
   ECT effects on, 147-148, 163, 166, 173, 180
   emotional and behavioral role of, 178-179
   functions of, changing view on, 175
Hypoxemia, 144, 169
Hypoxia
   in brain damage, 43-44
   in ECT, 144, 169
   oxygen inhalation in prevention of, 213
Hysteria, ECT contraindicated in, 218
Hysterical psychosis, as indication for ECT, 77

Iceland, ECT usgae in, 78
Imipramine
   cyclic AMP levels and, 144
   in deluded patients, 27
   in depressed patients, 24, 27
   and ECT compared, 23-25
   patient adaptations with, 134
   risks of, 53
Incomplete seizures, see Partial seizures
Indoklon, see Flurothyl
Insulin; see also Insulin coma therapy
   in ECT modification, 210
Insulin coma therapy; see also Insulin
   in acute schizophrenia, 33
   characterized, 3-4
   in chronic schizophrenia, 35
   development, 7-8, 10, 15
   diencephalon in, 162-163
   ECT compared with, 33, 35, 163, 169
   EEG slow wave activity and, 168
   explanations, 162-163
   replaced by pharmacotherapy, 8, 15
   in schizophrenia, 185, 186
Intocostrin, see Curare
Intoxication, ECT in, 38
Iproniazid, 23, 24
Isocarboxazid, 23, 24

Kindling, epileptic, in seizures, 46

Lactate, blood levels and ECT, 144
Language changes, seizure induced
   amobarbital, 135, 137
   attitude changes, 134
   brain function changes, 134, 137
   denial of illness, 134, 135
   in speech, 124, 134-139
Learning and ECT, 108, 110-112, 128
Leucotomy
   characterized, 3-4
   replaced by pharmacotherapy, 15-16
   in schizophrenia, 11, 185-186
Lidocaine
   in ECT seizures, 26, 104, 210
   EEG effects of, 100, 104, 174
   memory performance and, 124
b-Lipotropin central effects, 177-178, 236
Lithium therapy
   cyclical AMP levels, 144
   ECT compared with, 31-32, 51, 183
   ECT replaced by, 15
   ECT in complication of, 124
   in depressive psychosis, 24
   maintenance ECT and, 231
   in mania treatment, 31-32, 54, 183, 237
   mineral metabolism and, 144
Lobotomy, see Leucotomy
Low-energy brief pulse (LEBS) stimulation, 195-196
Luteinizing hormone (LH) and ECT, 148
Lysergic acid diethylamide (LSD), 104

Magnesium ion levels, 145
Maintenance ECT
   efficacy, 207
   in depressive psychosis, 231
   drug modification, 231
   lithium therapy and, 231
   in manic-depressive patients, 40
Mania, see Manic-depressive psychosis;
      Manic psychosis
Manic-depressive psychosis; see also
      Manic psychosis
   catatonia and, 184
   characteristics of, 29-31
   ECT and antidepressant drugs, 23-24
   ECT efficacy, 21, 182-183
   ECT maintenance therapy, 40
   ECT prognosis, 70-71
   hormonal patterns in, 182
   vasopressin in, 178
Manic psychosis; see also Manic-depressive
      psychosis
   characteristics, 29-30, 182
   cyclic AMP in, 144
   ECT efficacy, 21, 30-32, 51, 54, 71-72, 182-183, 237-238
   ECT maintenance therapy, 40
   hormonal patterns, 182
   indications for ECT, 77, 216, 237
   lithium therapy and ECT compared, 31-32, 54, 183, 237
   pentylenetetrazol treatment, 30

Manic psychosis (*contd.*)
 phenothiazine treatment, 54
 schizophrenia and, 184, 186
 seizure number, 208
 treatment frequency, 230
Maryland, ECT usage, 74-75
Massachusetts, ECT usage, 73-74, 79-80
Mecholyl, 149
MECT, *see* Multiple electroconvulsive therapy
Memory
 auditory, 114-116
 barbiturate effects on, 124
 bilateral electrodes effects, 113-116, 122
 brain damage, 45
 current type and intensity, 117-118
 drug modified ECT, 124-125
 ECT effects, 45, 107-129
 electrode placement and, 113-117
 hormones and, 177
 impairment of, *see* Amnesia
 long-term, and electrode placement, 123-124
 restoration of, after ECT, 112
 self-assessment of, 121-122
 verbal, 108, 113
 visual, 108, 114-115
Mendels ECT prognosis score, 61, 62
Mental illness; *see also specific disorders by name*
 classification problems, 182
 indications for ECT, 215-216
 social stigma and treatment of, 55
Mephenesin, 212
Mescaline, 104
Met-enkephalin, 178
Methacholine, 149
Methohexital
 cardiac irregularities, 211
 as ECT premedication, 12, 49, 203, 211
 in fatality risk reduction, 49
Mianserin, 53
Milieu therapy
 in chronic schizophrenia, versus ECT, 35, 36
 risks of, versus ECT, 53
Mineral metabolism, in depression, 144
Modified ECT, *see* Drug modified ECT
Monoamine activity
 ECT effects, 151, 172-173, 175-176
 hypothalamic functions hormonal, 175-176, 180
Monoamine hypothesis, of depressive psychosis, 23, 151, 175-176
Monoamine oxidase inhibitors; *see also specific agents by name*
 in depressive psychosis therapy, 23
 ECT effects, 149, 172-173

 restrictions on use of, 53
 in schizophrenia, 185
Monoamine neurotransmitters, 172-176
Motor performance, ECT and, 125
Movement abnormalities, as ECT risks, 50
MSH-release inhibiting factor (MIF-1), 77
Multiple ECT (MECT)
 disruptive effects, 207, 231
 EEG, 207, 233
 frequency rate, 206-207, 231
 induction procedure, 232-233
 memory impairment, 112-113
 monitored (MMECT), 19, 93, 206
 number per session, 231
 organic mental syndrome, 131
 oxygen inhalation, 213-214
 risk reduction, 206
Multiple sclerosis, ECT efficacy, 38
Muscular dystrophy, ECT efficacy, 38
Muscular paralysis, in fracture reduction, 212
Mutism, ECT efficacy, 34
Myocardial infarction, risk, 222
Myxedema, ECT efficacy, 38

Neuroendocrine functions, ECT, 236
Neurohormones, 149, 180
Neurohumoral effects
 as ECT responses, 149-151, 169, 235
 hypothalamic activity and, 180
 in schizophrenia, 185
Neuroleptic drugs and ECT in chronic schizophrenia, 36-37
Neuronal tracts, electrical conductivity of, 202
Neurophysiological-adaptive hypothesis, 167-168, 173
Neuroses
 applicability of ECT in, 39, 57, 218
 in ECT prognosis, 59-64
Neurosyphilis and fever therapy, 6-7
Neurotic depression
 ECT contraindicated, 218
 low-wave brief pulse stimulation, 194, 195
 number of seizures, 208
Neurotransmitters, 175-176; *see also by name*
New York, ECT usage in, 74, 78, 79
Nobel Prize in Medicine, 7,
Nonconvulsive stimulation; *see also* Subconvulsive current stimulation
 in post-bilateral ECT, 234
Norepinephrine
 brain permeability, 145
 in ECT, 149, 169, 170, 225
Norway, ECT usage, 78
Nyström ECT prognosis, index, 61

Organic mental syndrome/psychosis, 41-42, 46

Organic mental syndrome/psychosis (contd.)
   characteristics of, 46-47, 131
   in drug modified ECT, 47, 211
   with ECT, unmodified, 47
   as ECT risk, 41-42
   in induced seizures, 47, 131, 165
   regressive ECT, 47, 234
Oxygen consumption, cerebral, during seizures, 143-144, 156
Oxygen inhalation
   administration of, 226
   in amnesia reduction, 108, 213-214, 226
   cardiac dysfunction, 211
   ECT efficacy, 169
   in ECT risk reduction, 41, 43, 49, 213
   in multiple ECT, 233
   seizure duration, 209-210

Pacemaker, cardiac, 219
Pain, intractable, 38
Panic mode of patient adaptation, 131-134
Paranoia, ECT contraindicated, 218
Paranoid-withdrawal mode in patient adaptation, 131, 133-134
Paresis, general, ECT efficacy, 38
Parkinsonism
   ECT efficacy, 38, 176
   as ECT risk, 50
Partial seizures, 12-13, 22, 49, 50, 233
Patient adaptation
   euphoric-hypomanic mode, 131-134
   language changes and, 135
   memory self-rating, 121-122
   modes, 132-134
   panic mode, 131-134
   self-reporting and treatment number, 139
   somatization mode, 132-134
Patient anxiety reactions
   toward ECT, 49, 50, 220-222
   in missed seizures, 49
   in pentylenetetrazol treatment, 189-190
   reduction of, 50, 210-214; *see also* Anesthetics
Patient consent
   assessment of, 73
   procedures, 219-221, 238
Patient improvement, *see* Patient adaptation
Pemoline, 124
Pentetrazol, *see* Pentylenetetrazol
Pentothal, *see* Thiopental
Pentylenetetrazol
   amnesia, 189
   blood pressure change, 156
   as convulsant, 189-190, 202, 234
   in depressive psychosis treatment, 10
   ECT compared with, 33, 190
   EEG wave patterns induced with, 86, 87, 89
   efficacy, 9-10, 189-190
   in mania treatment, 30
   missed seizures with, 40
   in pre-ECT treatment, 234
   risks of, 40
   in schizophrenia, 190
   seizure kindling by, 46
Peptide hormones
   antidepressant activity of, 177
   behavioral effects of, 177-178
   in ECT-induced amnesia, 124
Perception
   ECT effects on, testing of, 125-128
   hidden figure tests, 126-128
   language and changes in, 134-135
   recovery of, after seizures, 125-128
Pernicious anemia, 38
Personality disorders, ECT contra-indications, 39, 218
Petit mal seizures, 12-13, 233; *see also* Subconvulsive current seizures
Pharmacotherapy; *see also* Antidepressant therapy; Chemical induction seizure therapy; Drug modified ECT; *and specific pharamacological agents by name*
   in acute schizophrenia, 33-34, 185
   characterized, 3-4
   in chronic schizophrenia, 35-37
   development, historical, 15, 189-190
   ECT compared with, 16, 23-25, 33-37, 189-190
   efficacy, 53-54
   in maintenance after ECT, 231
   military use of, 39
   risks, 53-54
   in schizophrenia, *see* Schizophrenia
   tricyclic anitdepressants in, *see* Tricyclic antidepressants(TCAD)
Phenelzine, 23-28
Phenothiazine
   in acute schizophrenia, 33, 34
   ECT compared with, 31, 32, 34
   in hidden figure perception tests, 127-128
   in manic-depressive psychosis, 31, 54
   patient adaptations, 134
Phosphate ions, 144
Photic stimulation (photoshock), 25-26, 202
Piracetam, 126
Picrotoxin, 202
Pituitary glands, and ECT, 146-148, 175, 176
Plethysmography, 156
Porphyria, 38
Potassium ions, 144
Pregnancy, 217
Probenecid, 150
Procyclidine, 152
Prolactin and ECT, 148, 185

Protein synthesis, and ECT, 146, 147
Pseudodementia, 38
Psychological testing
  brain damage index, 45
  cerebral dysfunction, induced, and, 139
  in ECT prognosis, 65-70
  electrode placement and, 202
Psychomotor responses and ECT, 125
Psychosurgery, 4, 11 ; see also Leucotomy
Psychotherapy and ECT, 33, 35, 36, 53, 140-141
Psychotropic drugs
  in ECT, precluded, 223
  movement abnormalities and, 50
Public perception of convulsive therapies, 16, 50, 51, 55-56, 79
Punishment, in ECT efficacy, 164-165

Rapid eye movement sleep (REM) and ECT, 95, 168
Reaction time and ECT, 125
Recall; see also Learning; Memory
  ECT effects, 108-110, 123-124
  electrode placement, 114-115, 117
  emotion, 109
  hormones influencing, 176
  of temporal sequences, 123-124
  testing, 110, 116-117
Regressive ECT
  amnesia, 166
  characterized, 37, 47
  in chronic schizophrenia, 37, 231
  in dementia, 47
  in depressive psychosis, 166
  drug therapy, 37, 206
  efficacy, 234
  hyperoxygenation, 47
  memory performance after, 123
  organic mental syndrome, 57, 131, 234
  as schizophrenia therapy, 46, 166, 186
  seizure efficacy, 164
  seizure frequency rate, 206
Relapse, 232
Repression and ECT, 164-165
Reserpine, 15, 34
Risk-benefit analysis, 51
Risks, see under specific therapies and agents by name
Rohrschach test criteria, in ECT prognosis, 67-68

Safety of ECT, 11, 16, 52

Scandinavia, use of ECT, 78
Schizophrenia
  acute, 32-34, 37, 38, 230
  amnesia, 109, 122
  antidepressant drug risks, 54
  biochemical aspects, 185
  characterization, 32, 184, 186
  catatonia and, 34, 35, 183, 184, 185 237
  chronic, 32, 35-37
  convulsive therapy in, 12, 16, 21, 32-34, 57, 185-186
  drug therapy in, 34-37. 185
  ECT as contraindicated, 36-37, 54, 217, 218
  ECT efficacy, 12, 16, 21, 32-37, 52, 163, 184, 216
  electrode placement, 199-201
  EEG patterns in, 94
  β-endorphin, 178
  epilepsy and, as incompatible, 162
  epilepsy therapy in, 9, 189
  flurothyl treatment, 203
  insulin coma treatment in, 8, 15, 33, 35, 185, 186
  maintenance drug therapy in, 231
  Meduna's hypothesis of, 8-9
  memory, 122
  neurohormonal response to, 185, 186
  organic mental syndrome, 47
  pentylenetetrazol, 189, 190
  pharmacotherapy, 16, 34-37, 185
  psychosurgery, 11, 185-186
  regressive ECT, 37, 47, 176, 231, 234
  relapse rate, 36
  seizure duration, 29, 209
  seizure frequency, 37, 208
  types of, 32; see also specific types by name
Scopolamine
  as anesthetic in ECT, 210
  ECT efficacy, 152-153
  EEG effects, 102-103, 152
Sedation
  in ECT prognosis, 64
  in anxiety relief, 210
Seizure see also Convulsive therapy; Electroconvulsive therapy (ECT)
  aborted, 88
  acetylcholine levels in, 151-152
  biochemical effects, 143-153
  in brain, 29, 105-106, 143, 199
  brain damage, 43-44
  cardiovascular effects, 155-156, 213-214
  cell membrane permeability, 146
  cerebrovascular effects, 145-146, 147
  chemical induction of, see Chemical induction seizure therapy

Seizure (contd.)
  drug modified induction, see Drug modified ECT
  duration, 87-89, 206, 209-210
  EEG, 85-89, 94-97, 101, 105-106, 155, 227
  electrically induced, see Electroconvulsive therapy (ECT)
  electrophysiological equivalence of 86
  variously induced, 174
  epileptic, see Epilepsy
  failure of, 229
  flurothyl induced, 203; see also Flurothyl
  focal, epileptic kindling, 45-46, 197-198
  frequency rates, 205-207, 230-231
  grand mal, 85
  incomplete, see Partial seizures
  induction techniques, 29, 189-214, 232-234
  missed, 49, 50
  monitoring, 105, 225-227
  motor performance, 125
  multiple, see Multiple ECT
  number, therapeutic, 207-209, 230-231
  partial, see Partial seizures
  perception impairment, 125-128
  psychological consequences, 163-166
  psychomotor errors, 125
  risks, 41-50
  spontaneous, see Spontaneous seizures
  tardive, see Spontaneous
Senile agitation, and ECT, 38
Senile dementia and ECT, 38
Serotonin (5-HT; Hydroxytryptamine), ECT effects, 149-151, 169, 170
Shock-countershock, 234
Shock treatment; see also specific types by name
  public perceptions, 55
  term and usage, 3, 50
Sleep
  ECT efficacy, 169
  as therapy, 3, 4, 7
Sodium ions, 144
Somatization mode in patient adaptation, 132-134
Speech, see Language changes
Spontaneous seizures
  anesthetics in reduction of, 53
  characterization, 45
  as ECT risk, 42, 52
  epileptic convulsions, 45
  kindling, 46
  persistent, 96
Stress responses
  ECT effects, 147-149

  seizure equivalence, 164
  in schizophrenia, 185
Subconvulsive current stimulation
  attitudinal changes and, 139
  characterized, 194, 233
  in chronic schizophrenia, 35, 36
  of diencephalon, 197-198
  ECT compared with, 25-26, 35, 139
  efficacy, 193-195
  hand-held electrodes, 197
  hidden-figures test, 126-127
  induction, 233-234
  in schizophrenia, 194
  unidirectional, 197
Succinylcholine
  anesthetics and, 211
  blood pressure effects, 155
  in cardiac arrhythmias, 155, 157
  in cardiovascular effect reduction, 213
  as premedication, 12, 41, 49, 102, 203
  in ECT modification, 102, 211
  in fracture risk reduction, 41, 49, 211-212
  memory performance effects, 124
  respiratory effects, 211
  risks, 211-213, 223
  in subconvulsive current therapy, 1
Suicide rate, in depressive psychosis, 27, 54-55

Tactile perception and ECT, 125-126
Tardive seizures, see Spontaneous seizures
Task Force on Electroconvulsive therapy, 2-3, 16, 73, 74, 237
Therapeutic window, in ECT, 29, 230
Thiopental
  in ECT prognosis, 97-98, 181
  in ECT premedication, 12, 174, 210, 210
  EEG wave activity effects of, 96-97, 174, 181
  in psychotic depression, 98
Thioridazine and ECT compared in schizophrenia therapy, 34
Thyrotropin-releasing hormone (TRH)
  antidepressant effects, 236
  in depressive psychosis, 175
Thyroid-stimulating hormone (TSH) and ECT, 148, 175
Tourniquet method in ECT monitoring, 227 227
Toxic delirium and ECT, 38
Tricyclic antidepressants ; see also Antidepressant therapy, and specific agents by name
  and amnesia, 53-54
  brain permeability and ECT, 145
  ECT compared with, 62
  efficacy in depressive psychosis, 27, 216, 280

Tricyclic antidepressants (contd.)
  risks, 53
  in schizophrenia, 185
l-Tryptophan
  in depression therapy, 150
  in ECT modification, 24, 125, 149-150
  memory performance effects, 125
Twin study in mania, 31
Type-token ratio (TTR), 137
Tyrosine hydroxylase and ECT, 149

Unidirectional current stimulation; *see also* Electrical currents
  alternating current compared, 193
  brief stimulus compared, 193
  efficacy, 192,
  equipment producing, 191, 229
  patient effects, 192
  rectangular pulse, 191
  subconvulsive, 197
Unilateral electrode placement; *see also* Bilateral electrode placement; Electrode placement
  anesthetics, 211-212
  auditory memory effects, 114-116
  brain pathways, 202
  EEG monitoring, 105
  efficacy, 80-81, 166, 174, 198
  electrode positions, 228-229
  introduction, 197
  memory effects, 112-117, 122, 123
  nondominant, 156
  seizure duration, 209
  usage by localities, 78
United States ECT usage, 73-79

Valsalva effect in seizures, 155
Vasopressin in manic-depressive psychosis, 178
Verbal memory and electrode placement, 108, 113, 115
Veterans' administration hospitals, ECT usage, 73-75
Visual memory and electrode placement, 108, 114-115
Visual perception and ECT, 125, 126